The Latest Trends in Sleep Medicine

Edited by

Imran H. Iftikhar

*Division of Pulmonary, Allergy,
Critical Care & Sleep Medicine,
Emory University School of Medicine,
Atlanta, GA,
USA*

&

Ali I. Musani

*Division of Pulmonary Sciences and Critical Care,
University of Colorado School of Medicine,
Aurora, CO 80045,
USA*

The Latest Trends in Sleep Medicine

Editors: Imran H. Iftikhar and Ali I. Musani

ISBN (Online): 978-981-5051-03-2

ISBN (Print): 978-981-5051-04-9

ISBN (Paperback): 978-981-5051-05-6

need for a court order if at any point you breach any terms of this License Agreement. In no event will any delay or failure by Bentham Science Publishers in enforcing your compliance with this License Agreement constitute a waiver of any of its rights.

3. You acknowledge that you have read this License Agreement, and agree to be bound by its terms and conditions. To the extent that any other terms and conditions presented on any website of Bentham Science Publishers conflict with, or are inconsistent with, the terms and conditions set out in this License Agreement, you acknowledge that the terms and conditions set out in this License Agreement shall prevail.

Bentham Science Publishers Pte. Ltd.
80 Robinson Road #02-00
Singapore 068898
Singapore
Email: subscriptions@benthamscience.net

BENTHAM SCIENCE

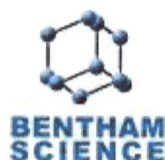

CONTENTS

CHAPTER 3 RESTLESS LEG SYNDROME MANAGEMENT 39
Shaden O. Qasrawi and *Ahmed S. BaHammam*

CHAPTER 4 SLEEP AND DRIVING SAFETY 64
Aneesa Das and *Nancy Collop*

PREFACE I

The field of sleep medicine has gone through tremendous evolution since the discovery of REM sleep in 1953 and remarkable research in recent years has led to multiple advances in sleep medicine. Among the most important improvements are the approval of the new medication for treating excessive daytime sleepiness in patients with obstructive sleep apnea and narcolepsy, treatment of central sleep apnea with phrenic nerve stimulation, treatment of obstructive sleep apnea with hypoglossal nerve stimulation, and emerging evidence on possible medication treatment of obstructive sleep apnea. These are exciting times in the field of sleep medicine, which is now a specialty in its own right. Technological advances are helping us break down diagnoses (e.g., further differentiating Narcolepsy into Type 1 and Type) and lead to novel ways of home sleep apnea testing (like peripheral arterial tonometry) and computerized interpretation of home sleep studies. We have potential tools in some areas of sleep medicine, such as obstructive sleep apnea, that can be used as part of a strategy for deep phenotyping of patients in precision medicine. Not only that, areas such as chronic insomnia and restless legs syndrome show promise for precision medicine application, especially after the identification of genetic markers and application of our understanding of the pharmacogenetics of commonly used medications in sleep medicine. Undoubtedly, much greater progress will be made in the coming years. We believe that the contributions of this book authored by international and respected experts will be useful to the respiratory and sleep medicine clinicians, whose efforts are still needed in treating and improving the quality and length of life in patients with complex sleep disorders.

Imran H. Iftikhar
Division of Pulmonary, Allergy, Critical Care & Sleep Medicine
Emory University School of Medicine,
Atlanta, GA, USA

PREFACE II

I am delighted to present a state-of-the-art, up-to-date, comprehensive sleep medicine textbook. You will recognize many world-renowned scholars and scientists in the list of authors in this book. The credit goes to Dr. Imran Iftikhar's vision and tireless work in compiling this well-rounded book covering all essential topics of sleep physiology, pathology, latest research, and interventions. Content experts have written each chapter in this book with extensive subject experience.

I thank and congratulate all authors and Dr. Iftikhar for putting together an enormous resource for new and seasoned sleep doctors alike. This book's format also lends itself nicely to non-sleep health care workers. Ultimately, this textbook will improve the standard of sleep medicine and benefit patients suffering from sleep disorders.

Ali I. Musani
Vice-Chair, Global Health. Department of Medicine
Professor of Medicine and Surgery
Director, Complex Airway Pillar of the Center for Lung and Breathing
Director, Bronchoscopy Service, Interventional Pulmonology Program and Interventional
Pulmonology Fellowship
Director, Global Health Pathway, Internal Medicine Residency Program
Division of Pulmonary Sciences & Critical Care Medicine
University of Colorado School of Medicine, Denver
USA

List of Contributors

Ahmed S. BaHammam	The University Sleep Disorders Center, College of Medicine, King Saud University, Box 225503, Riyadh 11324, Saudi Arabia National Plan for Science and Technology, College of Medicine, King Saud University, Riyadh, Saudi Arabia
Aneesa Das	Division of Pulmonary/Critical Care/Sleep Medicine, Ohio State University, Columbus, OH, USA
Alicia J. Roth	Sleep Disorders Center, Neurological Institute, Cleveland Clinic, Cleveland, OH 44124, USA
Ali I. Musani	Division of Pulmonary Sciences and Critical Care, University of Colorado School of Medicine, Aurora, CO 80045, USA
Cheryl Augenstein	Department of Medicine, Division of Pulmonary, Allergy, Critical Care & Sleep Medicine, Emory University School of Medicine, Atlanta, GA, USA
Emmanuel During	Department of Psychiatry, Division of Sleep Medicine, Department of Neurology, Stanford University, Palo Alto, CA, USA
Imran H. Iftikhar	Department of Medicine, Division of Pulmonary, Allergy, Critical Care & Sleep Medicine, Emory University School of Medicine and the Atlanta Veterans Affairs Medical Center, Atlanta, GA, USA
John DuBose	Atrium Health Sleep Medicine, Charlotte, NC, USA
Jennifer M. Mundt	Department of Neurology, Center for Circadian and Sleep Medicine, Northwestern University Feinberg School of Medicine, Chicago, IL 60611, USA
Lawrence Chan	Division of Pulmonary Critical Care and Sleep Medicine, Department of Internal Medicine, The Ohio State University Wexner Medical Center, Columbus, Ohio, USA
Meena Khan	Division of Pulmonary Critical Care and Sleep Medicine, Department of Internal Medicine, The Ohio State University Wexner Medical Center, Columbus, Ohio, USA
Michael Awad	Department of Otolaryngology, Division of Sleep Surgery, Feinberg School of Medicine, Northwestern University, USA
Nancy Collop	Department of Medicine, Division of Pulmonary, Allergy, Critical Care & Sleep Medicine, Emory University School of Medicine, USA Emory Sleep Center, Emory University, Atlanta, GA, USA
Rami Khayat	Division of Pulmonary and Critical Care Medicine, University of California-Irvine, Irvine, CA 92868, USA
Robson Capasso	Department of Otolaryngology-Head and Neck Surgery, Division of Sleep Surgery, Stanford Hospital and Clinics, Stanford, California, USA
Stanley Y.C. Liu	Department of Otolaryngology-Head and Neck Surgery, Division of Sleep Surgery, Stanford Hospital and Clinics, Stanford, California, USA
Sonia Ali Malik	Division of Family Medicine, USA University of Utah, Salt Lake City, Utah, USA
Shaden O. Qasrawi	Sleep Disorders Unit, Kingdom Hospital, Riyadh, Saudi Arabia

Sneha Giri   Department of Otolaryngology / Head & Neck Surgery, Northwestern University, Chicago, Illinois, USA

William J. Healy   Division of Pulmonary, Critical Care, and Sleep Medicine, The Medical College of Georgia at Augusta University, Augusta, GA 30912, USA

CHAPTER 1

Management of Non-Narcolepsy Hypersomnia and Excessive Daytime Sleepiness

Imran H. Iftikhar[1,*]

[1] *Department of Medicine, Division of Pulmonary, Allergy, Critical Care & Sleep Medicine, Emory University School of Medicine and the Atlanta Veterans Affairs Medical Center, Atlanta, GA, USA*

Abstract: The International Classification for Sleep Disorders- third edition (ICSD-3) has classified central disorders of hypersomnolence as, Narcolepsy type 1 and type 2, idiopathic hypersomnia (IH), Kleine–Levin syndrome (KLS), hypersomnia due to a medical or neurologic disorder, hypersomnia due to medication or substance, hypersomnia associated with psychiatric disorders, and insufficient sleep syndrome. A number of pharmacological treatment options are now available for Narcolepsy type 1 and type 2. However, for conditions like IH and KLS, much work is still being done to understand the underlying pathophysiologic mechanisms and consequently, these conditions have the least amount of high-grade evidence on pharmacologic options, and most medicines are used 'off-label'. This chapter focuses on treating non-narcoleptic hypersomnia syndromes- those commonly encountered in Sleep disorders clinics such as residual hypersomnia despite having a patient adherent to therapeutic positive airway pressure settings, to some uncommon conditions like IH and an exceedingly rare condition like KLS. New medications like solriamfetol and pitolisant and their possible use in some of these conditions is also discussed in this chapter.

Keywords: Hypersomnia, Idiopathic Hypersomnia, Kliene-Levin syndrome.

INTRODUCTION

Excessive daytime sleepiness (EDS) is the cardinal feature of several disorders of central hypersomnolence. This specific sub-field in Sleep Medicine has evolved significantly over time. The earliest known use of the word 'Narcolepsy' is believed to have been in a case report published in 1880 by Jean Baptiste Gélineau describing a 38-year-old wine merchant with > 200 sleep attacks per day [1]. Gélineau used the Greek word, 'νάρκη' (*narkē*), meaning "numbness" and λῆψις (*lepsis*) meaning 'attack', to coin the term we use now, 'Narcolepsy'.

* **Corresponding author Imran H. Iftikhar:** Department of Medicine, Division of Pulmonary, Allergy, Critical Care & Sleep Medicine, Emory University School of Medicine and the Atlanta Veterans Affairs Medical Center, Atlanta, GA, USA; Tel: 803-873-3193; E-mail: imran.hasan.iftikhar@emory.edu

Imran H. Iftikhar and Ali I. Musani (Eds.)

From the works of Bedrich Roth and colleagues [2] in the mid-1970s to 1980s, the term 'idiopathic hypersomnia (IH) was introduced, who actually subdivided non-narcoleptic functional hypersomnias into three types: (1) monosymptomatic IH, characterized by diurnal hypersomnia and long nocturnal sleep periods; (2) polysymptomatic hypersomnia characterized by the same symptoms as well as by prolonged confusion and disorientation upon awakening (sleep drunkenness); and (3) neurotic hypersomnia [3]. ICSD-1 then formally incorporated the term 'IH' [4]. This then evolved over time and the term was further sub-divided into 'IH with or without long sleep time' in ICSD-2 [5], only to be lumped back again into one category, 'IH' in ICSD-3 [6]. Recently, a new debate has emerged in literature on re-arranging this classification further and lumping in 'IH' with the Narcolepsy type 2 category, primarily because 'IH with long sleep time' appears to be an identifiable and meaningful disease subtype as seen by most experts in the field and because 'IH without long sleep time' and Narcolepsy type 2 share substantial phenotypic overlap and cannot reliably be distinguished with current testing [7].

As such, the management approach of Narcolepsy (especially Type 1) is well-established, extensively published with a continued supply of new pharmacologic treatment options to our armamentarium to manage this condition [8, 9]. However, not much is known about the non-narcoleptic disorders of hypersomnolence like Kleine–Levin syndrome, hypersomnia due to a medical or neurologic disorder, hypersomnia due to medication or substance, hypersomnia associated with psychiatric disorders, and insufficient sleep syndrome, and hence will be the focus of this chapter. Table **1** summarizes the diagnostic criteria of each category and the treatment options.

IDIOPATHIC HYPERSOMNIA

Current diagnostic criteria as laid out by ICSD-3 requires the presence of excessive daily sleepiness for at least 3 months, along with the absence of cataplexy, evidence of fewer than 2 sleep onset Rapid Eye Movements period of sleep (SOREMPs) on multiple sleep latency testing (MSLT) or none if the preceding overnight polysomnography (PSG) had one, and either having an MSL of less than 8 min on MSLT or evidence of sleeping > 660 minutes based on objective testing from either a 24 hour PSG or at least a 7-day wrist actigraphy aided with sleep log [6]. More often than not, patients with this condition will also have features of autonomic dysfunction (like orthostatic blood pressure changes or Raynaud's phenomenon) [10, 11], long sleep durations at night, long naps, a sense of unrefreshing sleep, and extreme difficulty in awakening, known as sleep drunkenness or pronounced sleep inertia [12], as well as fatigue and cognitive dysfunction [13].

Table 1. Summary of diagnostic criteria, treatment options and side effects.

Non-Narcoleptic Hypersomnias	Treatment Options	Possible Side Effects
Idiopathic Hypersomnia: Criteria A-F must be met A. Daily periods of irrepressible need to sleep or daytime lapses into sleep occurring for at least 3 months B. Cataplexy is absent C. An MSLT performed according to standard techniques shows < 2 SOREMPs or no sleep onset REM periods if the REM latency on the preceding PSG was $\leq$ 15 min D. The presence of at least 1 of the following: 1. The MSLT shows a MSL of $\leq$ 8 minutes 2. Total 24-hour sleep time is $\geq$ 660 minutes on 24 hour PSG monitoring, or by wrist actigraphy in association with a sleep log (averaged over at least 7 days with unrestricted sleep) E. Insufficient sleep syndrome is ruled out F. The hypersomnolence and/or MSLT findings are not better explained by another sleep disorder, other medical or psychiatric disorder or use of drugs or medications	1. Modafinil and Armodafinil	Headache, anxiety, and palpitations, insomnia, Stevens–Johnson syndrome, angioedema, psychosis, mania, hallucinations, suicidal ideation, and dependency or abuse, reduce the effectiveness of hormonal contraception
	2. Methylphenidate	Irritability, tachycardia/palpitations, anxiety, insomnia, and increases in blood pressure, dependence and abuse, psychosis, behavior changes, mood changes, arrhythmias, hypertension, other cardiac disease, seizures, hepatotoxicity, pancytopenia, and erythema multiforme
	3. Solriamfetol	Headache, anxiety, palpitations, and insomnia, risk of abuse and dependence
	4. Pitolisant	Headache, insomnia, nausea, and anxiety, QT prolongation, reduce the effectiveness of hormonal contraception
	5. Clarithromycin	GI upset and taste perversion, antibiotic resistance, superinfection with infections, QT prolongation
	6. Flumazenil, transdermal, sublingual, or subcutaneous	Side effects not well understood
	7. Sodium Oxybate	CNS and respiratory depression, psychosis, depression, suicidal ideation, and abuse or dependence

(Table 1) cont.....

Non-Narcoleptic Hypersomnias	Treatment Options	Possible Side Effects
Kleine-Levin Syndrome: Criteria A-E must be met A. The patient experiences at least 2 recurrent episodes of excessive sleepiness and sleep duration, each persisting for 2 days to five weeks. B. Episodes recur usually more than once a year and at least once every 18 months. C. The patient has normal alertness, cognitive function, behavior, and mood between episodes. D. The patient must demonstrate at least one of the following during episodes: 1. Cognitive dysfunction 2. Altered perception 3. Eating disorder (anorexia or hyperphagia) 4. Disinhibited behavior (such as hypersexuality) E. The hypersomnolence and related symptoms are not better explained by another sleep disorder, other medical, neurologic or psychiatric disorder or use of drugs or medications	**Medications During KLS Episodes** 1. IV methylprednisolone 1 g/day for 3 days 2. Clarithromycin 3. Psychostimulants may partially improve alertness, but have no effect on apathy, derealization, and confusion **Medications Preventing New KLS Episodes** 1. Lithium 2. Antiepileptic mood stabilizers (*e.g.*, valproate)	IV steroids found to be well tolerated in KLS population with a few minor (*e.g.*, insomnia) side effects Thyroid and kidney insufficiency
Hypersomnia due to a medical disorder: Diagnostic criteria A-D must be met A. The patient has daily periods of irrepressible need to sleep or daytime lapses into sleep occurring for at least 3 months B. The daytime sleep occurs as a consequence of a significant underlying medical or neurological condition C. If an MSLT is performed, the MSL is $\leq$ 8 min, and < 2 SOREMPs are observed D. The symptoms are not better explained by another untreated sleep disorder, a mental disorder, or the effects of medications or drugs	**Residual sleepiness for OSA patients adherent on CPAP:** Modafinil, armodafinil, and solriamfetol **Parkinson's disease, myotonic dystrophy:** Modafinil	-

(Table 1) cont.....

Non-Narcoleptic Hypersomnias	Treatment Options	Possible Side Effects
Hypersomnia associated with a Psychiatric condition: Diagnostic criteria A-C must be met A. The patient has daily periods of irrepressible need to sleep or daytime lapses into sleep occurring for at least 3 months B. The daytime sleepiness occurs in association with a concurrent psychiatric disorder C. The symptoms are not better explained by another untreated sleep disorder, a medical or neurologic condition, or the effects of medications or drugs	**Depression with hypersomnia symptoms** Modafinil	-
Hypersomnia due to a Medication or Substance: Diagnostic criteria A-C must be met A. The patient has daily periods of irrepressible need to sleep or daytime lapses into sleep B. The daytime sleep occurs as a consequence of current medication or substance use or withdrawal from a wake-promoting medication or substance C. The symptoms are not better explained by another untreated sleep disorder, a medical or neurologic condition, or mental disorder	Minimize or discontinue the offending agent	-

(Table 1) cont.....

Non-Narcoleptic Hypersomnias	Treatment Options	Possible Side Effects
Insufficient Sleep Syndrome: Diagnostic criteria A-F must be met A. The patient has daily periods of irrepressible need to sleep or daytime lapses into sleep, or in the case of pre-pubertal children there is a complaint of behavioral abnormalities attributable to sleepiness B. The patient's sleep time established by personal or collateral history, sleep logs or actigraphy, is usually shorter than for expected age C. The curtailed sleep duration is present for most days for at least 3 months D. The patient curtails sleep time by measures such as an alarm clock or being awakened by another person and generally sleeps longer when such measures are not used such as on weekends or vacations E. Extension of total sleep time results in resolution of the symptoms of the sleepiness F. The symptoms are not better explained by another untreated sleep disorder, the effects of medications or drugs or other medical, neurologic condition, or mental disorder	Sleep extension	-

MSLT indicates multiple sleep latency testing, SOREMPs indicates sleep-onset REM periods, CNS indicates central nervous system, IV indicates intravenous; Diagnostic criteria are taken from American Academy of Sleep Medicine International Classification of Sleep Disorder- 3rd Edition available online to members at: https://learn.aasm.org/Users/LearningActivity

The exact pathophysiology of IH is not clear. Several theories exist in literature. One of them relates to the increased activity of the sedating GABA-A system, presumably by the presence of a trypsin-sensitive substance found in the CSF of these patients [14]. Circadian dysfunction is postulated as another theory because of the noted similarities in clinical phenotype, melatonin, and cortisol rhythms with a circadian phase delay condition [15]. Recently a study of magnetic resonance imaging (MRI) of IH patients showed that the Default-Mode Network (DMN)—a brain network key to alertness and sleep had strikingly distinct findings- specifically greater gray matter volume and cortical thickness in the posterior DMN and lowered regional cerebral blood flow and functional connectivity in the anterior DMN [16]. Lastly, some have proposed that IH patients may have a dysfunction of the parasympathetic activity during awake and sleep and an altered autonomic response to arousals, further suggesting that an impaired parasympathetic function may explain some vegetative symptoms in these patients [17].

Currently, there are no medications approved by the US Food and Drug Administration (FDA) for the treatment of IH. Most clinicians have resorted to "off-label" prescribing of drugs used in other disorders of excessive daytime sleepiness. Some of these drugs are discussed below.

Modafinil

Modafinil is approved by the US FDA for the excessive daytime sleepiness associated with Narcolepsy type 1, type 2, obstructive sleep apnea, and shift work sleep disorder in adults besides other non-sleep indications. Although it is not entirely clear how modafinil works but a major mechanism of its action seems to be the prevention of dopamine reuptake [18]. In a randomized controlled trial (RCT), though modafinil 200 mg/day over a 3 week period showed -6 points mean reduction in Epworth Sleepiness Scale (ESS) score compared with -1.5 points with placebo, MWT improvement when compared to placebo was not significant (+ 3 min *vs.* 0 min) [19]. In another double-blind cross-over RCT, modafinil, in a composite group of patients with IH and patients with narcolepsy, improved driving performance and improved MWT (from 19.7 ± 9.2 min under placebo to 30.8 ± 9.8 min) [20]. Another RCT showed similar results [21]. The latter two RCTs [20, 21] did not specifically assess the effects of modafinil in the IH group alone. Although these studies [20, 21] do not directly indicate a treatment benefit of modafinil for people with IH because the majority of patients in these 2 studies (31/54, 57%) had IH, it is conceivably possible that these significant treatment benefits were because of that in the IH group.

Like modafinil, armodafinil which is the r-enantiomer of modafinil, is also not labeled for use in IH. There are no RCTs todate on armodafinil in IH patients. Simply based on clinical experience and because of its pharmacology, it is presumed to have similar effectiveness to modafinil in people with IH. However, unlike modafinil, which is quite often prescribed in divided doses so that its wake-promoting effects can last until the afternoon and early evening, armodafinil is usually taken as a single morning dose.

Sympathomimetic Psychostimulants

Numerous sympathomimetic psychostimulants that are used for attention deficit hyperactivity disorder ADHD are also used for narcolepsy and are FDA-approved for both. However, none is FDA-approved for the treatment of IH. These include methylphenidate, dexmethylphenidate, dextroamphetamine, amphetamine, lisdexamfetamine, methamphetamine, and combinations of some of these. Despite the fact that not many RCTs have been performed testing this class of medications for the treatment of narcolepsy, its use is still endorsed by the American Academy of Sleep Medicine [22]. Methylphenidate is frequently used as a second-line medication in IH. In a single retrospective case series including 61 patients treated with a mean dose of 51 mg of methylphenidate, 51% of the patients took methylphenidate and the rest modafinil. Of those on methylphenidate, 95% had a complete or partial response, instead of the 88% on modafinil [23].

Solriamfetol

Solriamfetol, a dopamine and norepinephrine reuptake inhibitor, is a wake-promoting medication, approved by the FDA in March 2019 for the treatment of sleepiness associated with narcolepsy or obstructive sleep apnea only. Because narcolepsy and sleep apnea-associated daytime sleepiness would cover a broad range of pathophysiologic mechanisms, solriamfetol could be used 'off-label' in IH. In a 12-week RCT study on its effects on narcolepsy in adults, solriamfetol improved important measures of wakefulness and sleepiness without associated polysomnographic evidence of significant sleep disruption [24]. In another 12-week RCT study of solriamfetol in adult patients with EDS related to OSA, there was a dose-dependent improvement in measures of wakefulness [25]. Some notable side-effects seen with this medication include anxiety and elevated mood, as well as increases in blood pressure. A subsequent study of this medication found that it was efficacious at the maintenance of improvements at 6 months [26]. Given the theorized mechanism of action as a dopamine and norepinephrine reuptake inhibitor, which is similar to that of widely prescribed bupropion, future observation and studies could provide insights on its effect on depression as well. Solriamfetol is not approved for use in children because there is a risk of abuse and dependence, and this medication is FDA schedule 4.

Pitolisant

Pitolisant is another wakefulness-promoting drug for adult patients with narcolepsy and cataplexy. It acts as an inverse agonist and antagonist of histamine H3 receptors, resulting in a reduction of the usual feedback inhibition effected through the H3 receptor, thereby enhancing the central nervous system release of histamine and other neurotransmitters. It is not approved for IH as it has not been tested in a placebo-controlled trial of people with IH. In a small case series of IH patients whose symptoms could not be adequately controlled with modafinil, methylphenidate, or sodium oxybate, pitolisant was effective in reducing sleepiness- resulted in 3 points reduction in Epworth scores compared to baseline- in 37% of people with IH with long sleep times and 31% of people with IH without long sleep times [27].

Pitolisant is generally well tolerated, with headache, insomnia, nausea, and anxiety being the most common adverse reactions. It can also prolong the QT interval, so a baseline EKG is advised. There is a potential for interaction with hormonal birth control. Therefore,, additional or alternate methods of contraception should be used while taking pitolisant and for 28 days after discontinuation of pitolisant [28]. While pitolisant is a prescription medication, it is not a controlled substance and not a scheduled substance by the FDA. However, it is an expensive drug. Following FDA approval, its manufacturer Harmony Biosciences estimated an annual price tag of about $140,000 [29]. In a Swedish study, the cost per additional quality-adjusted life-year was estimated at SEK 356,337 (10 SEK ≈ 1 Euro) for pitolisant monotherapy and at SEK 491,128 for pitolisant as an adjunctive treatment [30].

Flumazenil

Following the discovery of a possible endogenous peptide enhancing GABA-A transmission in the CSF of patients with IH, flumazenil, commonly used as an antidote for benzodiazepine overdose, was tested in these patients. It is a negative allosteric modulator of GABA-A receptors, in addition to its role as a competitive antagonist at the benzodiazepine binding site. In an early proof-of-concept study, flumazenil was administered intravenously in a single-blind fashion to several hypersomnolent patients and was found to significantly improve subjective sleepiness, as measured by the Stanford Sleepiness Scale, and it also improved reaction times on the psychomotor vigilant testing [14]. Because of the large first-pass metabolism effect and short duration of action, if given intravenously or orally, it has been compounded as transdermal, sublingual, or subcutaneous for the treatment of IH. In a series of 153 patients with IH and similar other hypersomnolence disorders that were refractory to standard treatments, flumazenil was found to reduce symptoms of sleepiness in 62.8% [31]. Though serious side effects for intravenous flumazenil are well known, including seizures and arrhythmias, those of compounded flumazenil are not as well understood mainly because it has not been widely tested and used.

Clarithromycin

Clarithromycin is a macrolide antibiotic that has been shown to modulate the function of GABA-A receptors. In a randomized, crossover, double-blind, placebo-controlled study of patients with IH with evidence of endogenous GABA-A receptor activating peptide in the cerebrospinal fluid, clarithromycin given in a single morning dose of 500 to 1000 mg/d, reduced subjective sleepiness but did not change psychomotor vigilance testing results [32]. Caution is advised when prescribing clarithromycin as side effects include antibiotic resistance, superinfection with infections such as Clostridium difficile, QT prolongation, and potential for drug–drug interactions because of its actions as an inhibitor of CYP2C9, 3A4, P-gp, and OATP1B1.

Sodium Oxybate

It is FDA-approved for the treatment of narcolepsy in adults and children. When dosed at bedtime and during the night, it has been shown to improve nocturnal sleep quality and reduce daytime sleepiness as well as cataplexy in patients with narcolepsy [22]. But because nocturnal sleep quality is actually better in IH patients than in those with narcolepsy type 1 and also because sleep inertia could potentially worsen in healthy people with increasing amounts of N3 sleep, the concern remains that use of sodium oxybate could worsen 'sleep drunkenness' by increasing N3 [33, 34]. Since this risk with sodium oxybate seems theoretically possible, published evidence seems contradictory- a clinical series of 40 IH patients that showed a similar magnitude of reduction in subjective daytime sleepiness as in those with NT1, as well as showing that 71% of IH patients treated with sodium oxybate also demonstrated an improvement in sleep drunkenness [35]. However, the side effects from sodium oxybate were more common in those with IH, particularly nausea and dizziness [35].

Serious side effects of sodium oxybate include central nervous system and respiratory depression, psychosis depression, suicidal ideation, and abuse or dependence. Sodium oxybate must be dispensed under an FDA Risk Evaluation and Mitigation Strategy (REMS) program directly through a centralized pharmacy.

Other Strategies

Several other strategies have been proposed to cope with sleep inertia in IH. The French expert consensus statement includes melatonin at 3 mg (or 2 mg slow-release melatonin) to be taken at sleep onset to reduce sleep drunkenness upon waking up [36]. This is presumed to be because of melatonin's phase advance effects and we know that in IH patients, sleep inertia is exacerbated by the delayed sleep phase. Other strategies include taking a delayed-release stimulant at bedtime or taking a traditional stimulant after waking up an hour before the usual wakeup time, falling back asleep for an hour, and then waking up [12].

Reduction and/or adaptation of working time should be considered by employers of IH patients. Having the option to begin work at a later time (*e.g.*, to sleep an extra hour in the morning) or to telework from home on a few days of the week can be other helpful strategies for IH patients [37].

KLEINE–LEVIN SYNDROME

Kleine–Levin syndrome (KLS) is a rare disorder characterized by recurring but reversible periods of excessive sleep (up to 20 hours per day). Symptoms occur as episodes typically lasting a few days to a few weeks. The onset of an episode is often abrupt and may be associated with flu-like symptoms. During the episodes, caregivers may notice behaviors such as excessive food intake, irritability, childishness, disorientation, hallucinations, and an abnormally uninhibited sex drive. Derealization affects more than 9 in 10 patients and is strongly linked to hypoactivity of the right temporoparietal junction on functional imaging [38]. Affected individuals are completely normal between episodes, although they may not be able to remember afterward everything that happened during the episode. It may be weeks or more before symptoms reappear. Symptoms may be related to malfunction of the hypothalamus and thalamus, parts of the brain that govern appetite and sleep [39].

KLS prevalence is estimated at around 1 to 4 cases per million, with 5% of the cases being familial [40]. The cause of KLS is not entirely clear. Most KLS symptoms, specifically derealization, apathy, and disinhibition, are suggestive of transient alterations of the associative cortices. While not much is known about the cause of hypersomnia in KLS, it is believed that KLS patients are not hypocretin- or histamine-deficient [41]. Functional brain imaging studies during episodes are frequently abnormal, showing hypometabolism in the thalamus, hypothalamus, medial temporal lobe, and frontal lobe. Some of these abnormalities also persist during asymptomatic periods in half of the patients [38, 42].

No drug has been shown to be efficacious in the treatment of KLS. Primarily because the condition is so rare, there are no RCTs of any drugs on prevention or treatment of episodes. It is generally believed that once an episode starts, it cannot be stopped by any medication. In a case series, 26 KLS patients treated with methylprednisolone during the episodes were compared with 48 untreated KLS patients. Of the treated patients, about 40% experienced a shortening of the duration of the episode by at least 1 week compared to their baseline compared to only 10% of untreated patients with a similar shortening of episodes. When methylprednisolone was given during the first 10 days of the episode, 65% of the treated patients experienced shorter episodes [43]. Methylprednisolone may be considered in patients with a history of longer (> 30 days) duration of episodes and not in those with brief (7-10 days) duration of episodes.

There is some anecdotal evidence for clarithromycin in KLS, altogether describing 5 patients who not only noticed some improvement in symptoms after an episode was stopped by clarithromycin but also experienced a lengthening of inter-episode duration [44 - 46]. Psychostimulants have been used in KLS with some benefit in improving alertness, as expected, but with no effect on other KLS symptoms like apathy, derealization or confusion [47 - 49]. Targeted management of other symptoms like using neuroleptics for psychotic symptoms [47, 50] and benzodiazepines for anxiety can be of some help. Lastly, there is also some anecdotal evidence with amantadine in terminating KLS episodes [51].

In terms of preventing KLS episodes, lithium has been shown to be somewhat effective. A large prospective, open-label, controlled study of 71 KLS patients who were treated with lithium showed superior outcomes when compared with 49 KLS patients who were not treated with lithium. It was noted that serum lithium levels kept between 0.8 and 1.2 mmol/L (measured 12 h after the drug intake) completely terminated the episodes in 35% of patients and in 45% of lithium-treated patients, episodes were either less frequent or less severe, and episodes relapsed within 2 days when lithium was discontinued [52]. Other mood stabilizers and antiepileptics valproic acid, carbamazepine, phenytoin, gabapentin, and lamotrigine have been studied, but none of these have consistently demonstrated significant benefit [53].

HYPERSOMNIA DUE TO A MEDICAL OR NEUROLOGIC DISEASE

Excessive daytime sleepiness can also be secondary to neurodegenerative disorders like Parkinson's disease or dementia with Lewy bodies [54], or other neurologic conditions like Prader–Willi syndrome [55], muscular dystrophies, or tumoral pathologies like craniopharyngioma, and even vascular or inflammatory insults to the central nervous system. Additionally, around 10% of patients with severe obstructive sleep apnea (OSA) may also have residual sleepiness despite being adherent to therapeutic PAP settings [56], and there is some evidence to suggest that this may possibly be associated with long-term damage to arousal systems from intermittent hypoxemia [57]. Lastly, post-viral hypersomnia can also be seen, especially after infections with Epstein–Barr virus [58].

Of the conditions listed above, only hypersomnia associated with obstructive sleep apnea has specific pharmacologic options that are FDA-approved which include, modafinil [59], armodafinil [60], and solriamfetol [25]. Because of the association of Hypertension with OSA, and the risk of elevating blood pressure with these medications, caution is advised when using these medications in this specific subset of the population.

In Parkinson's patients, modafinil may have some clinical utility as a meta-analysis of several small RCTs showed a mean ESS reduction of 2.3 points compared to placebo [61]. A double-blind, placebo-controlled crossover trial of 12 patients with Parkinson's disease showed that sodium oxybate, compared with placebo, significantly improved daytime sleepiness as well as sleep quality both subjectively and objectively [62]. However, careful attention should be paid when prescribing as the risks of sodium oxybate could potentially be magnified in Parkinson's disease [41].

While subjective daytime sleepiness was not improved with armodafinil in an RCT of 117 patients with traumatic brain injury [63], modafinil, on the other hand, did show a modest effect (ESS reduction of 1.6 points) in a meta-analysis of a few studies of myotonic dystrophy [64].

HYPERSOMNIA SECONDARY TO PSYCHIATRIC CONDITIONS

Overall, most mood disorders are associated with insomnia than hypersomnolence. However, atypical depression can present with prolonged sleep time and sleep inertia. Bipolar disorder can also present with fluctuating sleep times, oscillating from reduced sleep time with absent daytime sleepiness for a few days followed by a progressive increase of sleep time. Patients with the seasonal affective disorder can also present with increased sleep time, apathy, and decreased mood during winters. Although the pathophysiological mechanisms underlying hypersomnolence in major depressive disorders is not entirely clear, it is believed that impairment in the thalamo-striatal connectivity may have a role [65].

Management of hypersomnolence in psychiatric disorders is not well-established due to the relative paucity of data. Even though modafinil is sometimes used as adjunctive therapy for depression with hypersomnolence symptoms, 2 RCTs of modafinil in hypersomnia associated with major depression did not show sustained evidence of benefit on subjective daytime sleepiness [66, 67].

HYPERSOMNIA DUE TO A MEDICATION OR SUBSTANCE AND INSUFFICIENT SLEEP SYNDROME

Management of hypersomnia due to a medication or substance with sedating properties mostly involves minimizing or discontinuing the medication.

Insufficient sleep syndrome, defined as sleepiness caused by failure to obtain the recommended amount of sleep expected for the age, is managed by sleep extension, which may include interventions targeted to address the barriers to obtaining sufficient sleep.

CONCLUSION

From the evidence presented in this chapter, it is clear that we need a better understanding of the underlying pathophysiological mechanisms of the non-narcoleptic hypersomnia conditions, which would then hopefully pave the way for more RCTs for targeted treatment of not just excessive daytime sleepiness but also other symptoms of hypersomnolence that contribute to disease burden and functional limitations in these disorders.

CONSENT FOR PUBLICATION

Not applicable.

CONFLICT OF INTEREST

The author declares no conflict of interest, financial or otherwise.

ACKNOWLEDGEMENTS

Declared none.

REFERENCES

[1]   Schenck CH, Bassetti CL, Arnulf I, Mignot E. English translations of the first clinical reports on narcolepsy and cataplexy by Westphal and Gélineau in the late 19th century, with commentary. J Clin Sleep Med 2007; 3(3): 301-11.
       [http://dx.doi.org/10.5664/jcsm.26804] [PMID: 17561602]

[2]   Roth B. Narcolepsy and hypersomnia: review and classification of 642 personally observed cases. Schweiz Arch Neurol Neurochir Psychiatr 1976; 119(1): 31-41.
       [PMID: 981985]

[3]   Roth B, Guilleminault C, Dement WC, Passouant P. Roth B (1976) Functional hypersomnia. In: Guilleminault C, Dement WC, Passouant P, eds Narcolepsy New York: Spectrum. 1976; pp. 333-49.

[4]   Diagnostic Classification Steering Committee; Thorpy MJ C (1990) International classification of sleep disorders: diagnostic and coding manual. Rochester, Minnesota: American Sleep Disorders Association.

[5]   2nd ed. Westchester, Illinois: American Academy of Sleep Medicine; 2005. The International Classification of Sleep Disorders, 2nd ed: Diagnostic and coding manual

[6]   American Academy of Sleep Medicine. International Classification of Sleep Disorders. 3rd ed., 2014.

[7]   Fronczek R, Arnulf I, Baumann CR, Maski K, Pizza F, Trotti LM. To split or to lump? Classifying the central disorders of hypersomnolence. Sleep 2020; 43(8): zsaa044.
       [http://dx.doi.org/10.1093/sleep/zsaa044] [PMID: 32193539]

[8]   Bogan RK, Thorpy MJ, Dauvilliers Y, *et al.* Efficacy and safety of calcium, magnesium, potassium, and sodium oxybates (lower-sodium oxybate [LXB]; JZP-258) in a placebo-controlled, double-blind, randomized withdrawal study in adults with narcolepsy with cataplexy. Sleep (Basel) 2020.
[http://dx.doi.org/10.1093/sleep/zsaa206] [PMID: 33184650]

[9]   Szakacs Z, Dauvilliers Y, Mikhaylov V, *et al.* Safety and efficacy of pitolisant on cataplexy in patients with narcolepsy: a randomised, double-blind, placebo-controlled trial. Lancet Neurol 2017; 16(3): 200-7.
[http://dx.doi.org/10.1016/S1474-4422(16)30333-7] [PMID: 28129985]

[10]   Maness C, Saini P, Bliwise DL, Olvera V, Rye DB, Trotti LM. Systemic exertion intolerance disease/chronic fatigue syndrome is common in sleep centre patients with hypersomnolence: A retrospective pilot study. J Sleep Res 2019; 28(3): e12689.
[http://dx.doi.org/10.1111/jsr.12689] [PMID: 29624767]

[11]   Miglis MG, Schneider L, Kim P, Cheung J, Trotti LM. Frequency and severity of autonomic symptoms in idiopathic hypersomnia. J Clin Sleep Med 2020; 16(5): 749-56.
[http://dx.doi.org/10.5664/jcsm.8344] [PMID: 32039754]

[12]   Trotti LM. Waking up is the hardest thing I do all day: Sleep inertia and sleep drunkenness. Sleep Med Rev 2017; 35: 76-84.
[http://dx.doi.org/10.1016/j.smrv.2016.08.005] [PMID: 27692973]

[13]   Vernet C, Leu-Semenescu S, Buzare MA, Arnulf I. Subjective symptoms in idiopathic hypersomnia: beyond excessive sleepiness. J Sleep Res 2010; 19(4): 525-34.
[http://dx.doi.org/10.1111/j.1365-2869.2010.00824.x] [PMID: 20408941]

[14]   Rye DB, Bliwise DL, Parker K, *et al.* Modulation of vigilance in the primary hypersomnias by endogenous enhancement of GABAA receptors. Sci Transl Med 2012; 4(161): 161ra151.
[http://dx.doi.org/10.1126/scitranslmed.3004685] [PMID: 23175709]

[15]   Landzberg D, Trotti LM. Is Idiopathic Hypersomnia a Circadian Rhythm Disorder? Curr Sleep Med Rep 2019; 5(4): 201-6.
[http://dx.doi.org/10.1007/s40675-019-00154-x] [PMID: 33312847]

[16]   Pomares FB, Boucetta S, Lachapelle F, *et al.* Beyond sleepy: structural and functional changes of the default-mode network in idiopathic hypersomnia. Sleep 2019; 42(11): zsz156.
[http://dx.doi.org/10.1093/sleep/zsz156] [PMID: 31328786]

[17]   Sforza E, Roche F, Barthélémy JC, Pichot V. Diurnal and nocturnal cardiovascular variability and heart rate arousal response in idiopathic hypersomnia. Sleep Med 2016; 24: 131-6.
[http://dx.doi.org/10.1016/j.sleep.2016.07.012] [PMID: 27810179]

[18]   Murillo-Rodríguez E, Barciela Veras A, Barbosa Rocha N, Budde H, Machado S. An Overview of the Clinical Uses, Pharmacology, and Safety of Modafinil. ACS Chem Neurosci 2018; 9(2): 151-8.
[http://dx.doi.org/10.1021/acschemneuro.7b00374] [PMID: 29115823]

[19]   Mayer G, Benes H, Young P, Bitterlich M, Rodenbeck A. Modafinil in the treatment of idiopathic hypersomnia without long sleep time--a randomized, double-blind, placebo-controlled study. J Sleep Res 2015; 24(1): 74-81.
[http://dx.doi.org/10.1111/jsr.12201] [PMID: 25196321]

[20]   Philip P, Chaufton C, Taillard J, *et al.* Modafinil improves real driving performance in patients with hypersomnia: a randomized double-blind placebo-controlled crossover clinical trial. Sleep 2014; 37(3): 483-7.
[http://dx.doi.org/10.5665/sleep.3480] [PMID: 24587570]

[21]   Sagaspe P, Micoulaud-Franchi JA, Coste O, *et al.* Maintenance of Wakefulness Test, real and simulated driving in patients with narcolepsy/hypersomnia. Sleep Med 2019; 55: 1-5.
[http://dx.doi.org/10.1016/j.sleep.2018.02.009] [PMID: 30735912]

[22]   Morgenthaler TI, Kapur VK, Brown T, *et al.* Practice parameters for the treatment of narcolepsy and

other hypersomnias of central origin. Sleep 2007; 30(12): 1705-11.
[http://dx.doi.org/10.1093/sleep/30.12.1705] [PMID: 18246980]

[23] Ali M, Auger RR, Slocumb NL, Morgenthaler TI. Idiopathic hypersomnia: clinical features and response to treatment. J Clin Sleep Med 2009; 5(6): 562-8.
[http://dx.doi.org/10.5664/jcsm.27658] [PMID: 20465024]

[24] Thorpy MJ, Shapiro C, Mayer G, *et al.* A randomized study of solriamfetol for excessive sleepiness in narcolepsy. Ann Neurol 2019; 85(3): 359-70.
[http://dx.doi.org/10.1002/ana.25423] [PMID: 30694576]

[25] Schweitzer PK, Rosenberg R, Zammit GK, *et al.* Solriamfetol for excessive sleepiness in obstructive sleep apnea (TONES 3). A randomized controlled trial. Am J Respir Crit Care Med 2019; 199(11): 1421-31.
[http://dx.doi.org/10.1164/rccm.201806-1100OC] [PMID: 30521757]

[26] Malhotra A, Shapiro C, Pepin JL, *et al.* Long-term study of the safety and maintenance of efficacy of solriamfetol (JZP-110) in the treatment of excessive sleepiness in participants with narcolepsy or obstructive sleep apnea. Sleep 2020; 43(2): zsz220.
[http://dx.doi.org/10.1093/sleep/zsz220] [PMID: 31691827]

[27] Leu-Semenescu S, Nittur N, Golmard JL, Arnulf I. Effects of pitolisant, a histamine H3 inverse agonist, in drug-resistant idiopathic and symptomatic hypersomnia: a chart review. Sleep Med 2014; 15(6): 681-7.
[http://dx.doi.org/10.1016/j.sleep.2014.01.021] [PMID: 24854887]

[28] Wakix (pitolisant) package insert https://wakix.com

[29] Emerson E. Newly approved narcolepsy product has a price tag exceeding 100K annually. Crumdale Partners 2020.

[30] Bolin K, Niska PA, Pirhonen L, Wasling P, Landtblom AM. The cost utility of pitolisant as narcolepsy treatment. Acta Neurol Scand 2020; 141(4): 301-10.
[http://dx.doi.org/10.1111/ane.13202] [PMID: 31838740]

[31] Trotti LM, Saini P, Koola C, LaBarbera V, Bliwise DL, Rye DB. Flumazenil for the treatment of refractory hypersomnolence: Clinical experience with 153 patients. J Clin Sleep Med 2016; 12(10): 1389-94.
[http://dx.doi.org/10.5664/jcsm.6196] [PMID: 27568889]

[32] Trotti LM, Saini P, Bliwise DL, Freeman AA, Jenkins A, Rye DB. Clarithromycin in γ-aminobutyric acid-Related hypersomnolence: A randomized, crossover trial. Ann Neurol 2015; 78(3): 454-65.
[http://dx.doi.org/10.1002/ana.24459] [PMID: 26094838]

[33] Takei Y, Komada Y, Namba K, *et al.* Differences in findings of nocturnal polysomnography and multiple sleep latency test between narcolepsy and idiopathic hypersomnia. Clin Neurophysiol 2012; 123(1): 137-41.
[http://dx.doi.org/10.1016/j.clinph.2011.05.024] [PMID: 21723190]

[34] Tassi P, Muzet A. Sleep inertia. Sleep Med Rev 2000; 4(4): 341-53.
[http://dx.doi.org/10.1053/smrv.2000.0098] [PMID: 12531174]

[35] Leu-Semenescu S, Louis P, Arnulf I. Benefits and risk of sodium oxybate in idiopathic hypersomnia *versus* narcolepsy type 1: a chart review. Sleep Med 2016; 17: 38-44.
[http://dx.doi.org/10.1016/j.sleep.2015.10.005] [PMID: 26847972]

[36] Lopez R, Arnulf I, Drouot X, Lecendreux M, Dauvilliers Y. French consensus. Management of patients with hypersomnia: Which strategy? Rev Neurol (Paris) 2017; 173(1-2): 8-18.
[http://dx.doi.org/10.1016/j.neurol.2016.09.018] [PMID: 27865546]

[37] Arnulf I, Leu-Semenescu S, Dodet P. Precision medicine for idiopathic hypersomnia. Sleep Med Clin 2019; 14(3): 333-50.
[http://dx.doi.org/10.1016/j.jsmc.2019.05.007] [PMID: 31375202]

[38]   Kas A, Lavault S, Habert MO, Arnulf I. Feeling unreal: a functional imaging study in patients with Kleine-Levin syndrome. Brain 2014; 137(Pt 7): 2077-87.
[http://dx.doi.org/10.1093/brain/awu112] [PMID: 24785943]

[39]   Arnulf I, Rico TJ, Mignot E. Diagnosis, disease course, and management of patients with Kleine-Levin syndrome. Lancet Neurol 2012; 11(10): 918-28.
[http://dx.doi.org/10.1016/S1474-4422(12)70187-4] [PMID: 22995695]

[40]   Lavault S, Golmard JL, Groos E, *et al.* Kleine-Levin syndrome in 120 patients: differential diagnosis and long episodes. Ann Neurol 2015; 77(3): 529-40.
[http://dx.doi.org/10.1002/ana.24350] [PMID: 25559212]

[41]   Trotti LM, Arnulf I. Idiopathic Hypersomnia and Other Hypersomnia Syndromes. Neurotherapeutics 2021; 18: 20-31.
[http://dx.doi.org/10.1007/s13311-020-00919-1] [PMID: 32901432]

[42]   Huang YS, Guilleminault C, Kao PF, Liu FY. SPECT findings in the Kleine-Levin syndrome. Sleep 2005; 28(8): 955-60.
[http://dx.doi.org/10.1093/sleep/28.8.955] [PMID: 16218078]

[43]   Léotard A, Groos E, Chaumereuil C, *et al.* IV steroids during long episodes of Kleine-Levin syndrome. Neurology 2018; 90(17): e1488-92.
[http://dx.doi.org/10.1212/WNL.0000000000005349] [PMID: 29572278]

[44]   [ICD-10 (International Classification of Diseases): a new way with speed bumps? Discussed on the example of depression, anxiety and sleep disorders] (1996). Psychiatr Prax 23 (1 Suppl):1-8

[45]   Rezvanian E, Watson NF. Kleine-levin syndrome treated with clarithromycin. J Clin Sleep Med 2013; 9(11): 1211-2.
[http://dx.doi.org/10.5664/jcsm.3176] [PMID: 24235906]

[46]   Trotti LM, Bliwise DL, Rye DB. Further experience using clarithromycin in patients with Kleine-Levin syndrome. J Clin Sleep Med 2014; 10(4): 457-8.
[http://dx.doi.org/10.5664/jcsm.3634] [PMID: 24733995]

[47]   Arnulf I, Lin L, Gadoth N, *et al.* Kleine-Levin syndrome: a systematic study of 108 patients. Ann Neurol 2008; 63(4): 482-93.
[http://dx.doi.org/10.1002/ana.21333] [PMID: 18438947]

[48]   Arnulf I, Zeitzer JM, File J, Farber N, Mignot E. Kleine-Levin syndrome: a systematic review of 186 cases in the literature. Brain 2005; 128(Pt 12): 2763-76.
[http://dx.doi.org/10.1093/brain/awh620] [PMID: 16230322]

[49]   Carpenter S, Yassa R, Ochs R. A pathologic basis for Kleine-Levin syndrome. Arch Neurol 1982; 39(1): 25-8.
[http://dx.doi.org/10.1001/archneur.1982.00510130027005] [PMID: 6948538]

[50]   Hegarty A, Merriam AE. Autonomic events in Kleine-Levin syndrome. Am J Psychiatry 1990; 147(7): 951-2.
[http://dx.doi.org/10.1176/ajp.147.7.951] [PMID: 2356886]

[51]   El Otmani H, Amzil R, Abdoh Rafai M, El Moutawakil B. Excellent response to amantadine in Kleine Levin syndrome. Sleep Med 2020; 75: 540-1.
[http://dx.doi.org/10.1016/j.sleep.2020.07.018] [PMID: 32917543]

[52]   Leu-Semenescu S, Le Corvec T, Groos E, Lavault S, Golmard JL, Arnulf I. Lithium therapy in Kleine-Levin syndrome: An open-label, controlled study in 130 patients. Neurology 2015; 85(19): 1655-62.
[http://dx.doi.org/10.1212/WNL.0000000000002104] [PMID: 26453648]

[53]   Miglis MG, Guilleminault C. Kleine-Levin syndrome: a review. Nat Sci Sleep 2014; 6: 19-26.
[http://dx.doi.org/10.2147/NSS.S44750] [PMID: 24470783]

[54]   Arnulf I. Excessive daytime sleepiness in parkinsonism. Sleep Med Rev 2005; 9(3): 185-200.
[http://dx.doi.org/10.1016/j.smrv.2005.01.001] [PMID: 15893249]

[55]   Ghergan A, Coupaye M, Leu-Semenescu S, *et al.* Prevalence and Phenotype of Sleep Disorders in 60 Adults With Prader-Willi Syndrome. Sleep 2017; 40: 12.
[http://dx.doi.org/10.1093/sleep/zsx162] [PMID: 29294134]

[56]   Pépin JL, Viot-Blanc V, Escourrou P, *et al.* Prevalence of residual excessive sleepiness in CPAP-treated sleep apnoea patients: the French multicentre study. Eur Respir J 2009; 33(5): 1062-7.
[http://dx.doi.org/10.1183/09031936.00016808] [PMID: 19407048]

[57]   Vernet C, Redolfi S, Attali V, *et al.* Residual sleepiness in obstructive sleep apnoea: phenotype and related symptoms. Eur Respir J 2011; 38(1): 98-105.
[http://dx.doi.org/10.1183/09031936.00040410] [PMID: 21406511]

[58]   Sforza E, Hupin D, Roche F. Mononucleosis: A Possible Cause of Idiopathic Hypersomnia. Front Neurol 2018; 9: 922.
[http://dx.doi.org/10.3389/fneur.2018.00922] [PMID: 30429823]

[59]   Kingshott RN, Vennelle M, Coleman EL, Engleman HM, Mackay TW, Douglas NJ. Randomized, double-blind, placebo-controlled crossover trial of modafinil in the treatment of residual excessive daytime sleepiness in the sleep apnea/hypopnea syndrome. Am J Respir Crit Care Med 2001; 163(4): 918-23.
[http://dx.doi.org/10.1164/ajrccm.163.4.2005036] [PMID: 11282766]

[60]   Roth T, White D, Schmidt-Nowara W, *et al.* Effects of armodafinil in the treatment of residual excessive sleepiness associated with obstructive sleep apnea/hypopnea syndrome: a 12-week, multicenter, double-blind, randomized, placebo-controlled study in nCPAP-adherent adults. Clin Ther 2006; 28(5): 689-706.
[http://dx.doi.org/10.1016/j.clinthera.2006.05.013] [PMID: 16861091]

[61]   Sheng P, Hou L, Wang X, *et al.* Efficacy of modafinil on fatigue and excessive daytime sleepiness associated with neurological disorders: a systematic review and meta-analysis. PLoS One 2013; 8(12): e81802.
[http://dx.doi.org/10.1371/journal.pone.0081802] [PMID: 24312590]

[62]   Büchele F, Hackius M, Schreglmann SR, *et al.* Sodium Oxybate for Excessive Daytime Sleepiness and Sleep Disturbance in Parkinson Disease: A Randomized Clinical Trial. JAMA Neurol 2018; 75(1): 114-8.
[http://dx.doi.org/10.1001/jamaneurol.2017.3171] [PMID: 29114733]

[63]   Menn SJ, Yang R, Lankford A. Armodafinil for the treatment of excessive sleepiness associated with mild or moderate closed traumatic brain injury: a 12-week, randomized, double-blind study followed by a 12-month open-label extension. J Clin Sleep Med 2014; 10(11): 1181-91.
[http://dx.doi.org/10.5664/jcsm.4196] [PMID: 25325609]

[64]   Annane D, Moore DH, Barnes PR, Miller RG. Psychostimulants for hypersomnia (excessive daytime sleepiness) in myotonic dystrophy. Cochrane Database Syst Rev 2006; (3): CD003218.
[http://dx.doi.org/10.1002/14651858.CD003218.pub2] [PMID: 16855999]

[65]   Plante DT, Birn RM, Walsh EC, Hoks RM, Cornejo MD, Abercrombie HC. Reduced resting-state thalamostriatal functional connectivity is associated with excessive daytime sleepiness in persons with and without depressive disorders. J Affect Disord 2018; 227: 517-20.
[http://dx.doi.org/10.1016/j.jad.2017.11.054] [PMID: 29161673]

[66]   Dunlop BW, Crits-Christoph P, Evans DL, *et al.* Coadministration of modafinil and a selective serotonin reuptake inhibitor from the initiation of treatment of major depressive disorder with fatigue and sleepiness: a double-blind, placebo-controlled study. J Clin Psychopharmacol 2007; 27(6): 614-9.
[http://dx.doi.org/10.1097/jcp.0b013e31815abefb] [PMID: 18004129]

[67]   DeBattista C, Doghramji K, Menza MA, Rosenthal MH, Fieve RR. Adjunct modafinil for the short-term treatment of fatigue and sleepiness in patients with major depressive disorder: a preliminary double-blind, placebo-controlled study. J Clin Psychiatry 2003; 64(9): 1057-64.
[http://dx.doi.org/10.4088/JCP.v64n0911] [PMID: 14628981]

CHAPTER 2

Circadian Sleep Disorders

Lawrence Chan[1,*] and **Meena Khan**[1]

[1] *Division of Pulmonary Critical Care and Sleep Medicine, Department of Internal Medicine, The Ohio State University Wexner Medical Center, Columbus, Ohio, USA*

Abstract: Circadian rhythm disorders are a group of sleep disorders where one's endogenous circadian clock for sleep does not align with one's environmental sleep wake schedule. The misalignment leads to complaints of poor sleep and wake time consequences such as excessive sleepiness, poor concentration, and even mood symptoms. Treatments vary depending on the disorder, but consist of re-entraining the circadian sleep clock using bright light and melatonin as well as developing sleep promoting behaviors.

Keywords: Advanced sleep phase disorder, Circadian clock, Circadian rhythm disorders, Delayed sleep phase disorder, Dim light melatonin onset, Irregular sleep-wake disorder, Jet lag disorder, Minimum body temperature, Non-24 hour disorder, Shift work disorder.

INTRODUCTION

The circadian rhythm is an internal pacemaker that monitors one's level of alertness throughout the day. It is housed in the suprachiasmatic nucleus (SCN) of the hypothalamus. There are several circadian clock genes. Mutations of these genes can alter one's circadian rhythm.

The human circadian clock for alertness runs a little over 24 hours. It can be entrained to a 24 hour cycle by certain environmental factors called zeitgebers. Light is the strongest zeitgeber. Meal times, temperature, and social cues are other zeitgebers. The human circadian rhythm for alertness can be determined by the minimum body temperature (Tmin) and the dim light melatonin onset (DLMO). Tmin is 2 hours before one's habitual wake up time, and DLMO is 2 hours before one's habitual sleep time.

* **Corresponding author Lawrence Chan:** Division of Pulmonary Critical Care and Sleep Medicine, Department of Internal Medicine, The Ohio State University Wexner Medical Center, Columbus, Ohio, USA; Fax: 614- 293-5503; Tel: 614-293-4925; E-mail: Lawrence.Chan@osumc.edu

Imran H. Iftikhar and Ali I. Musani (Eds.)

Circadian rhythm disorders occur when one's endogenous circadian sleepy rhythm is not in line with their environmental sleep/wake cycle leading to clinical symptoms of inability to sleep with subsequent daytime consequences such as sleepiness, fatigue, poor concentration, or mood. For instance, in the delayed sleep phase, one's natural circadian rhythm would have a preferred sleep time of 2 AM - 10 AM, but the person needs to get up at 7 AM for work. As a result, they go to bed at 10-11 PM but cannot sleep until 2 AM and then have to get up at 7 AM for work and feel sleepy and tired. In this chapter, we explore the different circadian rhythm disorders.

Delayed Sleep Phase

Clinical Presentation

Delayed sleep-wake phase disorder (DSWPD) occurs when an individual's sleep schedule is significantly delayed compared to typical patterns. Usually, the delay is by two or more hours with sleep onset between 1am to 6am and wake up times in the late morning or afternoon. As a result of this misalignment, patients will report difficulty falling asleep at earlier times and difficulty waking up in the morning. As they struggle to fall asleep, maladaptive perpetuating behaviors may develop into an insomnia disorder. Confusion and sleep inertia may occur upon awakening as their sleep period is shortened. Chronic sleep deprivation can lead to excessive daytime sleepiness. When allowed to follow their habitual sleep schedule, they sleep better and sufficiently. Prevalence estimates range from 0.2 – 10%, up to 7-16% among adolescents and young adults [1].

Diagnostic Criteria

The diagnostic criteria as determined by the International Classification of Sleep Disorders (edition 3) are: Criteria A-E must be met.

A. There is a significant delay in the phase of the major sleep episode in relation to the desired or required sleep time and wake-up time, as evidenced by a chronic or recurrent complaint by the patient or a caregiver of inability to fall asleep and difficulty awakening at a desired or required clock time.
B. The symptoms are present for at least three months.
C. When patients are allowed to choose their ad libitum schedule, they will exhibit improved sleep quality and duration for age and maintain a delayed phase of the 24-hour sleep-wake pattern
D. Sleep log and, whenever possible, actigraphy monitoring for at least seven days (preferably 14 days) demonstrate a delay in the timing of the habitual

sleep period. Both work/school days and free days must be included within this monitoring.

E. The sleep disturbance is not better explained by another current sleep disorder, medical or neurological disorder, mental disorder, medication use, or substance use disorder.

Pathophysiology

Physiological markers of circadian rhythm, including core body temperature minimum (CBTmin) and melatonin levels are delayed in DSWPD [2]. CBTmin can be delayed for up to 2 hours [3], and dim light melatonin onset up to 2.5 hours [4]. While the exact cause of DSWPD is unknown, there are a number of hypothesized mechanisms, including differences in circadian period length, the phase angle of entrainment, sleep drive, and responsiveness to light [5].

DSWPD patients have longer endogenous circadian periods (τ) compared to controls. Small studies have shown these differences ranging from an additional 25 to 57 min [5, 6]. As it takes patients longer to complete their daily period, their sleep onset and wake-up times tend to occur later, creating ongoing momentum toward further phase delay.

Phase angle of entrainment refers to the relationship between physiological markers (CBTmin, DLMO) and patients sleep. DSWPD patients were found to have a longer interval between CBTmin and wake up times (3.78 *vs* 2.86 hours) [3]. Since light-driven phase advancement occurs in the time period after CBTmin [7], this limits the window for corrective phase advancement.

Differences in how quickly patients accumulate and dissipate homeostatic sleep drive may also play a role in DSWPD. With sleep deprivation, delayed patients have a slower increase in sleep drive and therefore take longer to reach sleep onset [8]. It is also hypothesized that sleep drive is also less efficiently reduced with the loss of slow wave sleep and higher stage 1 and total sleep time [9]. With the impaired quality of sleep, patients tend to sleep longer, further contributing to delay.

Given light's role as a potent zeitgieber, the response to light is also considered a factor in DSWPD. Evening light exposure has been shown to suppress melatonin salivary concentration to a greater degree in DSWPD patients [10], while morning light may have less phase advancing effects [11].

Genetic Associations

Polymorphisms in the human PER3 gene has been associated with DSWPD. Shorter alleles and specifically allele -320T and -319A and combination TA2G are more common in DSWPD [12, 13]. Mutations in circadian clock gene CRY1 has also been suspected of playing a role as variants lengthen the period of circadian molecular rhythms [14].

Management

The evidence for treatment options in DSWPD is limited, however, as per the American Academy of Sleep Medicine (AASM) Clinical Practice Guidelines strategically timed melatonin can be used in adults, children and adolescents while post-awakening light therapy in conjunction with behavioral treatments can be used in children and adolescents [15].

The melatonin recommendation was based on two studies that showed improved total sleep time and initial sleep latency [4, 16] while a meta-analysis of 5 trials supported the improvements in sleep latency [17]. In children and adolescents, melatonin improved sleep latency for participants aged 6-12 years old [18]. Due to the limited data, the precise dosage and timing have not been well established, but it is commonly used at 0.5-3 mg 2-4 hours before dim light melatonin onset (DLMO) [19]. Melatonin is generally considered well tolerated. Studies looking at up to 4 years of observational data did not identify any safety concerns or serious adverse events [20, 21].

The light therapy recommendation is based on a single study that showed benefits in subjective total sleep time and sleep latency in adolescents aged 13-18 [22]. Due to insufficient evidence, this recommendation was not extended to adults. Light and melatonin therapy may be synergistically beneficial as two studies showed increased benefit in combination compared to either therapy alone [23, 24]. The dosage and timing of light generally used is 1000-10,000 lux right after CBTmin.

Chronotherapy is a behavioral treatment for DSWPD aimed at realigning a patient's sleep schedule [25]. The goal is to use gradual shifts until it is more optimally aligned to their environment. However, instead of advancing the sleep phase, the approach synchronizes with the tendency of patients with DSWPD toward delaying sleep. In Stage I of the treatment, by progressively delaying their sleep cycle by 3 hours, patients were able to obtain their ideal phase position in approximately 6 days. In Stage II, this schedule was maintained by emphasizing the importance of adhering to the new cycle without even temporary shifts.

Unfortunately, there have been no randomized controlled trials, and the therapy is not currently recommended in the guidelines due to insufficient evidence [15].

Advanced Sleep Phase

Clinical Presentation

Advanced sleep-wake phase disorder (ASWPD) occurs when an individual's sleep schedule is significantly advanced compared to typical patterns. Typically the advance is two or more hours with average sleep onset from 6-9 pm and awake time of 2 to 5 am. As a result of this misalignment, patients report excessive sleepiness in the evening and earlier than desired wake up times or sleep maintenance insomnia. As they struggle to stay asleep, maladaptive perpetuating behaviors may develop into an insomnia disorder. When allowed to follow their habitual sleep schedule, they experience an improved amount and quality of sleep. Prevalence has been estimated at 1% [1].

Diagnostic Criteria

The diagnostic criteria as determined by the International Classification of sleep disorders (edition 3) are: Criteria A-E must be met.

A. There is an advance (early timing) in the phase of the major sleep episode in relation to the desired or required sleep time and wake-up time, as evidenced by a chronic or recurrent complaint of difficulty staying awake until the required or desired conventional bedtime, together with an inability to remain asleep until the required or desired time for awakening.
B. The symptoms are present for at least three months.
C. When patients are allowed to sleep in accordance with their internal biological clock, sleep quality and duration are improved with a consistent but advanced timing of the major sleep episode.
D. Sleep log and, whenever possible, actigraphy monitoring for at least seven days (preferably 14 days) demonstrate a stable advance in the timing of the habitual sleep period. Both work/school days and free days must be included within this monitoring.
E. The sleep disturbance is not better explained by another current sleep disorder, medical or neurological disorder, mental disorder, medication use, or substance use disorder.

Pathophysiology/Genetic Associations

The primary proposed mechanism for ASWPD is a shortened endogenous circadian period (τ) and several gene mutations have been suspected as the cause.

Missense mutations on either cryptochrome 2 (CRY2) or two regions on the period gene (HPER2) involving casein kinase I delta (CK1δ) or epsilon (CK1ε) result in a shortened τ [26 - 28]. Additionally the CRY2 mutation may decrease the phase delay response to evening light [26].

Management

The evidence for treatment options in ASWPD is very limited, however, per AASM Clinical Practice Guidelines, evening light therapy can be used in adults. This recommendation is based on the review of a few studies, most of which examined light therapy in sleep maintenance insomnia. One randomized study specifically in ASWPD showed primarily subjective benefit however did not show significant differences in objective measures [29]. While a study looking at light therapy and sleep maintenance insomnia did show delayed circadian phase, increased TST and improved sleep efficiency [30]. Dosage and timing are not well established but is generally used for 2-4 hours during the evening at a strength of at least 2500 lux [31].

Non-24 Hour Sleep Phase

Clinical Presentation

Non-24-hour sleep-wake rhythm disorder (N24SWD) occurs when an individual's sleep schedule is completely disconnected from environmental light and dark cues, mostly due to total blindness. As a consequence, the patient sleeps based on their free-running endogenous circadian period which is generally longer than 24 hours. Gradual progression of phase delay results in alternating periods where patients can be asymptomatic or have difficulties drifting in and out alignment. Symptoms can mimic DSWPD or ASWPD depending on their current misalignment with the environment. When their schedule is completely opposite to their surroundings, it may be difficult to stay awake during the daytime and fall asleep during nighttime [1]. The estimated prevalence in blind individuals is between 50-63% [32, 33].

Diagnostic Criteria

The diagnostic criteria as determined by the International Classification of sleep disorders (edition 3) are: Criteria A-D must be met.

A. There is a history of insomnia, excessive daytime sleepiness, or both, which alternate with asymptomatic episodes due to misalignment between the 24-hour light-dark cycle and the non-entrained endogenous circadian rhythm of sleep-wake propensity.

B. The symptoms are present for at least three months.
C. Daily sleep logs and actigraphy for at least 14 days, preferably longer for blind persons, demonstrate a pattern of sleep and wake times that typically delay each day, with a circadian period that is usually longer than 24 hours.
D. The sleep disturbance is not better explained by another current sleep disorder, medical or neurological disorder, mental disorder, medication use or substance use disorder.

Pathophysiology

Most patients with (N24SWD) are completely blind and therefore cannot use light to entrain their sleep/wake schedule. However, some blind patients maintain light sensitivity in retinal ganglion cells within the retinohypothalamic pathway and do not develop the disorder. Additional zeitgebers such as meals and physical activity can also be used to remain connected to environmental schedules [1].

A small percentage of patients with N24SWD do not have a visual impairment. The exact pathophysiology is unclear but thought to be the combination of several hypothesized factors that notably overlap with DSWPD. Sighted patients have extended τ and sleep duration [34], producing progressive delays characteristic of N24SWD. Similar to pts with DSWPD, they may also have abnormal phase angles between CBTmin and sleep offset limiting corrective phase advancement [35] Additionally, they fall asleep later in relation to melatonin onset, promoting further exposure to evening light and signaling slower accumulation of homeostatic sleep drive [36]. Differing from DSWPD, patients may have decreased phase shift response to bright light [37]. Some may be socially isolated and have limited daytime light exposure thus behaviorally limiting contact to zeitgebers [38]. There is also a case report of N24SWD developing after head trauma [39].

Genetic Associations

Polymorphism in PER3 and the minor allele of rs228697 is more prevalent in N24SWD [40]. Alleles in the BHLHE40 gene have also been associated with the disorder [41].

Management

The evidence for treatment options in N24SWD is limited, however per AASM Clinical Practice Guidelines, strategically timed melatonin can be used in blind adults. The recommendation was based on 3 small studies where doses from 0.5 - 10mg were used 1 hour before preferred bedtime for 26-81 days [15]. Tasimelteon, a dual-melatonin receptor agonist, is the only FDA approved medication for N24SWD. In a study of 84 blind patients, 20% took tasimelteon entrained to a normal sleep –wake cycle compared to 3% in the placebo group [42].

Irregular Sleep-wake Rhythm Disorder

Clinical Presentation

Irregular sleep wake rhythm disorder (ISWRD) is a disorder where one does not have a clearly defined sleep wake pattern. Sleep occurs at variable times in a 24 hour period. The sleep periods are brief, with the longest being less than four hours, although if added up, the total sleep time is likely normal for their age [1, 43, 44]. Patients may complain of difficulty sleeping and/or daytime sleepiness [44]. Children with neurodevelopmental disorders or who have autism spectrum disorder, as well as adults with neurodegenerative diseases such as Alzheimer or Parkinson's disease are at risk to develop ISWRD [1, 43, 45]. It can also be behaviorally induced in those who do not have a daily structured routine or a hectic lifestyle.

Diagnostic Criteria

The diagnostic criteria as determined by the International Classification of sleep disorders (edition 3) are: (must have A-D):

A. Patient or caregiver reports a chronic or recurrent pattern of irregular sleep and wake episodes throughout the 24 hour period characterized by insomnia during the sleep time, excessive sleepiness during the day (in the form of naps) or both.
B. Symptoms present for 3 months or more
C. Sleep log (and actigraphy if possible) for at least 7 days (14 is preferred) shows at least 3 irregular sleep periods in a 24 hour period without a major sleep period.
D. The sleep disturbance is not better explained by another disorder, medication use, or substance use.

Pathophysiology

The pathophysiology is not completely understood, but it may be a combination of factors. There could be dysfunction of central processes that control circadian rhythm, issues with the suprachiasmatic nucleus (SCN), and zeitgebers not being used to entrain the circadian rhythm (an example would be limited light exposure during desired wake time, irregular social schedules, or limited activity and interactions during wake periods, and daytime napping) [44].

Management

Bright light therapy in the elderly with dementia can improve symptoms of nocturnal wandering, restlessness and delirium [15, 46]. White broad spectrum light therapy of 2500-5000 lux for 1-2 hours between 9 -11 am for 4-10 weeks can be tried [15, 46, 47]. This is based on one study showing that this amount of light improved symptoms reported by caregivers though total sleep time was not changed. It is recommended to not use sleep-promoting medications – including melatonin, in the demented elderly population due to possible adverse side effects such as daytime sleepiness, confusion, and cognitive impairment [15]. Melatonin could be used in children with ISWRD and neurological disorders [15]. Combination treatment of light therapy during the day and melatonin at night did not show improvement in total sleep time in the elderly demented population. Also, melatonin was associated with increased daytime sleepiness and daytime behavioral changes in this group [48 - 50]. There may be a role to use a combination of bright light with a prescribed sleep-wake schedule and physical activity, but more studies need to be done to further explore the efficacy of this in elderly demented patients.

Shift Work Syndrome

Clinical Presentation

Shift work disorder is a disorder with symptoms of insomnia when trying to sleep or excessive sleepiness during work hours. The work shift falls at least partly during the usual sleep period. About 15-30% of the European and American workforce have a job that involves shift work (night, early morning, late afternoon/early evening, or rotating shift). The prevalence of shift work also seems to be increasing [51]. This syndrome is mainly reported by those working night shifts, early morning shifts, and rotating shifts. Commonly these patients lose 1 to 4 hours of sleep a night and have an inadequate sleep [51]. Sleepiness impairs job performance and can also lead to safety concerns at work as well as driving to and/or from work [1, 51]. The actual prevalence is not known, but it is estimated that 10-38% of those on the night or rotating shift have shift work disorder [1]. There are health consequences associated with shift work. Many of the body's physiologic systems have a circadian timer that can be disrupted by shift work which may lead to metabolic and health consequences. Shift work has been associated with obesity, reduced glucose tolerance, diabetes, and some cancers such as breast cancer in nurses [51 - 56]. Cognitive impairment with regards to decreased attention, trouble learning new tasks, and difficulty with task completion have been seen in shift workers [57 - 61]. This can lead to errors in the workplace and pose a risk for accidents. Increased depression, poorer mental health, and decreased level of social and family engagement have also been reported in shift workers compared to their daytime counterparts [62, 63].

Diagnostic Criteria

The diagnostic criteria for as determined by the International Classification of Sleep Disorders (edition 3) are: (must have A-D):

A. There is a report of insomnia and/or excessive daytime sleepiness, accompanied by a reduction of total sleep time, which is associated with a recurring work schedule that overlaps the usual time for sleep.
B. The symptoms have been present and associated with the shift work schedule for 3 months or longer.
C. Sleep long and actigraphy (when possible and preferably with concurrent light exposure measurement) for at least 14 days (work and free days) demonstrate a disturbed sleep and wake pattern.
D. The sleep/wake disturbance is not better explained by another disorder, medication use, substance use, or poor sleep hygiene.

Pathophysiology

The disorder is a result of misalignment between one's circadian rhythm and their work shift leading to sleep loss [1, 51]. In addition, sleep pressure builds due to prolonged wake time and insufficient sleep [51]. In general, the circadian alertness level is high when the individual needs to sleep and sleepiness during the shift is due to increased sleep pressure and low alertness level when the individual needs to be awake for their shift and the commute to and from work. The ability to adapt to the work shift varies greatly and is also influenced by social and environmental factors.

Management

If possible, changing the shift to match the circadian rhythm of the individual is ideal but not always feasible. There are pharmacologic and non-pharmacological ways to treat shift work disorders. The mainstay of treatment is to improve the quality of sleep and then address any residual alertness issues that may continue after that. The optimization of sleep includes behavioral interventions to optimize sleep through behavioral techniques such as sleep hygiene and stimulus control. Ensuring an optimal setting for sleep with the use of blackout curtains, minimal environmental disturbance, and a regular bed and wake up time that is followed on work and non-work days would be suggested. The major sleep period could be a 7-8 hour block or 3-4 hour block that is regular and another second block that can be variable depending on the day [51]. A short acting hypnotic could help one enter into sleep faster as well. There needs to be awareness of grogginess upon awakening and any effects that may carry over into that person's work hours. Hypnotics such as zolpidem, triazolam, and temazepam have shown improved sleep duration but can have increased side effects compared to placebo [64 - 66]. Melatonin in doses of 1-10mg right before sleep have been shown to improve total sleep time [67].

Continued sleepiness during the shift can still occur even if sleep is improved and may require wake-promoting agents. Modafinil and armodafinil are approved by the Food and Drug Administration (FDA) for the treatment of sleepiness related to shift work disorders. Both have randomized controlled studies that show improvement in sleepiness, alertness, and driving performance using a simulator [68 - 70]. Caffeine at the start of a shift and naps before or during the shift have also been shown to improve sleepiness [51, 71, 72]. A nap of less than 60 minutes is recommended to avoid entering slow-wave sleep and waking with sleep inertia.

Altering the circadian clock can also be attempted. Bright light (2000-10,000 lux) during the shift can help improve alertness and shift the circadian clock. Light blocking glasses for the ride home can help as well as blackout shades during the sleep period [51].

Jet Lag Disorder

Clinical Presentation

Jet lag disorder is a condition where there is a temporary mismatch between the environmental sleep/wake cycle and one's circadian rhythm due to changes in time zones. Symptoms tend to be of difficulty in sleeping and daytime fatigue or sleepiness. In addition to sleep difficulties, those with the jet lag disorder may have gastrointestinal symptoms, feeling of malaise, memory difficulties, and impaired concentration [1]. Symptoms tend to occur within 1-2 days of travel and are more significant with an increased number of time zones crossed. They are also self-limiting and resolve once the endogenous circadian rhythm adjusts to the new time zone (about one time zone per day) [1, 73].

Due to the human circadian clock being slightly over 24 hours, the physiologic tendency for most is to go to bed later and get up later every day if left to their own endogenous clock. Due to this, traveling east is more difficult than traveling westward, although if there is a person whose endogenous circadian rhythm is less than 24 hours, it will be easier to adjust to eastward travel [1].

When one travels eastward, they are, in essence, needing to advance their sleep/wake cycle in the new time zone (go to bed earlier and wake up earlier), which is difficult to do. The typical issues are difficulty waking up in the morning and daytime sleepiness. When traveling westward, one has to delay their sleep/wake cycle to adjust to the new time zone (go to bed later and wake up later). This is a little easier than advancing their sleep/wake cycle. Common complaints on westward travel are evening sleepiness and early morning awakenings with difficulty going back to sleep [1, 74].

Diagnostic Criteria

The diagnostic criteria per the ICSD 3 are: (must have A-C):

A. Complaint of insomnia or excessive daytime sleepiness, accompanied by a reduction of total sleep time, associated with transmeridian jet travel across at least 2 time zones.
B. There is associated impairment of daytime function, general malaise, or somatic symptoms within 1-2 days after travel.
C. The sleep disorder is not better explained by another sleep, medical, mental disorder, medication use, or substance use disorder.

Pathophysiology

There is not a specific demographic that is affected by Jet Lag Disorder. There are individual variations in the ability to adjust to travel across time zones, but all ages, genders, and racial groups can develop the jet lag disorder.

Management

As stated earlier, due to the human circadian clock being slightly over 24 hours, the physiologic tendency for most is to go to bed later and get up later every day if left to our endogenous clock. Due to this, traveling east is more difficult than traveling westward for most people. The treatment of jet lag disorder centers around good sleep hygiene, the strategic use of bright light, and melatonin. In terms of sleep hygiene, when traveling, one should have a set sleep-wake schedule, have a dark environment when sleeping, avoid excessive alcohol and caffeine, and drink plenty of water [73]. During the flight to the destination, sleeping as much as possible and keeping meal times to the appropriate time according to the destination time zone can be helpful. If the duration at the new time zone will just be a day or two, temporary treatment with hypnotics may be helpful if insomnia is an issue. For a longer time at the destination, adjusting the endogenous circadian rhythm to the new time zone can be started even before travel. The phase shift techniques will depend on whether travel is eastward or westward [75].

If traveling eastward, one's endogenous circadian clock is "delayed" compared to the destination time zone. Therefore, the traveler will need to advance their circadian clock to the new time zone. One can start adjusting their circadian clock before travel by adjusting their sleep/wake cycle and strategically using bright light and melatonin up to 3 days before travel. A strategy can be to go to bed earlier and wake up earlier by an hour, expose themselves to bright light (5000 lux for 30 minutes) and use low dose melatonin (1-3mg) 5 hours before the typical bedtime [73, 76]. Once at the destination time zone, one should avoid bright morning light and should expose themselves to afternoon bright light. Melatonin before bed can be helpful as well as other hypnotics (zolpidem 10mg and ramelteon 1mg) [77 - 79].

If traveling westward, one's endogenous circadian rhythm is "advanced" compared to the destination time zone. Therefore, the person has to delay their circadian clock to align with the new time zone. To adjust the circadian clock before travel, one can delay the sleep/wake routine by 4 hours and use 2 hours of bright light at 4000 lux before bedtime. At the travel destination, one should avoid morning light and expose themselves to evening light [73, 80, 81].

CONCLUSION

Circadian rhythm disorders are a group of sleep disorders that occur when one's circadian or biological sleep clock is not in cinq with their desired sleep wake schedule. This can lead to symptoms of difficulty sleeping or excessive sleepiness during their wake time. The approach to treatment is typically a combination of behavioral changes and entraining the circadian clock to the desired sleep-wake timing if possible. At times the use of sleep-promoting and or wake-promoting medication may be helpful depending on the disorder.

CONSENT FOR PUBLICATION

Not applicable.

CONFLICT OF INTEREST

The author declares no conflict of interest, financial or otherwise.

ACKNOWLEDGEMENT

Declared none.

REFERENCES

[1]   Medicine, A.A.o.S. International Classification of Sleep Disorders. 3rd editin 2014.

[2]   Oren DA, Turner EH, Wehr TA. Abnormal circadian rhythms of plasma melatonin and body temperature in the delayed sleep phase syndrome. J Neurol Neurosurg Psychiatry 1995; 58(3): 379.
[http://dx.doi.org/10.1136/jnnp.58.3.379] [PMID: 7897427]

[3]   Ozaki S, Uchiyama M, Shirakawa S, Okawa M. Prolonged interval from body temperature nadir to sleep offset in patients with delayed sleep phase syndrome. Sleep 1996; 19(1): 36-40.
[PMID: 8650460]

[4]   Rahman SA, Kayumov L, Tchmoutina EA, Shapiro CM. Clinical efficacy of dim light melatonin onset testing in diagnosing delayed sleep phase syndrome. Sleep Med 2009; 10(5): 549-55.
[http://dx.doi.org/10.1016/j.sleep.2008.03.020] [PMID: 18725185]

[5]   Micic G, Lovato N, Gradisar M, Ferguson SA, Burgess HJ, Lack LC. The etiology of delayed sleep phase disorder. Sleep Med Rev 2016; 27: 29-38.
[http://dx.doi.org/10.1016/j.smrv.2015.06.004] [PMID: 26434674]

[6]   Campbell SS, Murphy PJ. Delayed sleep phase disorder in temporal isolation. Sleep 2007; 30(9): 1225-8.
[http://dx.doi.org/10.1093/sleep/30.9.1225] [PMID: 17910395]

[7]   Rosenthal NE, Joseph-Vanderpool JR, Levendosky AA, *et al.* Phase-shifting effects of bright morning light as treatment for delayed sleep phase syndrome. Sleep 1990; 13(4): 354-61.
[PMID: 2267478]

[8]   Uchiyama M, Okawa M, Shibui K, *et al.* Poor recovery sleep after sleep deprivation in delayed sleep phase syndrome. Psychiatry Clin Neurosci 1999; 53(2): 195-7.
[http://dx.doi.org/10.1046/j.1440-1819.1999.00481.x] [PMID: 10459687]

[9]   Watanabe T, Kajimura N, Kato M, *et al.* Sleep and circadian rhythm disturbances in patients with delayed sleep phase syndrome. Sleep 2003; 26(6): 657-61.
[http://dx.doi.org/10.1093/sleep/26.6.657] [PMID: 14572116]

[10]   Aoki H, Ozeki Y, Yamada N. Hypersensitivity of melatonin suppression in response to light in patients with delayed sleep phase syndrome. Chronobiol Int 2001; 18(2): 263-71.
[http://dx.doi.org/10.1081/CBI-100103190] [PMID: 11379666]

[11]   Crowley SJ, Carskadon MA. Modifications to weekend recovery sleep delay circadian phase in older adolescents. Chronobiol Int 2010; 27(7): 1469-92.
[http://dx.doi.org/10.3109/07420528.2010.503293] [PMID: 20795887]

[12]   Archer SN, Carpen JD, Gibson M, *et al.* Polymorphism in the PER3 promoter associates with diurnal preference and delayed sleep phase disorder. Sleep 2010; 33(5): 695-701.
[http://dx.doi.org/10.1093/sleep/33.5.695] [PMID: 20469812]

[13]   Archer SN, Robilliard DL, Skene DJ, *et al.* A length polymorphism in the circadian clock gene Per3 is linked to delayed sleep phase syndrome and extreme diurnal preference. Sleep 2003; 26(4): 413-5.
[http://dx.doi.org/10.1093/sleep/26.4.413] [PMID: 12841365]

[14]   Patke A, Murphy PJ, Onat OE, *et al.* Mutation of the Human Circadian Clock Gene CRY1 in Familial Delayed Sleep Phase Disorder. Cell 2017; 169(2): 203-215.e13.
[http://dx.doi.org/10.1016/j.cell.2017.03.027] [PMID: 28388406]

[15]   Auger RR, Burgess HJ, Emens JS, Deriy LV, Thomas SM, Sharkey KM. Clinical Practice Guideline for the Treatment of Intrinsic Circadian Rhythm Sleep-Wake Disorders: Advanced Sleep-Wake Phase Disorder (ASWPD), Delayed Sleep-Wake Phase Disorder (DSWPD), Non-24-Hour Sleep-Wake Rhythm Disorder (N24SWD), and Irregular Sleep-Wake Rhythm Disorder (ISWRD). An Update for 2015: An American Academy of Sleep Medicine Clinical Practice Guideline. J Clin Sleep Med 2015; 11(10): 1199-236.
[http://dx.doi.org/10.5664/jcsm.5100] [PMID: 26414986]

[16] Kayumov L, Brown G, Jindal R, Buttoo K, Shapiro CM. A randomized, double-blind, placebo-controlled crossover study of the effect of exogenous melatonin on delayed sleep phase syndrome. Psychosom Med 2001; 63(1): 40-8.
[http://dx.doi.org/10.1097/00006842-200101000-00005] [PMID: 11211063]

[17] van Geijlswijk IM, Korzilius HP, Smits MG. The use of exogenous melatonin in delayed sleep phase disorder: a meta-analysis. Sleep 2010; 33(12): 1605-14.
[http://dx.doi.org/10.1093/sleep/33.12.1605] [PMID: 21120122]

[18] van Geijlswijk IM, van der Heijden KB, Egberts AC, Korzilius HP, Smits MG. Dose finding of melatonin for chronic idiopathic childhood sleep onset insomnia: an RCT. Psychopharmacology (Berl) 2010; 212(3): 379-91.
[http://dx.doi.org/10.1007/s00213-010-1962-0] [PMID: 20668840]

[19] Burgess HJ, Revell VL, Molina TA, Eastman CI. Human phase response curves to three days of daily melatonin: 0.5 mg *versus* 3.0 mg. J Clin Endocrinol Metab 2010; 95(7): 3325-31.
[http://dx.doi.org/10.1210/jc.2009-2590] [PMID: 20410229]

[20] Hoebert M, van der Heijden KB, van Geijlswijk IM, Smits MG. Long-term follow-up of melatonin treatment in children with ADHD and chronic sleep onset insomnia. J Pineal Res 2009; 47(1): 1-7.
[http://dx.doi.org/10.1111/j.1600-079X.2009.00681.x] [PMID: 19486273]

[21] Carr R, Wasdell MB, Hamilton D, *et al.* Long-term effectiveness outcome of melatonin therapy in children with treatment-resistant circadian rhythm sleep disorders. J Pineal Res 2007; 43(4): 351-9.
[http://dx.doi.org/10.1111/j.1600-079X.2007.00485.x] [PMID: 17910603]

[22] Gradisar M, Dohnt H, Gardner G, *et al.* A randomized controlled trial of cognitive-behavior therapy plus bright light therapy for adolescent delayed sleep phase disorder. Sleep 2011; 34(12): 1671-80.
[http://dx.doi.org/10.5665/sleep.1432] [PMID: 22131604]

[23] Paul MA, Gray GW, Lieberman HR, *et al.* Phase advance with separate and combined melatonin and light treatment. Psychopharmacology (Berl) 2011; 214(2): 515-23.
[http://dx.doi.org/10.1007/s00213-010-2059-5] [PMID: 21069516]

[24] Burke TM, Markwald RR, Chinoy ED, *et al.* Combination of light and melatonin time cues for phase advancing the human circadian clock. Sleep 2013; 36(11): 1617-24.
[http://dx.doi.org/10.5665/sleep.3110] [PMID: 24179293]

[25] Czeisler CA, Richardson GS, Coleman RM, *et al.* Chronotherapy: resetting the circadian clocks of patients with delayed sleep phase insomnia. Sleep 1981; 4(1): 1-21.
[http://dx.doi.org/10.1093/sleep/4.1.1] [PMID: 7232967]

[26] Hirano A, Shi G, Jones CR, *et al.* A Cryptochrome 2 mutation yields advanced sleep phase in humans. eLife 2016; 5: 5.
[http://dx.doi.org/10.7554/eLife.16695] [PMID: 27529127]

[27] Toh KL, Jones CR, He Y, *et al.* An hPer2 phosphorylation site mutation in familial advanced sleep phase syndrome. Science 2001; 291(5506): 1040-3.
[http://dx.doi.org/10.1126/science.1057499] [PMID: 11232563]

[28] Xu Y, Padiath QS, Shapiro RE, *et al.* Functional consequences of a CKIdelta mutation causing familial advanced sleep phase syndrome. Nature 2005; 434(7033): 640-4.
[http://dx.doi.org/10.1038/nature03453] [PMID: 15800623]

[29] Palmer CR, Kripke DF, Savage HC Jr, Cindrich LA, Loving RT, Elliott JA. Efficacy of enhanced evening light for advanced sleep phase syndrome. Behav Sleep Med 2003; 1(4): 213-26.
[http://dx.doi.org/10.1207/S15402010BSM0104_4] [PMID: 15602801]

[30] Campbell SS, Dawson D, Anderson MW. Alleviation of sleep maintenance insomnia with timed exposure to bright light. J Am Geriatr Soc 1993; 41(8): 829-36.
[http://dx.doi.org/10.1111/j.1532-5415.1993.tb06179.x] [PMID: 8340561]

[31]   Lack L, Wright H, Kemp K, Gibbon S. The treatment of early-morning awakening insomnia with 2 evenings of bright light. Sleep 2005; 28(5): 616-23.
[http://dx.doi.org/10.1093/sleep/28.5.616] [PMID: 16171276]

[32]   Sack RL, Auckley D, Auger RR, *et al.* Circadian rhythm sleep disorders: part II, advanced sleep phase disorder, delayed sleep phase disorder, free-running disorder, and irregular sleep-wake rhythm. An American Academy of Sleep Medicine review. Sleep 2007; 30(11): 1484-501.
[http://dx.doi.org/10.1093/sleep/30.11.1484] [PMID: 18041481]

[33]   Flynn-Evans EE, Tabandeh H, Skene DJ, Lockley SW. Circadian Rhythm Disorders and Melatonin Production in 127 Blind Women with and without Light Perception. J Biol Rhythms 2014; 29(3): 215-24.
[http://dx.doi.org/10.1177/0748730414536852] [PMID: 24916394]

[34]   Hayakawa T, Uchiyama M, Kamei Y, *et al.* Clinical analyses of sighted patients with non-24-hour sleep-wake syndrome: a study of 57 consecutively diagnosed cases. Sleep 2005; 28(8): 945-52.
[http://dx.doi.org/10.1093/sleep/28.8.945] [PMID: 16218077]

[35]   Uchiyama M, Okawa M, Shibui K, *et al.* Altered phase relation between sleep timing and core body temperature rhythm in delayed sleep phase syndrome and non-24-hour sleep-wake syndrome in humans. Neurosci Lett 2000; 294(2): 101-4.
[http://dx.doi.org/10.1016/S0304-3940(00)01551-2] [PMID: 11058797]

[36]   Uchiyama M, Shibui K, Hayakawa T, *et al.* Larger phase angle between sleep propensity and melatonin rhythms in sighted humans with non-24-hour sleep-wake syndrome. Sleep 2002; 25(1): 83-8.
[http://dx.doi.org/10.1093/sleep/25.1.83] [PMID: 11833864]

[37]   McArthur AJ, Lewy AJ, Sack RL. Non-24-hour sleep-wake syndrome in a sighted man: circadian rhythm studies and efficacy of melatonin treatment. Sleep 1996; 19(7): 544-53.
[http://dx.doi.org/10.1093/sleep/19.7.544] [PMID: 8899933]

[38]   Malkani RG, Abbott SM, Reid KJ, Zee PC. Diagnostic and Treatment Challenges of Sighted Non-2--Hour Sleep-Wake Disorder. J Clin Sleep Med 2018; 14(4): 603-13.
[http://dx.doi.org/10.5664/jcsm.7054] [PMID: 29609703]

[39]   Boivin DB, James FO, Santo JB, Caliyurt O, Chalk C. Non-24-hour sleep-wake syndrome following a car accident. Neurology 2003; 60(11): 1841-3.
[http://dx.doi.org/10.1212/01.WNL.0000061482.24750.7C] [PMID: 12796546]

[40]   Hida A, Kitamura S, Katayose Y, *et al.* Screening of clock gene polymorphisms demonstrates association of a PER3 polymorphism with morningness-eveningness preference and circadian rhythm sleep disorder. Sci Rep 2014; 4(1): 6309.
[http://dx.doi.org/10.1038/srep06309] [PMID: 25201053]

[41]   Kripke DF, Klimecki WT, Nievergelt CM, *et al.* Circadian polymorphisms in night owls, in bipolars, and in non-24-hour sleep cycles. Psychiatry Investig 2014; 11(4): 345-62.
[http://dx.doi.org/10.4306/pi.2014.11.4.345] [PMID: 25395965]

[42]   Lockley SW, Dressman MA, Licamele L, *et al.* Tasimelteon for non-24-hour sleep-wake disorder in totally blind people (SET and RESET): two multicentre, randomised, double-masked, placebo-controlled phase 3 trials. Lancet 2015; 386(10005): 1754-64.
[http://dx.doi.org/10.1016/S0140-6736(15)60031-9] [PMID: 26466871]

[43]   Pavlova M. Circadian Rhythm Sleep-Wake Disorders Continuum (Minneap Minn) 2017; 23(4, Sleep Neurology): 1051-63.
[http://dx.doi.org/10.1212/CON.0000000000000499]

[44]   Oyegbile T, Videnovic A. Irregular Sleep-Wake Rhythm Disorder. Neurol Clin 2019; 37(3): 553-61.
[http://dx.doi.org/10.1016/j.ncl.2019.04.002] [PMID: 31256789]

[45]   Zee PC, Vitiello MV. Circadian Rhythm Sleep Disorder: Irregular Sleep Wake Rhythm Type. Sleep

Med Clin 2009; 4(2): 213-8.
[http://dx.doi.org/10.1016/j.jsmc.2009.01.009] [PMID: 20160950]

[46]   Mishima K, Okawa M, Hishikawa Y, Hozumi S, Hori H, Takahashi K. Morning bright light therapy for sleep and behavior disorders in elderly patients with dementia. Acta Psychiatr Scand 1994; 89(1): 1-7.
[http://dx.doi.org/10.1111/j.1600-0447.1994.tb01477.x] [PMID: 8140901]

[47]   Dowling GA, Burr RL, Van Someren EJ, *et al.* Melatonin and bright-light treatment for rest-activity disruption in institutionalized patients with Alzheimer's disease. J Am Geriatr Soc 2008; 56(2): 239-46.
[http://dx.doi.org/10.1111/j.1532-5415.2007.01543.x] [PMID: 18070004]

[48]   Riemersma-van der Lek RF, Swaab DF, Twisk J, Hol EM, Hoogendijk WJ, Van Someren EJ. Effect of bright light and melatonin on cognitive and noncognitive function in elderly residents of group care facilities: a randomized controlled trial. JAMA 2008; 299(22): 2642-55.
[http://dx.doi.org/10.1001/jama.299.22.2642] [PMID: 18544724]

[49]   Serfaty M, Kennell-Webb S, Warner J, Blizard R, Raven P. Double blind randomised placebo controlled trial of low dose melatonin for sleep disorders in dementia. Int J Geriatr Psychiatry 2002; 17(12): 1120-7.
[http://dx.doi.org/10.1002/gps.760] [PMID: 12461760]

[50]   Singer C, Tractenberg RE, Kaye J, *et al.* A multicenter, placebo-controlled trial of melatonin for sleep disturbance in Alzheimer's disease. Sleep 2003; 26(7): 893-901.
[http://dx.doi.org/10.1093/sleep/26.7.893] [PMID: 14655926]

[51]   Cheng P, Drake C. Shift Work Disorder. Neurol Clin 2019; 37(3): 563-77.
[http://dx.doi.org/10.1016/j.ncl.2019.03.003] [PMID: 31256790]

[52]   Grundy A, Cotterchio M, Kirsh VA, Nadalin V, Lightfoot N, Kreiger N. Rotating shift work associated with obesity in men from northeastern Ontario. Health Promot Chronic Dis Prev Can 2017; 37(8): 238-47.
[http://dx.doi.org/10.24095/hpcdp.37.8.02] [PMID: 28800293]

[53]   Scheer FA, Hilton MF, Mantzoros CS, Shea SA. Adverse metabolic and cardiovascular consequences of circadian misalignment. Proc Natl Acad Sci USA 2009; 106(11): 4453-8.
[http://dx.doi.org/10.1073/pnas.0808180106] [PMID: 19255424]

[54]   Knutsson A, Kempe A. Shift work and diabetes--a systematic review. Chronobiol Int 2014; 31(10): 1146-51.
[http://dx.doi.org/10.3109/07420528.2014.957308] [PMID: 25290038]

[55]   Pan A, Schernhammer ES, Sun Q, Hu FB. Rotating night shift work and risk of type 2 diabetes: two prospective cohort studies in women. PLoS Med 2011; 8(12): e1001141.
[http://dx.doi.org/10.1371/journal.pmed.1001141] [PMID: 22162955]

[56]   Yuan X, Zhu C, Wang M, Mo F, Du W, Ma X. Night Shift Work Increases the Risks of Multiple Primary Cancers in Women: A Systematic Review and Meta-analysis of 61 Articles. Cancer Epidemiol Biomarkers Prev 2018; 27(1): 25-40.
[http://dx.doi.org/10.1158/1055-9965.EPI-17-0221] [PMID: 29311165]

[57]   Graw P, Kräuchi K, Knoblauch V, Wirz-Justice A, Cajochen C. Circadian and wake-dependent modulation of fastest and slowest reaction times during the psychomotor vigilance task. Physiol Behav 2004; 80(5): 695-701.
[http://dx.doi.org/10.1016/j.physbeh.2003.12.004] [PMID: 14984804]

[58]   Horowitz TS, Cade BE, Wolfe JM, Czeisler CA. Searching night and day: a dissociation of effects of circadian phase and time awake on visual selective attention and vigilance. Psychol Sci 2003; 14(6): 549-57.
[http://dx.doi.org/10.1046/j.0956-7976.2003.psci_1464.x] [PMID: 14629685]

[59]   Cheng P, Tallent G, Bender TJ, Tran KM, Drake CL. Shift Work and Cognitive Flexibility: Decomposing Task Performance. J Biol Rhythms 2017; 32(2): 143-53.
       [http://dx.doi.org/10.1177/0748730417699309] [PMID: 28470121]

[60]   Belcher R, Gumenyuk V, Roth T. Insomnia in shift work disorder relates to occupational and neurophysiological impairment. J Clin Sleep Med 2015; 11(4): 457-65.
       [http://dx.doi.org/10.5664/jcsm.4606] [PMID: 25665690]

[61]   Gumenyuk V, Roth T, Korzyukov O, *et al.* Shift work sleep disorder is associated with an attenuated brain response of sensory memory and an increased brain response to novelty: an ERP study. Sleep 2010; 33(5): 703-13.
       [http://dx.doi.org/10.1093/sleep/33.5.703] [PMID: 20469813]

[62]   Jensen HI, Larsen JW, Thomsen TD. The impact of shift work on intensive care nurses' lives outside work: A cross-sectional study. J Clin Nurs 2018; 27(3-4): e703-9.
       [http://dx.doi.org/10.1111/jocn.14197] [PMID: 29193498]

[63]   Zhao Y, Richardson A, Poyser C, Butterworth P, Strazdins L, Leach LS. Shift work and mental health: a systematic review and meta-analysis. Int Arch Occup Environ Health 2019; 92(6): 763-93.
       [http://dx.doi.org/10.1007/s00420-019-01434-3] [PMID: 31055776]

[64]   Morgenthaler TI, Lee-Chiong T, Alessi C, *et al.* Practice parameters for the clinical evaluation and treatment of circadian rhythm sleep disorders. An American Academy of Sleep Medicine report. Sleep 2007; 30(11): 1445-59.
       [http://dx.doi.org/10.1093/sleep/30.11.1445] [PMID: 18041479]

[65]   Buscemi N, Vandermeer B, Friesen C, *et al.* The efficacy and safety of drug treatments for chronic insomnia in adults: a meta-analysis of RCTs. J Gen Intern Med 2007; 22(9): 1335-50.
       [http://dx.doi.org/10.1007/s11606-007-0251-z] [PMID: 17619935]

[66]   Balkin TJ, O'Donnell VM, Wesensten N, McCann U, Belenky G. Comparison of the daytime sleep and performance effects of zolpidem *versus* triazolam. Psychopharmacology (Berl) 1992; 107(1): 83-8.
       [http://dx.doi.org/10.1007/BF02244970] [PMID: 1589566]

[67]   Liira J, Verbeek J, Ruotsalainen J. Pharmacological interventions for sleepiness and sleep disturbances caused by shift work. JAMA 2015; 313(9): 961-2.
       [http://dx.doi.org/10.1001/jama.2014.18422] [PMID: 25734738]

[68]   Czeisler CA, Walsh JK, Roth T, *et al.* Modafinil for excessive sleepiness associated with shift-work sleep disorder. N Engl J Med 2005; 353(5): 476-86.
       [http://dx.doi.org/10.1056/NEJMoa041292] [PMID: 16079371]

[69]   Czeisler CA, Walsh JK, Wesnes KA, Arora S, Roth T. Armodafinil for treatment of excessive sleepiness associated with shift work disorder: a randomized controlled study. Mayo Clin Proc 2009; 84(11): 958-72.
       [http://dx.doi.org/10.1016/S0025-6196(11)60666-6] [PMID: 19880686]

[70]   Erman MK, Seiden DJ, Yang R, Dammerman R. Efficacy and tolerability of armodafinil: effect on clinical condition late in the shift and overall functioning of patients with excessive sleepiness associated with shift work disorder. J Occup Environ Med 2011; 53(12): 1460-5.
       [http://dx.doi.org/10.1097/JOM.0b013e318237a17e] [PMID: 22104981]

[71]   Ker K, Edwards PJ, Felix LM, Blackhall K, Roberts I. Caffeine for the prevention of injuries and errors in shift workers. Cochrane Database Syst Rev 2010; (5): CD008508.
       [http://dx.doi.org/10.1002/14651858.CD008508] [PMID: 20464765]

[72]   Schweitzer PK, Randazzo AC, Stone K, Erman M, Walsh JK. Laboratory and field studies of naps and caffeine as practical countermeasures for sleep-wake problems associated with night work. Sleep 2006; 29(1): 39-50.
       [http://dx.doi.org/10.1093/sleep/29.1.39] [PMID: 16453980]

[73]   Reid KJ, Abbott SM. Jet Lag and Shift Work Disorder. Sleep Med Clin 2015; 10(4): 523-35.
       [http://dx.doi.org/10.1016/j.jsmc.2015.08.006] [PMID: 26568127]

[74]   Auger RR, Morgenthaler TI. Jet lag and other sleep disorders relevant to the traveler. Travel Med
       Infect Dis 2009; 7(2): 60-8.
       [http://dx.doi.org/10.1016/j.tmaid.2008.08.003] [PMID: 19237139]

[75]   Burgess HJ, Crowley SJ, Gazda CJ, Fogg LF, Eastman CI. Preflight adjustment to eastward travel: 3
       days of advancing sleep with and without morning bright light. J Biol Rhythms 2003; 18(4): 318-28.
       [http://dx.doi.org/10.1177/0748730403253585] [PMID: 12932084]

[76]   Revell VL, Burgess HJ, Gazda CJ, Smith MR, Fogg LF, Eastman CI. Advancing human circadian
       rhythms with afternoon melatonin and morning intermittent bright light. J Clin Endocrinol Metab
       2006; 91(1): 54-9.
       [http://dx.doi.org/10.1210/jc.2005-1009] [PMID: 16263827]

[77]   Suhner A, Schlagenhauf P, Höfer I, Johnson R, Tschopp A, Steffen R. Effectiveness and tolerability of
       melatonin and zolpidem for the alleviation of jet lag. Aviat Space Environ Med 2001; 72(7): 638-46.
       [PMID: 11471907]

[78]   Jamieson AO, Zammit GK, Rosenberg RS, Davis JR, Walsh JK. Zolpidem reduces the sleep
       disturbance of jet lag. Sleep Med 2001; 2(5): 423-30.
       [http://dx.doi.org/10.1016/S1389-9457(00)00073-3] [PMID: 14592392]

[79]   Zee PC, Wang-Weigand S, Wright KP Jr, Peng X, Roth T. Effects of ramelteon on insomnia
       symptoms induced by rapid, eastward travel. Sleep Med 2010; 11(6): 525-33.
       [http://dx.doi.org/10.1016/j.sleep.2010.03.010] [PMID: 20483660]

[80]   Canton JL, Smith MR, Choi HS, Eastman CI. Phase delaying the human circadian clock with a single
       light pulse and moderate delay of the sleep/dark episode: no influence of iris color. J Circadian
       Rhythms 2009; 7(0): 8.
       [http://dx.doi.org/10.1186/1740-3391-7-8] [PMID: 19615064]

[81]   Smith MR, Eastman CI. Phase delaying the human circadian clock with blue-enriched polychromatic
       light. Chronobiol Int 2009; 26(4): 709-25.
       [http://dx.doi.org/10.1080/07420520902927742] [PMID: 19444751]

CHAPTER 3

Restless Leg Syndrome Management

Shaden O. Qasrawi[1] and **Ahmed S. BaHammam**[2,3,*]

[1] *Sleep Disorders Unit, Kingdom Hospital, Riyadh, Saudi Arabia*

[2] *The University Sleep Disorders Center, College of Medicine, King Saud University, Box 225503, Riyadh 11324, Saudi Arabia*

[3] *National Plan for Science and Technology, College of Medicine, King Saud University, Riyadh, Saudi Arabia*

Abstract: Restless legs syndrome (RLS) is a common disorder of unknown cause. The management of RLS is directed at relieving its symptoms. Secondary causes and factors associated with increased symptoms should be recognized and treated whenever possible. Iron stores should be assessed in everyone with RLS, and iron replacement is recommended for iron deficiency patients.

Patients with mild intermittent symptoms may be treated with non-pharmacological therapy, but when this is not effective, pharmacological treatment should be selected based on the timing of the symptoms and patients' needs. Patients with moderate to severe RLS usually need medications on a daily basis to control their symptoms.

A range of medications is now available for the management of RLS. Dopaminergic agonists are currently the first-line drugs for patients with moderate to severe RLS; however, drug-related problems like augmentation could restrict their use for long-term therapy. Alpha-2-delta calcium channel ligands are also considered first-line drugs for moderate to severe RLS patients. Opioids can be considered as a treatment option for RLS patients who have failed other therapies. When monitored properly, they can be safe and suitable for long-term therapy.

In conclusion, the therapeutic strategy should be tailored to accommodate each patient's presentation and needs.

Keywords: Alpha, Augmentation, Benzodiazepines, Calcium channel, Delta, Dopamine agents, Intermittent, Opioids, Iron, Pharmacologic therapy, Refractory, Restless legs, RLS, Syndrome, Willis–Ekbom.

---

[*] **Corresponding author Ahmed S. BaHammam:** University Sleep Disorders Center, College of Medicine, King Saud University, Riyadh, Saudi Arabia; Fax: +966114679495; E-mails: ashammam2@gmail.com, ashammam@ksu.edu.sa, ORCID: 0000-0002-1706-6167

Imran H. Iftikhar and Ali I. Musani (Eds.)

INTRODUCTION

Restless legs syndrome (RLS), also known as Willis-Ekbom disease (WED), describes an irresistible desire to move the legs typically combined with or caused by unpleasant sensations in the legs [1]. Diagnosis of RLS is based predominantly on history and physical examination to rule out other diagnoses [2].

Restless legs syndrome (RLS) has been accompanied by a considerable negative impact on overall well-being, daily activities, and life quality [3]. This effect is generally considered to be secondary to RLS symptoms effects on sleep [4 - 6]. Sleep deficit itself could lead to daytime sleepiness, poor concentration, and low mood [6]. RLS symptoms during daytime are common among patients with moderate to severe symptoms and can also have a negative impact on the quality of life [6].

RLS is a condition that can be treated and would usually respond to non-pharmacologic and pharmacologic treatment. Several agents have been investigated in randomized, controlled trials; the main classes of agents comprised dopaminergic agents, alpha-2-delta calcium channel ligands, benzodiazepines, and opioids [7 - 10].

RLS therapy aims to eliminate or decrease RLS symptoms and improve sleep quality, quality of life, and daytime function. Choosing a specific therapy varies according to multiple factors, including patient age, disease severity, presence of comorbidities, drug side effects, and patient preferences.

This chapter will review the treatment of RLS in adults.

RESTLESS LEG SYNDROME (RLS) MANAGEMENT

Non-pharmacological Therapy

Some activities and lifestyle behaviors are associated with RLS. Non-pharmacological treatments may be adequate for symptom alleviation when used in patients with mild symptoms. Even among patients with severe symptoms, non-pharmacological treatment might benefit as it may reduce the need for medications.

There are many behavioral strategies and interventions that can be useful in RLS management, such as [11 - 16]:

- Mental activities involving concentration, like video games or crossword puzzles, may also decrease RLS symptoms during rest.

- Reduction of caffeine and alcohol intake [11 - 13].
- Moderate regular exercise [17].
- For symptomatic relief: moving, bicycling, immersing the affected limbs, and massage of the legs [18].
- Avoiding exacerbating factors like predisposing medications: Certain medications are known to aggravate RLS symptoms, and therefore the need for those medications should be reviewed when possible. Those medications include antihistamines, dopamine antagonists, antinausea medications, anxiolytics, neuroleptics, beta-blockers, anticonvulsants, and lithium [19]. The majority of antidepressants have been associated with RLS, including tricyclics, selective serotonin reuptake inhibitors, and serotonin-norepinephrine reuptake inhibitors [20].
- However, it is important to keep in mind that discontinuing antidepressants is not always possible and may cause more harm. If antidepressants cannot be stopped, then secondary RLS symptoms can generally be managed in the same approach as primary RLS.
- There have been some studies investigating the use of specific interventions like complementary and alternative medical therapies such as yoga and acupuncture [21], pneumatic compression [22, 23], and near-infrared light [24] for the treatment of RLS. However, those treatments are still investigational, and the quality of the data endorsing any single therapy is low at the present time [25].
- Maintaining sleep hygiene is essential as it is known that sleep deprivation can provoke RLS symptoms in many patients.
- Any causes for sleep disturbances, like comorbid sleep disorders, *e.g.*, obstructive sleep apnea (OSA), need to be investigated and treated [26].

Iron Replacement

The altered brain iron homeostasis is a critical factor in developing a hyperdopaminergic state which is currently considered to be the primary RLS pathogenetic mechanism [27]. Low serum iron levels in 25% of patients with RLS were first reported by Ekbom [28], and many papers since then have shown a strong connection between the incidence and severity of RLS and peripheral iron deficiency, with or without the presence of anemia [29, 30].

Replacing iron is advised in RLS patients whose fasting serum ferritin level is ≤75 mcg/L [15, 31, 32]. Iron can be provided *via* oral or intravenous (IV) routes. The IV route has the benefit of restoring iron stores in a shorter period compared with oral therapy. However, sometimes it is cumbersome and less accessible than oral therapy and carries a low risk of serious infusion reactions, such as anaphylaxis. There are no direct comparisons between the efficacy of the IV and oral iron routes in RLS patients, and current evidence does not show the apparent advantage of one therapeutic route over the other.

- Oral iron: For most RLS patients, oral iron is preferred over parenteral because it is easier and safer. Ferrous Sulfate (325 mg orally twice daily) can be started as the initial therapy [31].
- IV iron: IV iron therapy is typically used in RLS patients who have a serum ferritin level ≤100 mcg/L and transferrin saturation <45 percent, accompanied by malabsorption or are intolerant to oral iron preparations, and for RLS patients with moderate to severe symptoms who did not respond to a trial of oral iron, or to those who require a faster improvement in iron levels because of symptoms severity [32]. Studies of IV iron indicate that it is effective in nearly 50% to 60% of the patients designated for this therapy [32].

There are many available IV iron preparations with differences mainly related to cost and the number of visits/times needed to receive the total dose. If ferric carboxymaltose is being used, a dose of 1000 mg rather than 500 mg should be administered by slow IV injection over 10 to 15 min. In case low molecular weight iron dextran is chosen, a test dose of 25 mg should be given initially, followed by 975 mg administered over 1 hour in a normal saline solution. It might need 12 weeks for the effects of IV iron therapy to be noticed [33, 34].

It is recommended to check the iron levels after 3-4 months of therapy and subsequently every 3-6 months till the serum ferritin level is >75 mcg/L, and iron saturation is greater than 20 percent. It is essential to monitor iron levels to prevent the uncommon but serious complications of iron overload in patients with hemochromatosis genes [35, 36].

The administration of iron can be stopped when target levels are achieved if a persistent cause for iron deficiency has not been identified.

Patients who fail to respond to iron replacement should be considered for pharmacotherapy for RLS.

Overview of Pharmacological Therapy for RLS

The choice of pharmacological therapy for RLS varies upon whether the condition is primary (idiopathic) or secondary (symptomatic). Those with primary RLS are expected to need treatment for the rest of their lives, especially if their symptoms are persistent. While in patients with secondary RLS, symptoms generally remit when the primary causes (*e.g.*, iron deficiency, chronic renal disease) are fixed [37, 38].

Therapeutic agents used to treat RLS include the following:

- Dopaminergic agents.
- Alpha-2-delta calcium channel ligand agonists.
- Benzodiazepines.
- Opioids.

In primary RLS with clinically significant symptoms, it is essential to review symptoms severity and frequency to plan treatment. The International Restless Legs Syndrome Study Group (IRLSSG) rating scale (IRLS) is used to determine RLS severity. The scale comprises 10 questions; each question is scored into one of five severity categories (from 0 to 4), with the maximum total score being 40 [39]. The severity of RLS symptoms is categorized as mild (1–10), moderate (11–20), severe (21–30), and very severe (31–40). The symptoms severity score can be used to determine if pharmacological therapy would be useful.

Intermittent RLS is defined as RLS with a frequency of symptoms that do not require daily treatment. Nonpharmacologic therapies can be tried in patients with mild or intermittent symptoms. However, some patients might still require treatment if the symptoms are clinically significant or disabling, even if they do not occur frequently enough. For these patients, the use of dopamine agonists on when needed basis can be suggested. Alternative treatment modalities for this group of patients include intermittent use of levodopa, a benzodiazepine, or a low-potency opioid [15].

Chronic persistent RLS is specified by RLS that is frequent and negatively impacts daily living to necessitate regular treatment, with symptoms typically happening at least twice a week causing moderate or severe distress [15].

Both dopamine agonists and alpha-2-delta calcium channel ligands are recommended as first-line therapy. Many agents from each of these drug groups are efficient compared to placebo in multiple randomized controlled trials [7 - 9].

However, there is only one head-to-head study comparing the two classes [40]. Therefore, the initial therapy should be chosen considering symptoms severity, comorbidities, drug side effect profiles, patient age, and preferences [15].

In most patients, an alpha-2-delta calcium channel ligand can be started initially due to the higher risk of augmentation associated with dopamine agonists. Alpha-2-delta calcium channel ligand agonists can be considered the first choice in patients with polyneuropathy (*e.g.*, diabetic polyneuropathy), insomnia or anxiety, or patients who have a history of impulse control disorders or addiction associated with dopamine agonist use. In contrast, Dopamine-receptor agonists should be considered as the first choice in patients with very severe symptoms, excessive weight, comorbid depression, increased risk of falls, or cognitive impairment [41].

The long-term risk of developing augmentation symptoms while using dopaminergic agents must be balanced against other short- and long-term adverse events of each agent alone; actions should be taken to ensure using the minimum possible dose in RLS patients chosen for dopaminergic agents [41].

If the first selected drug is unsuccessful or not tolerated, then a prescription from another class should be attempted. Drug dosages must be used at the lowest dose needed to control RLS symptoms [41].

Refractory restless legs syndrome (RLS) is defined as RLS that is unsuccessfully treated with monotherapy with adequate doses of a dopamine agonist or alpha-2-delta ligand due to lower efficacy, augmentation, or adverse events [15]. Iron stores should be re-checked in patients with resistant symptoms, and iron replacement commenced if the levels are low. Lifestyle, habits, medications, and compliance with treatment should also be assessed. Augmentation should be suspected in patients on dopamine agonists, mainly in those demanding increased daily doses [42]. The main therapeutic pharmacologic alternatives include using a grouping of agents, such as a dopamine agonist, alpha-2 delta ligand, and/or a benzodiazepine. Using a low-dose opioid is another option for refractory RLS [42, 43].

Dopaminergic Agents

Dopamine Precursor

Levodopa

Although Levodopa (Table 1) was the first drug to be officially investigated in RLS, and its ability to improve RLS symptoms was identified a long time ago, its use in RLS management has faded over time because of the risk of augmentation, which can appear in up to 50% of the patients during treatment [44]; a problem which has been recognized more in levodopa compared to other dopaminergic agents. However, levodopa continues to be an acceptable option for patients with intermittent RLS who do not need daily treatment as for when needed treatment is required [8, 15, 41].

Table 1. Pharmacological agents of restless legs syndrome (RLS) with their recommended doses, the time needed to reach the therapeutic effect, half-life, and possible adverse events [61, 83 - 88].

Medication		Starting Dose - Maximum Recommended Dose	Time to the Full Effect of the Therapeutic Dose	Half-Life	Adverse Effects
Dopaminergic Agents					
Non-ergot dopamine agonists	Ropinirole	0.25–4.0 mg	4–10 days	6 hours	Augmentation, impulse control disorder, fatigue, nausea, low blood pressure, dizziness, headache, nasal congestion, constipation, insomnia, lower limbs edema, and changes in mental condition
-	Pramipexole	0.125–0.75 mg	at first dose	8–12 hours	Augmentation, impulse control disorder, fatigue, nausea, low blood pressure, dizziness, headache, nasal congestion, constipation, insomnia, lower limbs edema, and changes in mental condition
-	Rotigotine (transdermal patch)	1–3 mg/24 hours	1 week	5–7 hours	Skin irritation, low risk of augmentation, nausea, low blood pressure, dizziness, headache, nasal congestion, sleepiness in susceptible patients
Levodopa formulation	Levodopa / carbidopa or levodopa / carbidopa CR	50/12.5 mg –200/50 mg	At first dose	1.5–2 hours	High rates of augmentation and loss of efficacy with rebound phenomena, dizziness, nausea, and sleepiness
Alpha-2-Delta Calcium Channel Ligands					
-	Pregabalin	75–300 mg	3–6 days	10 hours	Dizziness, sleepiness, peripheral edema, fatigue, headache, and weight gain
-	Gabapentin	300–2400 mg	3–6 days	5–7 hours	Sleepiness, dizziness, fluid retention, gait instability
-	Gabapentin enacarbil	600mg	3–6 days	5–9 hours	Sleepiness, dizziness, and weight gain
Benzodiazepines					

(Table 1) cont.....

Medication		Starting Dose - Maximum Recommended Dose	Time to the Full Effect of the Therapeutic Dose	Half-Life	Adverse Effects
-	Clonazepam	0.5–2.0 mg	First dose: effect mainly on sleep	30–40 hours	Cognitive impairment in the morning, instability, drowsiness, impotence and exacerbation of sleep apnea [43].
Opioids					
-	Oxycodone-immediate or extended-release	5 –30mg	7 days	1 hour	Constipation, nausea, dizziness, addiction and tolerance, increased sleep apnea, fatigue, somnolence, pruritus, dry mouth
-	Tramadol immediate release	50–100 mg	At first dose	6.3±1.4 hours	Constipation, nausea, dizziness, addiction and tolerance, increased sleep apnea, fatigue, somnolence, pruritus, dry mouth, augmentation
-	Methadone	2.5–40 mg	At first dose	15–60 hours	Constipation, fatigue, sedation, flush, depression, and anxiety

When levodopa is used for a short time, it is usually well-tolerated; side effects are typically mild and tend to improve with time; the most common side effects are dizziness, nausea, and sleepiness. Other challenges that patients on levodopa might encounter include symptom rebound in the early morning or the second half of the night [45, 46]. The use of controlled-release (CR) carbidopa-levodopa combined with standard carbidopa-levodopa may benefit this problem (Table **1**) [47].

- Carbidopa-levodopa 25 mg/100 mg can be started with one-half or one tablet for intermittent RLS that occurs during the evening, at bedtime, or on waking during the night. In addition, this medication may help with RLS, which can be triggered by certain situations like lengthy travel or lengthy sitting. Levodopa doses higher than 200 mg per day should be avoided [47].

- Carbidopa-levodopa CR, which can be started at 25 mg/100 mg before bed, may be helpful for RLS symptoms that disturb the patient during sleep [47].

Non-Ergot-Derived Dopamine-Receptor Agonists

Pramipexole and Ropinirole

Pramipexole and ropinirole are non-ergot dopamine agonists that are efficacious in treating RLS and are less frequently to cause adverse events than other dopamine agonists. Those agents are considered the first-line dopamine agonists for RLS treatment [8, 15, 31].

Pramipexole and ropinirole action start 90 to 120 minutes after consumption. Therefore, those medications should be taken two hours before the expected onset of RLS symptoms because once the symptoms have started, the medication is less effective [15].

Below are the recommended doses for both drugs (Table **1**) [15]:

* Pramipexole is recommended to be started at 0.125 mg once daily. This dose may be boosted by 0.125 mg every 2-3 days until the disappearance of symptoms is achieved [48, 49].
* Ropinirole is started at 0.25 mg once daily. This dose can later be increased by 0.25 mg every two to three days until symptoms are relieved. The majority of patients require a minimum 2 mg, and the doses can go up to 4 mg [50]. However, in patients with end-stage renal disease who are on hemodialysis, the maximum recommended dose is 3 mg [51].

Pramipexole and ropinirole are available as long-acting oral formations, but those formations are not well studied in RLS. Side effects are generally minor, temporary, and limited to lightheadedness, fatigue, and nausea; those side effects usually settle within 10 to 14 days. There are less common side effects like constipation, insomnia, nasal stuffiness, lower limb edema, and mental conditions like confusion and psychosis; those changes are reversible with the cessation of the medication. At higher doses, excessive daytime sleepiness and rarely sudden, unexpected sleep attacks can occur [52].

Dopamine agonist therapy in RLS patients might be accompanied by a higher risk of impulsive disorders like pathologic gambling, compulsive eating, compulsive shopping, and compulsive inappropriate hypersexuality [53, 54].

To avoid and reduce the risk of augmentation, which is a common side effect observed with long-term dopaminergic treatment in RLS, doses of ropinirole and pramipexole should not normally be increased more than the above doses.

Early morning rebound symptoms have also been reported on some occasions and need to be handled similarly to augmentation.

After sudden discontinuation of dopamine agonist therapy, withdrawal syndrome can arise with symptoms including sweating, nausea, pain, anxiety, panic attacks, depression, fatigue, dizziness, and drug craving [55].

Rotigotine

Rotigotine is a 24-hour transdermal patch non-ergot dopamine agonist.

Rotigotine (Table **1**) is usually started at 1 mg/24 hours and gradually increased to a maximum dose of 3 mg/24 hours. The most common side effect is related to application site reaction and is not related to the rotigotine itself. This is reported by 40 to 50 percent of patients [56]. To reduce this, the manufacturer advises alternating application sites, refraining from direct sun exposure, and removing the patch during magnetic resonance imaging [57]. Other side effects and risks are like those seen with other oral dopamine agonists [58].

Alpha-2 Delta Calcium Channel Ligands

This class of drugs includes gabapentin, gabapentin enacarbil, and pregabalin, which have been reported to improve RLS symptoms and seems to be as effective as dopaminergic drugs. Alpha-2-delta calcium channel ligand drugs are now considered first-line therapy and an alternative to dopamine agonists [15, 59, 60].

The alpha-2-delta calcium channel ligands are primarily helpful for treating RLS symptoms in those patients with painful peripheral neuropathy, insomnia, or sleep disturbances that are disproportionate to other RLS symptoms [61]. They are also favored over dopamine agonists in patients who had impulse control disorders (ICD) and are possibly more useful than dopamine agonists in patients with a comorbid anxiety disorder [61].

Alpha-2-delta calcium channel ligands can also be used to treat RLS in patients with Parkinson's disease, who are usually on dopaminergic therapy, or in addition to the dopamine agonist therapy in patients with incomplete response who cannot tolerate higher doses of a dopamine agonist [61].

Alpha-2-delta calcium channel ligands are not associated with augmentation, but patients should be carefully monitored for possible suicidal ideations and depression [62]. There is also increasing awareness of the possible abuse of those drugs [63].

Pregabalin

It is recommended to start pregabalin (Table **1**) at a dose of 75 mg per day, which can gradually be increased to reach the effective dose, which is typically 150 to 450 mg. The side effects that are most commonly reported with pregabalin include dizziness, sleepiness, peripheral edema, fatigue, headache, and weight gain [40, 64, 65].

Gabapentin

There is also data suggesting that gabapentin (Table **1**) might be helpful in RLS treatment.

It is recommended that gabapentin is started at 300 mg two hours before bedtime and titrated slowly up because of the possibility of the drug causing sleepiness, dizziness, fluid retention, and gait instability, mainly in older adults [15]. The effective dose is usually 300 to 2400 mg daily, given in a single dose or divided doses (one-third at midday and two-thirds in the evening for maintenance doses ≥600 mg daily) [66].

Gabapentin Enacarbil

The initial recommended dose for gabapentin enacarbil (Table **1**) for RLS is 600 mg and is advised to be taken early evening. The most common side effects related to gabapentin enacarbil include sleepiness, dizziness, and weight gain; those side effects are usually mild to moderate and resolve over time [67 - 69]. Augmentation was not identified in a retrospective review of adverse events among patients [67 - 69].

Benzodiazepines

Benzodiazepines (Table **1**) can be helpful in mild cases of RLS, especially when used in young patients [70, 71]. Clonazepam is the best-researched benzodiazepine in RLS [72 - 74]. The clinical practice indicates that clonazepam is beneficial at 0.5 mg daily in some patients. If clonazepam is used for a long duration, it may cause more adverse effects like cognitive impairment in the morning, instability, drowsiness, impotence, and exacerbation of sleep apnea [43].

Long-term treatment with benzodiazepines is restricted by the risk of tolerance in many patients; however, clonazepam abuse seems to be minimal in this disorder. For these reasons, the use of benzodiazepines for RLS is usually limited to those patients who need the treatment intermittently or as an add-on therapy for patients who have refractory symptoms.

Zolpidem and short-acting benzodiazepine receptor agonists should usually be avoided because of the risk of side effects like somnambulism and sleep-related eating disorder which have been described in patients with RLS (up to 80 percent in a study of 15 patients) [75 - 78].

Opioids

Opioids (Table **1**) can be useful in the treatment of chronic and refractory RLS. Although the mechanism of action is not well understood, drug interaction between spinal opioids and dopamine receptors has been hypothesized [79].

Many studies have shown that the use of opioids, even those with lower potency, can alleviate paresthesias or dysesthesias, motor restlessness, and sleep disturbances associated with RLS [80, 81]. Opioid therapy's potential side effects include constipation, nausea, fatigue, itchiness, sweating, unsteadiness, depression, and exacerbation of sleep apnea *via* respiratory depression; also, there is always a risk of opioid addiction among RLS patients. Augmentation is also reported [81].

Low-potency opioids like tramadol and codeine have been tried, but generally, patients with persistent symptoms will commonly need a high-strength opioid like oxycodone or methadone [82].

Just like benzodiazepines, tolerance to high-potency opioids can build with long-term maintenance therapy, and augmentation is also reported. Although the risk for opioid abuse appears to be low in patients with RLS who do not have a history of substance abuse, nevertheless there is always a risk of opioid addiction among RLS patients [81]. Therefore, opioid use is typically restricted to patients with severe refractory symptoms who do not respond to other therapies, and they need to keep regular follow-up and monitoring for response and potential toxicity [82].

When opioid therapy is decided, the preference for a particular drug need to be tailored according to patient needs and preferences. An initial trial of a low-potency opioid is always recommended. Notably, the usual effective doses for RLS are significantly lower than those used for chronic pain [51].

Treatment should be started with the minimal possible dose described below, with the typical effective dose ranges for RLS given in brackets [43, 61, 82 - 88].

- Low-potency opioids or opioid agonists:
- Codeine 30 mg (60 to 180 mg)
- Tramadol (immediate release) 50 mg (50 to 100 mg)
- Tramadol (extended release) 100 mg (100 to 200 mg)

- High-potency opioids:
- Morphine controlled release 10 or 15 mg (15 to 45 mg)
- Oxycodone (immediate or extended release) 5 mg (10 to 30 mg)
- Hydrocodone (immediate or extended release) 10 mg (20 to 45 mg)
- Methadone 2.5 mg (5 to 40 mg)

Other Drugs

There are other drugs that could be beneficial in RLS but have been investigated in only limited studies, such as carbamazepine (mean dose 236 mg/day) [89], clonidine (0.05 mg/day) [90], and amantadine (up to 300 mg/day) [91].

Vitamin D deficiency has also been linked to a higher risk of developing RLS in some observational studies [92, 93]. However, it is unknown if vitamin D supplements would improve symptoms [93].

Duration of Therapy and Follow-up

RLS is usually a lifetime disorder; however, the best and safe duration of pharmacologic treatment has not yet been identified [61]. Most of the available data are based on comparatively short duration (≤12-week) randomized trials, with a small number of long-term studies supporting the effectiveness of 6 to 12 months of therapy with either a dopamine agonist or alpha-2-delta calcium channel ligand agonists. Patients on long-term therapy should be assessed regularly and evaluated for adverse effects and complications such as augmentation and lack of efficacy [8, 15, 31, 41].

The European Restless Legs Study Group (EURLSSG) advises that patients need to be assessed by their physician every 6–12 months, even in the absence of complications. The patient is advised to provide a symptom diary completed over 7–14 days before the consultation to give the physician information about symptom severity and treatment effects [83].

If there is worsening of RLS symptoms despite treatment, the physician should check patient compliance, the addition of medications that might exacerbate symptoms, or new lifestyle changes (*e.g.*, more sedentary behavior) [83]. It is also imperative to assess iron levels during follow-up visits as iron deficiency is involved in the onset and the severity of RLS [30].

Treatment Complications

Augmentation

Augmentation is the major problem of prolonged dopaminergic therapy for RLS

[41]. It describes the general increase in RLS symptoms severity with medication doses increase, which includes the earlier onset of symptoms, higher symptoms intensity, shorter drug action duration, or topographic spread of symptoms to other parts of the body, such as the arms and trunk [41].

Augmentation should be suspected if there is an increase in symptom severity despite appropriate treatment or if the increase in symptom severity is maintained despite an increase in the dose increase, especially if a dose reduction results in an improvement in symptoms [41, 94]. Augmentation should also be suspected with an earlier start of symptoms (*e.g.*, in the afternoon or evening or if there is a spread of symptoms to previously unaffected parts of the body (*e.g.*, trunk and arms) [41, 94].

The differential diagnosis of augmentation includes tolerance, natural disease progression, end-of-dose rebound, and exacerbating factors [41].

Differentiation can be made according to symptom characteristics and reaction to dose adjustments. For example, the end-of-dose rebound can worsen early morning symptoms but does not generally cause spread to the arms.

Augmentation was first documented in patients taking levodopa [44]. Although the risk of augmentation is less with other dopamine agonists, it is still not insignificant and has been reported in pramipexole, ropinirole, and rotigotine [40, 95 - 97].

The risk of augmentation rises with increased daily doses, the duration of use, and the low level of iron stores [40, 98]. There are other less-known risk factors for augmentation, including an increase in the risk in patients with a family history of RLS and those with no evidence of neuropathy on studies [99].

Using dopaminergic drugs intermittently instead of continuously using them may reduce the risk of augmentation, although there are not enough studies about this. This is most likely the justification for using levodopa in patients with intermittent symptoms [100, 101]. Tramadol has also been shown to cause augmentation in some patients [19].

As per consensus guideline for the management of augmentation in patients on dopamine agonists, it is important to do the following [15, 41]:

• Checking Iron stores and replacing iron if its stores are low.
• Reviewing any new lifestyle changes or new medications that could exacerbate symptoms.
• In Mild augmentation, dopamine agonist dose can be divided between nighttime

and early morning doses. If this intervention is not sufficient, the dose can be increased with caution not to exceed the maximum advised total daily dose. It is important to monitor patients to make sure that augmentation is not deteriorating.

- In severe cases, shifting from pramipexole or ropinirole to rotigotine, the extended-release transdermal form, can sometimes improve symptoms, as rotigotine is associated with less significant augmentation [102].
- Otherwise, dopamine agonists can be stopped and switched to alpha-2-delta calcium channel ligands. It is recommended that when the new drug is introduced, its dose be gradually increased to the effective level before gradually withdrawing the dopamine agonist and discontinuing it. Some specialists promote a wash-out period before initiating the alpha-2-delta ligand in order to determine disease severity, but this can cause an increase in RLS symptoms and intense insomnia during the wash-out period.
- A low dose of a long-acting opioid could be considered in certain patients with severe, continuous symptoms persistent after the above measures.

End-of-Dose Rebound

Early morning rebound is defined as the recurrence of RLS symptoms early in the morning as the treatment effects wear off. Symptoms become worse than anticipated if no treatment is administered, but they resolve a few hours later. Early morning rebound often happens with short half-life drugs like levodopa [46]. It is essential to exclude coexisting disorders, such as depression or sleep apnea, that may affect sleep before adjusting the existing medications. To solve this problem, the dose of the used drug can be increased, the time of ingestion can be altered, or a different drug with a longer half-life can be recommended [103].

Tolerance and Loss of Efficacy

Tolerance refers to a reduced response to a drug over time, necessitating an increment in dosage to reach the initial improvement in symptoms. It is important to differentiate this from the disease progression and deterioration of RLS symptoms, which would likewise require higher drug doses [83]. Although tolerance is unlike rebound or augmentation, symptoms related to tolerance are not worse compared to before treatment commencement. However, it is unknown if tolerance will inevitably precede and lead to augmentation [83].

Impulse Control Disorders

Impulse control disorders (ICD) are well-recognized side effects of dopaminergic agents in patients with Parkinson's disease [104]. ICDs have also been documented in RLS, despite the lower doses of dopaminergic agents used by RLS patients. ICDs include obsessive-compulsive behavior, hypersexuality, binge eating, pathologic gambling, and compulsive shopping [52, 54, 105].

ICDs during RLS treatment are expected to affect between 3% and 17% of patients. The rate of ICDs is dose-dependent and ends when dopaminergic treatment is discontinued [83]. If ICDs arise during treatment with a dopaminergic agent, the drug should be either stopped or gradually decreased until the side effect resolves or until the medication is switched to another non-dopaminergic drug [83].

Weight Gain

Sleep loss is known to be associated with weight gain and obesity [106]. Weight gain is also a common side effect of Alpha 2 delta calcium ligands, which seem to be dose-dependent. Water retention might also happen with dopaminergic agents [83]. However, it is vital to differentiate weight gain, fluid retention (edema), and binge eating. It is estimated that between 20% and 30% of RLS patients eat during the night [83].

Mood Changes

Depression and anxiety are well-recognized comorbid conditions that are associated with RLS [107]. Patients with RLS, especially those on Alpha 2 delta calcium ligands, are at a higher risk of developing depression compared to healthy individuals [83]. Moreover, augmentation is considered to be a trigger of anxiety [83]. If depression occurs, it is important to avoid, if possible, dispensing antidepressants that are known to increase or trigger RLS symptoms, such as selective norepinephrine reuptake inhibitors or selective serotonin reuptake inhibitors. Other possible appropriate antidepressants include duloxetine, bupropion, lamictal, trazodone, and desipramine [83, 107]. Cognitive-behavioral therapy can also be of value [83].

Special Populations

Pregnancy and Lactation

The management of RLS in pregnancy should be tailored according to the severity of the patient's symptoms, mental comorbidities (*e.g.*, depression or anxiety), and patient preferences [108 - 110].

Many patients can be managed effectively without using pharmacological agents through patient education, reassurance, and iron supplements if indicated [108, 109]. Pharmacologic agents like Clonazepam or carbidopa-levodopa can be reserved for patients with severe symptoms who want to use medications [108 - 110].

End-stage Renal Disease

Managing RLS in patients with end-stage renal disease is not different from managing it in those with normal renal function. However, doses of different medications may need adjustment, particularly if the patient is still not on dialysis, as the majority of dopamine agonists, apart from transdermal rotigotine and alpha-2-delta ligands, are excreted by the kidneys. Monitoring iron status is also particularly crucial in patients with renal failure [111].

CONCLUSION

RLS is a common sleep disorder that can have a significant impact on patients' quality of life, primarily because of disrupted nighttime sleep and daytime symptoms. RLS generally responds well to a variety of pharmacologic and nonpharmacologic treatments. The aim of therapy is to decrease or eliminate RLS symptoms.

Secondary causes that exacerbate RLS symptoms should be detected and treated whenever possible. Iron stores should be assessed in all patients with RLS, and iron replacement is recommended for patients with iron deficiency.

Choosing a specific treatment for RLS depends on the severity and the frequency of symptoms. Mild and intermittent RLS may respond well to nonpharmacologic options, including lifestyle changes, avoiding aggravating drugs and substances, complex mental activities, moderate exercise, leg massage, and applied heat.

Moderate to severe cases require pharmacological treatment in addition to nonpharmacologic treatment; dopamine agonists or alpha-2-delta calcium channel ligands are usually recommended as first-line drugs. The choice of the suitable class for treatment depends on the severity of the symptoms, age of the patient age, coexisting morbidities, adverse events of the drug, and patient preferences. Refractory RLS symptoms can be treated with combination therapy and opioids.

CONSENT FOR PUBLICATION

Not applicable.

CONFLICT OF INTEREST

The author declares no conflict of interest, financial or otherwise.

ACKNOWLEDGEMENTS

Declared none.

REFERENCES

[1] Allen RP, Picchietti D, Hening WA, Trenkwalder C, Walters AS, Montplaisi J. Restless legs syndrome: diagnostic criteria, special considerations, and epidemiology. A report from the restless legs syndrome diagnosis and epidemiology workshop at the National Institutes of Health. Sleep Med 2003; 4(2): 101-19.
[http://dx.doi.org/10.1016/S1389-9457(03)00010-8] [PMID: 14592341]

[2] Allen RP, Picchietti DL, Garcia-Borreguero D, *et al.* Restless legs syndrome/Willis-Ekbom disease diagnostic criteria: updated International Restless Legs Syndrome Study Group (IRLSSG) consensus criteria--history, rationale, description, and significance. Sleep Med 2014; 15(8): 860-73.
[http://dx.doi.org/10.1016/j.sleep.2014.03.025] [PMID: 25023924]

[3] Kushida C, Martin M, Nikam P, *et al.* Burden of restless legs syndrome on health-related quality of life. Qual Life Res 2007; 16(4): 617-24.
[http://dx.doi.org/10.1007/s11136-006-9142-8] [PMID: 17268935]

[4] Allen RP, Bharmal M, Calloway M. Prevalence and disease burden of primary restless legs syndrome: results of a general population survey in the United States. Mov Disord 2011; 26(1): 114-20.
[http://dx.doi.org/10.1002/mds.23430] [PMID: 21322022]

[5] Kushida CA, Allen RP, Atkinson MJ. Modeling the causal relationships between symptoms associated with restless legs syndrome and the patient-reported impact of RLS. Sleep Med 2004; 5(5): 485-8.
[http://dx.doi.org/10.1016/j.sleep.2004.04.004] [PMID: 15341894]

[6] Hening W, Walters AS, Allen RP, Montplaisir J, Myers A, Ferini-Strambi L. Impact, diagnosis and treatment of restless legs syndrome (RLS) in a primary care population: the REST (RLS epidemiology, symptoms, and treatment) primary care study. Sleep Med 2004; 5(3): 237-46.
[http://dx.doi.org/10.1016/j.sleep.2004.03.006] [PMID: 15165529]

[7] Scholz H, Trenkwalder C, Kohnen R, Riemann D, Kriston L, Hornyak M. Dopamine agonists for restless legs syndrome. Cochrane Database Syst Rev 2011; (3): CD006009.
[PMID: 21412893]

[8] Aurora RN, Kristo DA, Bista SR, *et al.* The treatment of restless legs syndrome and periodic limb movement disorder in adults--an update for 2012: practice parameters with an evidence-based systematic review and meta-analyses: an American Academy of Sleep Medicine Clinical Practice Guideline. Sleep (Basel) 2012; 35(8): 1039-62.
[http://dx.doi.org/10.5665/sleep.1986] [PMID: 22851801]

[9] Wilt TJ, MacDonald R, Ouellette J, *et al.* Pharmacologic therapy for primary restless legs syndrome: a systematic review and meta-analysis. JAMA Intern Med 2013; 173(7): 496-505.
[http://dx.doi.org/10.1001/jamainternmed.2013.3733] [PMID: 23460396]

[10] Trotti LM, Becker LA. Iron for the treatment of restless legs syndrome. Cochrane Database Syst Rev 2019; 1(1): CD007834.
[http://dx.doi.org/10.1002/14651858.CD007834.pub3] [PMID: 30609006]

[11] Lutz EG. Restless legs, anxiety and caffeinism. J Clin Psychiatry 1978; 39(9): 693-8.
[PMID: 690085]

[12] Aldrich MS, Shipley JE. Alcohol use and periodic limb movements of sleep. Alcohol Clin Exp Res 1993; 17(1): 192-6.
[http://dx.doi.org/10.1111/j.1530-0277.1993.tb00747.x] [PMID: 8452202]

[13] Terao T, Terao M, Yoshimura R, Abe K. Restless legs syndrome induced by lithium. Biol Psychiatry 1991; 30(11): 1167-70.

[http://dx.doi.org/10.1016/0006-3223(91)90185-O] [PMID: 1777530]

[14]   Russell M. M R. Massage therapy and restless legs syndrome. J Bodyw Mov Ther 2007; 11(2): 146-50.
       [http://dx.doi.org/10.1016/j.jbmt.2006.12.001]

[15]   Silber MH, Becker PM, Earley C, Garcia-Borreguero D, Ondo WG. Willis-Ekbom Disease Foundation revised consensus statement on the management of restless legs syndrome. Mayo Clin Proc 2013; 88(9): 977-86.
       [http://dx.doi.org/10.1016/j.mayocp.2013.06.016] [PMID: 24001490]

[16]   Mitchell UH. Nondrug-related aspect of treating Ekbom disease, formerly known as restless legs syndrome. Neuropsychiatr Dis Treat 2011; 7: 251-7.
       [http://dx.doi.org/10.2147/NDT.S19177] [PMID: 21654870]

[17]   Aukerman MM, Aukerman D, Bayard M, Tudiver F, Thorp L, Bailey B. Exercise and restless legs syndrome: a randomized controlled trial. J Am Board Fam Med 2006; 19(5): 487-93.
       [http://dx.doi.org/10.3122/jabfm.19.5.487] [PMID: 16951298]

[18]   Lettieri CJ, Eliasson AH. Pneumatic compression devices are an effective therapy for restless legs syndrome: a prospective, randomized, double-blinded, sham-controlled trial. Chest 2009; 135(1): 74-80.
       [http://dx.doi.org/10.1378/chest.08-1665] [PMID: 19017878]

[19]   Hoque R, Chesson AL Jr. Pharmacologically induced/exacerbated restless legs syndrome, periodic limb movements of sleep, and REM behavior disorder/REM sleep without atonia: literature review, qualitative scoring, and comparative analysis. J Clin Sleep Med 2010; 6(1): 79-83.
       [http://dx.doi.org/10.5664/jcsm.27716] [PMID: 20191944]

[20]   Rottach KG, Schaner BM, Kirch MH, *et al.* Restless legs syndrome as side effect of second generation antidepressants. J Psychiatr Res 2008; 43(1): 70-5.
       [http://dx.doi.org/10.1016/j.jpsychires.2008.02.006] [PMID: 18468624]

[21]   Xu XM, Liu Y, Jia SY, Dong MX, Cao D, Wei YD. Complementary and alternative therapies for restless legs syndrome: An evidence-based systematic review. Sleep Med Rev 2018; 38: 158-67.
       [http://dx.doi.org/10.1016/j.smrv.2017.06.003] [PMID: 28886918]

[22]   Rajaram SS, Shanahan J, Ash C, Walters AS, Weisfogel G. Enhanced external counter pulsation (EECP) as a novel treatment for restless legs syndrome (RLS): a preliminary test of the vascular neurologic hypothesis for RLS. Sleep Med 2005; 6(2): 101-6.
       [http://dx.doi.org/10.1016/j.sleep.2004.10.012] [PMID: 15716213]

[23]   Eliasson AH, Lettieri CJ. Sequential compression devices for treatment of restless legs syndrome. Medicine (Baltimore) 2007; 86(6): 317-23.
       [http://dx.doi.org/10.1097/MD.0b013e31815b1319] [PMID: 18004176]

[24]   Mitchell UH, Myrer JW, Johnson AW, Hilton SC. Restless legs syndrome and near-infrared light: An alternative treatment option. Physiother Theory Pract 2011; 27(5): 345-51.
       [http://dx.doi.org/10.3109/09593985.2010.511440] [PMID: 20977377]

[25]   Trenkwalder C, Hening WA, Montagna P, *et al.* Treatment of restless legs syndrome: an evidence-based review and implications for clinical practice. Mov Disord 2008; 23(16): 2267-302.
       [http://dx.doi.org/10.1002/mds.22254] [PMID: 18925578]

[26]   Silva C, Peralta AR, Bentes C. The urge to move and breathe - the impact of obstructive sleep apnea syndrome treatment in patients with previously diagnosed, clinically significant restless legs syndrome. Sleep Med 2017; 38: 17-20.
       [http://dx.doi.org/10.1016/j.sleep.2017.06.023] [PMID: 29031750]

[27]   Earley CJ, Connor J, Garcia-Borreguero D, *et al.* Altered brain iron homeostasis and dopaminergic function in Restless Legs Syndrome (Willis-Ekbom Disease). Sleep Med 2014; 15(11): 1288-301.
       [http://dx.doi.org/10.1016/j.sleep.2014.05.009] [PMID: 25201131]

[28]   Ekbom KA. Restless legs syndrome. Neurology 1960; 10(9): 868-73.
[http://dx.doi.org/10.1212/WNL.10.9.868] [PMID: 13726241]

[29]   Aul EA, Davis BJ, Rodnitzky RL. The importance of formal serum iron studies in the assessment of restless legs syndrome. Neurology 1998; 51(3): 912.
[http://dx.doi.org/10.1212/WNL.51.3.912] [PMID: 9748060]

[30]   Sun ER, Chen CA, Ho G, Earley CJ, Allen RP. Iron and the restless legs syndrome. Sleep 1998; 21(4): 371-7.
[http://dx.doi.org/10.1093/sleep/21.4.381] [PMID: 9646381]

[31]   Winkelman JW, Armstrong MJ, Allen RP, *et al.* Practice guideline summary: Treatment of restless legs syndrome in adults: Report of the Guideline Development, Dissemination, and Implementation Subcommittee of the American Academy of Neurology. Neurology 2016; 87(24): 2585-93.
[http://dx.doi.org/10.1212/WNL.0000000000003388] [PMID: 27856776]

[32]   Allen RP, Picchietti DL, Auerbach M, *et al.* Evidence-based and consensus clinical practice guidelines for the iron treatment of restless legs syndrome/Willis-Ekbom disease in adults and children: an IRLSSG task force report. Sleep Med 2018; 41: 27-44.
[http://dx.doi.org/10.1016/j.sleep.2017.11.1126] [PMID: 29425576]

[33]   Trenkwalder C, Winkelmann J, Oertel W, Virgin G, Roubert B, Mezzacasa A. Ferric carboxymaltose in patients with restless legs syndrome and nonanemic iron deficiency: A randomized trial. Mov Disord 2017; 32(10): 1478-82.
[http://dx.doi.org/10.1002/mds.27040] [PMID: 28643901]

[34]   Cho YW, Allen RP, Earley CJ. Efficacy of ferric carboxymaltose (FCM) 500 mg dose for the treatment of Restless Legs Syndrome. Sleep Med 2018; 42: 7-12.
[http://dx.doi.org/10.1016/j.sleep.2017.11.1134] [PMID: 29458749]

[35]   Barton JC, Wooten VD, Acton RT. Hemochromatosis and iron therapy of Restless Legs Syndrome. Sleep Med 2001; 2(3): 249-51.
[http://dx.doi.org/10.1016/S1389-9457(01)00081-8] [PMID: 11311689]

[36]   Garcia-Malo C, Miranda C, Novo Ponte S, *et al.* Low risk of iron overload or anaphylaxis during treatment of restless legs syndrome with intravenous iron: a consecutive case series in a regular clinical setting. Sleep Med 2020; 74: 48-55.
[http://dx.doi.org/10.1016/j.sleep.2020.06.002] [PMID: 32841843]

[37]   Lee KA, Zaffke ME, Baratte-Beebe K. Restless legs syndrome and sleep disturbance during pregnancy: the role of folate and iron. J Womens Health Gend Based Med 2001; 10(4): 335-41.
[http://dx.doi.org/10.1089/152460901750269652] [PMID: 11445024]

[38]   Molnar MZ, Novak M, Ambrus C, *et al.* Restless Legs Syndrome in patients after renal transplantation. Am J Kidney Dis 2005; 45(2): 388-96.
[http://dx.doi.org/10.1053/j.ajkd.2004.10.007] [PMID: 15685518]

[39]   Walters AS, LeBrocq C, Dhar A, *et al.* Validation of the International Restless Legs Syndrome Study Group rating scale for restless legs syndrome. Sleep Med 2003; 4(2): 121-32.
[http://dx.doi.org/10.1016/S1389-9457(02)00258-7] [PMID: 14592342]

[40]   Allen RP, Chen C, Garcia-Borreguero D, *et al.* Comparison of pregabalin with pramipexole for restless legs syndrome. N Engl J Med 2014; 370(7): 621-31.
[http://dx.doi.org/10.1056/NEJMoa1303646] [PMID: 24521108]

[41]   Garcia-Borreguero D, Silber MH, Winkelman JW, *et al.* Guidelines for the first-line treatment of restless legs syndrome/Willis-Ekbom disease, prevention and treatment of dopaminergic augmentation: a combined task force of the IRLSSG, EURLSSG, and the RLS-foundation. Sleep Med 2016; 21: 1-11.
[http://dx.doi.org/10.1016/j.sleep.2016.01.017] [PMID: 27448465]

[42]   Rinaldi F, Galbiati A, Marelli S, Ferini Strambi L, Zucconi M. Treatment Options in Intractable

Restless Legs Syndrome/Willis-Ekbom Disease (RLS/WED). Curr Treat Options Neurol 2016; 18(2): 7.
[http://dx.doi.org/10.1007/s11940-015-0390-1] [PMID: 26874840]

[43]   Silber MH, Ehrenberg BL, Allen RP, *et al.* An algorithm for the management of restless legs syndrome. Mayo Clin Proc 2004; 79(7): 916-22.
[http://dx.doi.org/10.4065/79.7.916] [PMID: 15244390]

[44]   Högl B, García-Borreguero D, Kohnen R, *et al.* Progressive development of augmentation during long-term treatment with levodopa in restless legs syndrome: results of a prospective multi-center study. J Neurol 2010; 257(2): 230-7.
[http://dx.doi.org/10.1007/s00415-009-5299-8] [PMID: 19756826]

[45]   Earley CJ, Allen RP. Pergolide and carbidopa/levodopa treatment of the restless legs syndrome and periodic leg movements in sleep in a consecutive series of patients. Sleep 1996; 19(10): 801-10.
[http://dx.doi.org/10.1093/sleep/19.10.801] [PMID: 9085489]

[46]   Guilleminault C, Cetel M, Philip P. Dopaminergic treatment of restless legs and rebound phenomenon. Neurology 1993; 43(2): 445.
[http://dx.doi.org/10.1212/WNL.43.2.445] [PMID: 8094897]

[47]   Collado-Seidel V, Kazenwadel J, Wetter TC, *et al.* A controlled study of additional sr-L-dopa in L-dopa-responsive restless legs syndrome with late-night symptoms. Neurology 1999; 52(2): 285-90.
[http://dx.doi.org/10.1212/WNL.52.2.285] [PMID: 9932945]

[48]   Jama L, Hirvonen K, Partinen M, *et al.* A dose-ranging study of pramipexole for the symptomatic treatment of restless legs syndrome: polysomnographic evaluation of periodic leg movements and sleep disturbance. Sleep Med 2009; 10(6): 630-6.
[http://dx.doi.org/10.1016/j.sleep.2008.05.014] [PMID: 19171500]

[49]   Partinen M, Hirvonen K, Jama L, *et al.* Efficacy and safety of pramipexole in idiopathic restless legs syndrome: a polysomnographic dose-finding study--the PRELUDE study. Sleep Med 2006; 7(5): 407-17.
[http://dx.doi.org/10.1016/j.sleep.2006.03.011] [PMID: 16815748]

[50]   Kushida CA. Ropinirole for the treatment of restless legs syndrome. Neuropsychiatr Dis Treat 2006; 2(4): 407-19.
[http://dx.doi.org/10.2147/nedt.2006.2.4.407] [PMID: 19412490]

[51]   Trenkwalder C, Garcia-Borreguero D, Montagna P, *et al.* Ropinirole in the treatment of restless legs syndrome: results from the TREAT RLS 1 study, a 12 week, randomised, placebo controlled study in 10 European countries. J Neurol Neurosurg Psychiatry 2004; 75(1): 92-7.
[PMID: 14707315]

[52]   Lipford MC, Silber MH. Long-term use of pramipexole in the management of restless legs syndrome. Sleep Med 2012; 13(10): 1280-5.
[http://dx.doi.org/10.1016/j.sleep.2012.08.004] [PMID: 23036265]

[53]   Tippmann-Peikert M, Park JG, Boeve BF, Shepard JW, Silber MH. Pathologic gambling in patients with restless legs syndrome treated with dopaminergic agonists. Neurology 2007; 68(4): 301-3.
[http://dx.doi.org/10.1212/01.wnl.0000252368.25106.b6] [PMID: 17242339]

[54]   Cornelius JR, Tippmann-Peikert M, Slocumb NL, Frerichs CF, Silber MH. Impulse control disorders with the use of dopaminergic agents in restless legs syndrome: a case-control study. Sleep 2010; 33(1): 81-7.
[PMID: 20120624]

[55]   Nirenberg MJ. Dopamine agonist withdrawal syndrome: implications for patient care. Drugs Aging 2013; 30(8): 587-92.
[http://dx.doi.org/10.1007/s40266-013-0090-z] [PMID: 23686524]

[56]   Sixel-Döring F, Trenkwalder C. Rotigotine transdermal delivery for the treatment of restless legs

syndrome. Expert Opin Pharmacother 2010; 11(4): 649-56.
[http://dx.doi.org/10.1517/14656561003621257] [PMID: 20163275]

[57]   Chen JJ, Swope DM, Dashtipour K, Lyons KE. Transdermal rotigotine: a clinically innovative dopamine-receptor agonist for the management of Parkinson's disease. Pharmacotherapy 2009; 29(12): 1452-67.
[http://dx.doi.org/10.1592/phco.29.12.1452] [PMID: 19947805]

[58]   A controlled trial of rotigotine monotherapy in early Parkinson's disease. Arch Neurol 2003; 60(12): 1721-8.
[http://dx.doi.org/10.1001/archneur.60.12.1721] [PMID: 14676046]

[59]   Kushida CA, Becker PM, Ellenbogen AL, Canafax DM, Barrett RW, Group XPS. Randomized, double-blind, placebo-controlled study of XP13512/GSK1838262 in patients with RLS. Neurology 2009; 72(5): 439-46.
[http://dx.doi.org/10.1212/01.wnl.0000341770.91926.cc] [PMID: 19188575]

[60]   Kushida CA, Walters AS, Becker P, *et al.* A randomized, double-blind, placebo-controlled, crossover study of XP13512/GSK1838262 in the treatment of patients with primary restless legs syndrome. Sleep 2009; 32(2): 159-68.
[http://dx.doi.org/10.1093/sleep/32.2.159] [PMID: 19238802]

[61]   Garcia-Borreguero D, Kohnen R, Silber MH, *et al.* The long-term treatment of restless legs syndrome/Willis-Ekbom disease: evidence-based guidelines and clinical consensus best practice guidance: a report from the International Restless Legs Syndrome Study Group. Sleep Med 2013; 14(7): 675-84.
[http://dx.doi.org/10.1016/j.sleep.2013.05.016] [PMID: 23859128]

[62]   Garcia-Borreguero D, Patrick J, DuBrava S, *et al.* Pregabalin *versus* pramipexole: effects on sleep disturbance in restless legs syndrome. Sleep 2014; 37(4): 635-43.
[http://dx.doi.org/10.5665/sleep.3558] [PMID: 24899755]

[63]   Goodman CW, Brett AS. A Clinical Overview of Off-label Use of Gabapentinoid Drugs. JAMA Intern Med 2019; 179(5): 695-701.
[http://dx.doi.org/10.1001/jamainternmed.2019.0086] [PMID: 30907944]

[64]   Garcia-Borreguero D, Larrosa O, Williams AM, *et al.* Treatment of restless legs syndrome with pregabalin: a double-blind, placebo-controlled study. Neurology 2010; 74(23): 1897-904.
[http://dx.doi.org/10.1212/WNL.0b013e3181e1ce73] [PMID: 20427750]

[65]   Allen RP. Pregabalin *versus* pramipexole for restless legs syndrome. N Engl J Med 2014; 370(21): 2050-1.
[PMID: 24849090]

[66]   Garcia-Borreguero D, Larrosa O, de la Llave Y, Verger K, Masramon X, Hernandez G. Treatment of restless legs syndrome with gabapentin: a double-blind, cross-over study. Neurology 2002; 59(10): 1573-9.
[http://dx.doi.org/10.1212/WNL.59.10.1573] [PMID: 12451200]

[67]   Ellenbogen AL, Thein SG, Winslow DH, *et al.* A 52-week study of gabapentin enacarbil in restless legs syndrome. Clin Neuropharmacol 2011; 34(1): 8-16.
[http://dx.doi.org/10.1097/WNF.0b013e3182087d48] [PMID: 21242741]

[68]   Imamura S, Kushida C. Gabapentin enacarbil (XP13512/GSK1838262) as an alternative treatment to dopaminergic agents for restless legs syndrome. Expert Opin Pharmacother 2010; 11(11): 1925-32.
[http://dx.doi.org/10.1517/14656566.2010.494598] [PMID: 20629607]

[69]   Hayes WJ, Lemon MD, Farver DK. Gabapentin enacarbil for treatment of restless legs syndrome in adults. Ann Pharmacother 2012; 46(2): 229-39.
[http://dx.doi.org/10.1345/aph.1Q578] [PMID: 22298601]

[70]   Schenck CH, Mahowald MW. Long-term, nightly benzodiazepine treatment of injurious parasomnias

and other disorders of disrupted nocturnal sleep in 170 adults. Am J Med 1996; 100(3): 333-7.
[http://dx.doi.org/10.1016/S0002-9343(97)89493-4] [PMID: 8629680]

[71]   Montplaisir J, Godbout R, Boghen D, DeChamplain J, Young SN, Lapierre G. Familial restless legs
       with periodic movements in sleep: electrophysiologic, biochemical, and pharmacologic study.
       Neurology 1985; 35(1): 130-4.
       [http://dx.doi.org/10.1212/WNL.35.1.130] [PMID: 3965987]

[72]   Roshi, Tandon VR, Mahajan A, Sharma S, Khajuria V. Comparative Efficacy and Safety of
       Clonazepam *versus* Nortriptyline in Restless Leg Syndrome among Forty Plus Women: A Prospective,
       Open-Label Randomized Study. J Midlife Health 2019; 10(4): 197-203.
       [http://dx.doi.org/10.4103/jmh.JMH_26_18] [PMID: 31942156]

[73]   Montagna P, Sassoli de Bianchi L, Zucconi M, Cirignotta F, Lugaresi E. Clonazepam and vibration in
       restless legs syndrome. Acta Neurol Scand 1984; 69(6): 428-30.
       [http://dx.doi.org/10.1111/j.1600-0404.1984.tb07826.x] [PMID: 6380197]

[74]   Read DJ, Feest TG, Nassim MA. Clonazepam: effective treatment for restless legs syndrome in
       uraemia. Br Med J (Clin Res Ed) 1981; 283(6296): 885-6.
       [http://dx.doi.org/10.1136/bmj.283.6296.885-a] [PMID: 6793161]

[75]   Howell MJ, Schenck CH. Restless nocturnal eating: a common feature of Willis-Ekbom Syndrome
       (RLS). J Clin Sleep Med 2012; 8(4): 413-9.
       [http://dx.doi.org/10.5664/jcsm.2036] [PMID: 22893772]

[76]   Lauerma H. Nocturnal wandering caused by restless legs and short-acting benzodiazepines. Acta
       Psychiatr Scand 1991; 83(6): 492-3.
       [http://dx.doi.org/10.1111/j.1600-0447.1991.tb05581.x] [PMID: 1679281]

[77]   Morgenthaler TI, Silber MH. Amnestic sleep-related eating disorder associated with zolpidem. Sleep
       Med 2002; 3(4): 323-7.
       [http://dx.doi.org/10.1016/S1389-9457(02)00007-2] [PMID: 14592194]

[78]   Carlos K, Prado GF, Teixeira CD, *et al.* Benzodiazepines for restless legs syndrome. Cochrane
       Database Syst Rev 2017; 3: CD006939.
       [PMID: 28319266]

[79]   Trenkwalder C, Zieglgänsberger W, Ahmedzai SH, Högl B. Pain, opioids, and sleep: implications for
       restless legs syndrome treatment. Sleep Med 2017; 31: 78-85.
       [http://dx.doi.org/10.1016/j.sleep.2016.09.017] [PMID: 27964861]

[80]   Walters AS, Winkelmann J, Trenkwalder C, *et al.* Long-term follow-up on restless legs syndrome
       patients treated with opioids. Mov Disord 2001; 16(6): 1105-9.
       [http://dx.doi.org/10.1002/mds.1214] [PMID: 11748742]

[81]   Vetrugno R, La Morgia C, D'Angelo R, *et al.* Augmentation of restless legs syndrome with long-term
       tramadol treatment. Mov Disord 2007; 22(3): 424-7.
       [http://dx.doi.org/10.1002/mds.21342] [PMID: 17230457]

[82]   Silber MH, Becker PM, Buchfuhrer MJ, *et al.* The Appropriate Use of Opioids in the Treatment of
       Refractory Restless Legs Syndrome. Mayo Clin Proc 2018; 93(1): 59-67.
       [http://dx.doi.org/10.1016/j.mayocp.2017.11.007] [PMID: 29304922]

[83]   Klingelhoefer L, Cova I, Gupta S, Chaudhuri KR. A review of current treatment strategies for restless
       legs syndrome (Willis-Ekbom disease). Clin Med (Lond) 2014; 14(5): 520-4.
       [http://dx.doi.org/10.7861/clinmedicine.14-5-520] [PMID: 25301914]

[84]   Garcia-Borreguero D, Ferini-Strambi L, Kohnen R, *et al.* European guidelines on management of
       restless legs syndrome: report of a joint task force by the European Federation of Neurological
       Societies, the European Neurological Society and the European Sleep Research Society. Eur J Neurol
       2012; 19(11): 1385-96.
       [http://dx.doi.org/10.1111/j.1468-1331.2012.03853.x] [PMID: 22937989]

[85]   Trenkwalder C, Beneš H, Grote L, *et al.* Prolonged release oxycodone-naloxone for treatment of severe restless legs syndrome after failure of previous treatment: a double-blind, randomised, placebo-controlled trial with an open-label extension. Lancet Neurol 2013; 12(12): 1141-50.
[http://dx.doi.org/10.1016/S1474-4422(13)70239-4] [PMID: 24140442]

[86]   Lauerma H, Markkula J. Treatment of restless legs syndrome with tramadol: an open study. J Clin Psychiatry 1999; 60(4): 241-4.
[http://dx.doi.org/10.4088/JCP.v60n0407] [PMID: 10221285]

[87]   Silver N, Allen RP, Senerth J, Earley CJ. A 10-year, longitudinal assessment of dopamine agonists and methadone in the treatment of restless legs syndrome. Sleep Med 2011; 12(5): 440-4.
[http://dx.doi.org/10.1016/j.sleep.2010.11.002] [PMID: 21239226]

[88]   Ondo WG. Methadone for refractory restless legs syndrome. Mov Disord 2005; 20(3): 345-8.
[http://dx.doi.org/10.1002/mds.20359] [PMID: 15580610]

[89]   Telstad W, Sørensen O, Larsen S, Lillevold PE, Stensrud P, Nyberg-Hansen R. Treatment of the restless legs syndrome with carbamazepine: a double blind study. Br Med J (Clin Res Ed) 1984; 288(6415): 444-6.
[http://dx.doi.org/10.1136/bmj.288.6415.444] [PMID: 6419958]

[90]   Wagner ML, Walters AS, Coleman RG, Hening WA, Grasing K, Chokroverty S. Randomized, double-blind, placebo-controlled study of clonidine in restless legs syndrome. Sleep 1996; 19(1): 52-8.
[PMID: 8650464]

[91]   Evidente VG, Adler CH, Caviness JN, Hentz JG, Gwinn-Hardy K. Amantadine is beneficial in restless legs syndrome. Mov Disord 2000; 15(2): 324-7.
[http://dx.doi.org/10.1002/1531-8257(200003)15:2<324::AID-MDS1020>3.0.CO;2-4]   [PMID: 10752586]

[92]   Wali S, Alsafadi S, Abaalkhail B, *et al.* The Association Between Vitamin D Level and Restless Legs Syndrome: A Population-Based Case-Control Study. J Clin Sleep Med 2018; 14(4): 557-64.
[http://dx.doi.org/10.5664/jcsm.7044] [PMID: 29609719]

[93]   Oran M, Unsal C, Albayrak Y, *et al.* Possible association between vitamin D deficiency and restless legs syndrome. Neuropsychiatr Dis Treat 2014; 10: 953-8.
[http://dx.doi.org/10.2147/NDT.S63599] [PMID: 24899811]

[94]   Garcia-Borreguero D, Stillman P, Benes H, *et al.* Algorithms for the diagnosis and treatment of restless legs syndrome in primary care. BMC Neurol 2011; 11(1): 28.
[http://dx.doi.org/10.1186/1471-2377-11-28] [PMID: 21352569]

[95]   Winkelman JW, Johnston L. Augmentation and tolerance with long-term pramipexole treatment of restless legs syndrome (RLS). Sleep Med 2004; 5(1): 9-14.
[http://dx.doi.org/10.1016/j.sleep.2003.07.005] [PMID: 14725821]

[96]   Högl B, Oertel WH, Stiasny-Kolster K, *et al.* Treatment of moderate to severe restless legs syndrome: 2-year safety and efficacy of rotigotine transdermal patch. BMC Neurol 2010; 10(1): 86.
[http://dx.doi.org/10.1186/1471-2377-10-86] [PMID: 20920156]

[97]   Beneš H, García-Borreguero D, Ferini-Strambi L, Schollmayer E, Fichtner A, Kohnen R. Augmentation in the treatment of restless legs syndrome with transdermal rotigotine. Sleep Med 2012; 13(6): 589-97.
[http://dx.doi.org/10.1016/j.sleep.2011.09.016] [PMID: 22503658]

[98]   Frauscher B, Gschliesser V, Brandauer E, *et al.* The severity range of restless legs syndrome (RLS) and augmentation in a prospective patient cohort: association with ferritin levels. Sleep Med 2009; 10(6): 611-5.
[http://dx.doi.org/10.1016/j.sleep.2008.09.007] [PMID: 19200780]

[99]   Ondo W, Romanyshyn J, Vuong KD, Lai D. Long-term treatment of restless legs syndrome with dopamine agonists. Arch Neurol 2004; 61(9): 1393-7.

[http://dx.doi.org/10.1001/archneur.61.9.1393] [PMID: 15364685]

[100] Nagandla K, De S. Restless legs syndrome: pathophysiology and modern management. Postgrad Med J 2013; 89(1053): 402-10.
[http://dx.doi.org/10.1136/postgradmedj-2012-131634] [PMID: 23524988]

[101] Lesage S, Earley CJ. Restless Legs Syndrome. Curr Treat Options Neurol 2004; 6(3): 209-19.
[http://dx.doi.org/10.1007/s11940-004-0013-8] [PMID: 15043804]

[102] Maestri M, Fulda S, Ferini-Strambi L, *et al.* Polysomnographic record and successful management of augmentation in restless legs syndrome/Willis-Ekbom disease. Sleep Med 2014; 15(5): 570-5.
[http://dx.doi.org/10.1016/j.sleep.2014.01.016] [PMID: 24767724]

[103] Garcia-Borreguero D, Odin P, Schwarz C. Restless legs syndrome: an overview of the current understanding and management. Acta Neurol Scand 2004; 109(5): 303-17.
[http://dx.doi.org/10.1111/j.1600-0404.2004.00269.x] [PMID: 15080856]

[104] Antonini A, Cilia R. Behavioural adverse effects of dopaminergic treatments in Parkinson's disease: incidence, neurobiological basis, management and prevention. Drug Saf 2009; 32(6): 475-88.
[http://dx.doi.org/10.2165/00002018-200932060-00004] [PMID: 19459715]

[105] Schreglmann SR, Gantenbein AR, Eisele G, Baumann CR. Transdermal rotigotine causes impulse control disorders in patients with restless legs syndrome. Parkinsonism Relat Disord 2012; 18(2): 207-9.
[http://dx.doi.org/10.1016/j.parkreldis.2011.10.010] [PMID: 22030321]

[106] Chaput JP, Després JP, Bouchard C, Tremblay A. The association between sleep duration and weight gain in adults: a 6-year prospective study from the Quebec Family Study. Sleep 2008; 31(4): 517-23.
[http://dx.doi.org/10.1093/sleep/31.4.517] [PMID: 18457239]

[107] Winkelmann J, Prager M, Lieb R, *et al.* "Anxietas tibiarum". Depression and anxiety disorders in patients with restless legs syndrome. J Neurol 2005; 252(1): 67-71.
[http://dx.doi.org/10.1007/s00415-005-0604-7] [PMID: 15654556]

[108] Jahani Kondori M, Kolla BP, Moore KM, Mansukhani MP. Management of Restless Legs Syndrome in Pregnancy and Lactation. J Prim Care Community Health 2020; 11: 2150132720905950.
[http://dx.doi.org/10.1177/2150132720905950] [PMID: 32054396]

[109] Picchietti DL, Hensley JG, Bainbridge JL, *et al.* Consensus clinical practice guidelines for the diagnosis and treatment of restless legs syndrome/Willis-Ekbom disease during pregnancy and lactation. Sleep Med Rev 2015; 22: 64-77.
[http://dx.doi.org/10.1016/j.smrv.2014.10.009] [PMID: 25553600]

[110] Gupta R, Dhyani M, Kendzerska T, *et al.* Restless legs syndrome and pregnancy: prevalence, possible pathophysiological mechanisms and treatment. Acta Neurol Scand 2016; 133(5): 320-9.
[http://dx.doi.org/10.1111/ane.12520] [PMID: 26482928]

[111] Giannaki CD, Hadjigeorgiou GM, Karatzaferi C, Pantzaris MC, Stefanidis I, Sakkas GK. Epidemiology, impact, and treatment options of restless legs syndrome in end-stage renal disease patients: an evidence-based review. Kidney Int 2014; 85(6): 1275-82.
[http://dx.doi.org/10.1038/ki.2013.394] [PMID: 24107848]

CHAPTER 4

Sleep and Driving Safety

Aneesa Das[1] and **Nancy Collop**[2,*]

[1] *Division of Pulmonary/Critical Care/Sleep Medicine, Ohio State University, Columbus, OH, USA*

[2] *Emory Sleep Center, Emory University, Atlanta, GA, USA*

Abstract: Drowsy driving is a widespread problem that results in accidents and injuries, costing lives and money. Drowsy driving can occur due to inadequate sleep, circadian rhythm influences and sleep disorders. It is agnostic to the driver affecting any age, sex, amount of prior driving experience and can include those who drive cars, trucks, buses and motorcycles. Laws and regulations are spotty on drowsy driving in part due to the challenges in defining it and confirming it.

Keywords: Chronotype, Circadian rhythm, Commercial driver's license, Commercial driver medical examiner, Drowsy driving, Hours of service, Hypersomnia, Maggie's Law, Motor vehicle crash, Narcolepsy, Obstructive sleep apnea, Sleep deprivation, Standard deviation of lateral position.

INTRODUCTION

Insufficient quantity and quality of sleep and circadian timing can affect driving performance. While sleep is a factor in all forms of transportation, this chapter will focus on motor vehicles, including automobiles and trucks. It will not address the railroad and air transportation industries. Approximately one in twenty-five drivers report falling asleep at the wheel in the preceding month [1]. While falling asleep at the wheel can be deadly, drowsiness in and of itself can affect driving safety and performance. Even in the absence of truly falling asleep while at the wheel, drowsy driving can lead to motor vehicle crashes (MVC). Driving while drowsy leads to deficits similar to those seen when driving under the influence of alcohol, including reduced reaction time, attentiveness and decision-making ability [2, 3]. Although official government statistics from the National Highway Traffic Safety Administration (NHTSA), suggest drowsy driving was associated with 1.9-2.5% of overall injury or fatal crashes, they are potentially limited

* **Corresponding author Nancy Collop:** Emory Sleep Center, Emory University, Atlanta, GA, USA; Tel: 404-712-7533; Fax: 404-712-8145; E-mail: nancy.collop@emory.edu

Imran H. Iftikhar and Ali I. Musani (Eds.)

in their ability to collect comprehensive data; therefore this number is likely much higher [4]. The American Automobile Association (AAA) Foundation for Traffic Safety analyzed data from 14,268 crashes requiring the vehicle to be towed and reported a much higher association with drowsy drivers. They found that a drowsy driver was involved in 6% of all crashes in which a vehicle was towed from the scene, 7% of crashes causing injury requiring treatment, 13% of crashes requiring hospitalization, and 21% of fatal crashes [5].

SLEEP NEEDS AND CIRCADIAN INFLUENCES

Homeostatic Influence

Insufficient sleep is a common problem. Approximately one-third of Americans sleep less than 7 hours per night. Adults should sleep 7 or more hours of sleep consistently for optimal safety. Sleeping less than 7 hours is associated with an increased risk for errors, performance and accidents [6]. In survey data analyzed by the Center for Disease Control (CDC), drowsy driving was associated with a reported habitual sleep time of $\leq$ 6 hours, snoring, and unintentionally nodding off during the day [7]. In particular, sleeping 6 hours per night has been associated with a 33% increased crash risk when compared to 7-8 hours of sleep per night. This association was even noted in individuals who did not report significant sleepiness [8].

Extensive studies have been done assessing changes in performance with sleep deprivation, including simulated driving performance, vigilance, and reaction time. Sleep loss is most strongly associated with changes in sustained attention, decision making and working memory processes. Psychomotor vigilance testing (PVT) assesses both sustained visual attention and reaction time and is progressively affected by worsening sleep deprivation. However, several studies have suggested that sustained attention appears to affect high-level performance in the setting of sleep deprivation more significantly than the reaction time [9]. Therefore, improved sustained attentiveness has been the focus of safety advancements in the automotive industry for the prevention of drowsy driving-related crashes.

MVCs due to drowsy driving can affect all ages and gender, however, young men between the ages of 16 and 24 are at the greatest risk of motor vehicle crashes due to drowsy driving [5]. Furthermore, men aged 18 to 30 may be at a greater increase for worsened driving performance with moderate sleep deprivation when combined with even low levels of alcohol (0.025% blood alcohol level) that are well within the legal limits by most national standards [10].

Finally, chronic sleep deprivation can affect neurobehavioral changes as well as acute sleep deprivation. A single night of recovery sleep of up to 10 hours is insufficient to resolve all of the neurocognitive deficits back to baseline levels after chronic sleep deprivation [11]. However, banking sleep prior to chronic sleep deprivation can affect the rate of deterioration of alertness during sleep deprivation and improve the rate of improvement with recovery sleep [12].

Circadian Influence

MVCs from drowsy driving occur most frequently between midnight and six A.M. and are frequently associated with a single driver without passengers, according to the National Highway Traffic Safety Administration [13].

Subjective tools of sleepiness and daytime alertness that determine scoring in the current state of the patient typically reflect circadian variation, as opposed to those that reflect assessment over a longer period of time. It can be difficult to separate out the effects of the circadian and homeostatic influences in objective testing. The circadian changes in performance and cognitive ability are most prominent in the presence of sleep deprivation. Forced desynchrony protocols have been done to assess the changes in neurobehavioral functions that are attributed to endogenous circadian control and homeostatic drive. In a forced desynchrony protocol, a subject is given an artificial sleep and wake time in a controlled environment that is either longer or shorter than the traditional 24 hour day. In this setting, the subject is unable to entrain to the imposed schedule and therefore experiences sleep and wake distinctly from their unsynchronized circadian system. These protocols have shown that the consequence of chronic sleep deprivation is more prominent during the biological night, even if the wake period immediately preceding is short, supporting the importance of circadian timing [14].

Chronotype, or propensity towards morningness *versus* eveningness, may cause individual variation in circadian changes. Sex can affect chronotype, with more women having a morning preference than men. Additionally, age can affect chronotype with adolescents having a preference for an evening chronotype and older adults having a preference for a morning chronotype. Among adolescents, having an evening chronotype was independently associated with an increased prevalence for drowsy driving even when controlled for the duration of sleep [15]. This may be related to sleep deprivation, as evening chronotypes will have a later bedtime but may still have imposed societal wake times resulting in reduced sleep.

Techniques to Optimize Alertness and Safety While Driving

Individuals employ numerous counter activities in order to try to stay alert while driving. However, some of these activities, including listening to loud music, talking on the phone, and eating, are not effective alerting techniques and may actually serve to further distract the driver. Caffeine is the most commonly used psychoactive stimulant. It is an adenosine receptor agonist which can improve alertness, vigilance, attention, and reaction time. However, the effects are less consistent on higher-level cognitive functions such as decision making [16]. In a meta-analysis by Irwin *et al.,* eight trials evaluating car driving performance and caffeine were assessed. Driving assessments included lane crossing, the standard deviation of lateral position, crashes, and standard deviation of speed. All areas improved with caffeine [17]. Ultimately, it should be remembered that while caffeine may temporarily improve alertness, it cannot resolve the issue of sleep loss.

Planned naps can improve nighttime driving performance and may have greater improvement in younger *versus* older adults [18, 19]. These benefits have been noted more significantly in on-road driving performances as compared to simulated driving performances, which do not have the associated threat of injury from accident [20]. When naps are limited to 20-30 minutes, they are less likely to be associated with interruption of subsequent nighttime sleep.

An important facet of addressing the issue of drowsy driving is increasing the awareness of the driver to their symptoms in real-time. Vehicle safety advancements are emerging and drowsy driving assist systems are being incorporated into new automobile models. Crossing highway lines is a sign of decreased attentiveness and has been strongly associated with the risk of the accident [10]. Measures to determine risk of lane crossing have been tested as a way to determine early detection of drowsy driving for intervention. Eyelid closure parameters including prolonged eyelid closures, blink duration, the ratio of amplitude to the velocity of eyelid closure have been associated with increased lane crossing [11]. Eye closure monitoring can be performed *via* a camera mounted to the vehicle and provided real-time feedback to the driver regarding potential drowsiness. Alternatively, wearable devices can be purchased to provide similar feedback [21]. Standard deviation of lateral position (SDLP) of a vehicle within a lane is also a marker of alertness. While drivers who are alert make frequent, small adjustments to stay within the lane, drivers who are drowsy make less frequent larger adjustments yielding a greater SDLP. This can also be measured in steering wheel movement and has been incorporated into the drowsy driving assist systems by some automotive makers [22, 23].

Laws Regarding Driving Safety

While the actual number of driving accidents attributed to drowsy driving is unknown, it is estimated to be between 10-20% [5, 24]. Depending on the study, it is estimated that as many as 40% of drivers admit to falling asleep behind the wheel [25]. One of the first cases addressing drowsy driving was tried in 1925 in the state of Connecticut [26]. In this case of a husband and wife, the husband was driving a car that crashed with his wife as a passenger. She sued her husband because he fell asleep at the wheel and his side argued that sleep occurs without warning. The court ruled against Mr. Bushnell, noting that sleep is not a sudden "blackout" and that falling asleep will have precursors such as fatigue and "dulling of the senses." Further, he should have known that sleep was affecting his driving and stopped driving while he was awake and hence avoided the accident. Since this decision, many other court cases have addressed numerous issues related to drowsy driving, including those related to commercial drivers, driving to and from places of work, driving in the setting of sleep disorders, to name a few.

Overall, regulations about drowsy driving or driving with sleep disorders are scarce. Currently, only 2 states (Arkansas and New Jersey) have laws that directly classify drowsy driving as a punishable offence and 5 others have assigned a day or week to spread awareness about drowsy driving (Massachusetts, California, Alabama, Florida, Texas). In both Arkansas and New Jersey, the impetus for these laws was brought about by court cases. Maggie McDonnell, a 20 year old college student, was driving when her car was crashed into by a van that crossed 3 lanes of traffic and hit her car head on. The driver subsequently admitted to having been awake for 30 hours and had been using drugs. The jury deadlocked 9 *vs* 3, on a decision because there was no law in New Jersey against falling asleep while driving. The driver subsequently received a $200 fine and a suspended jail sentence. Maggie's mother, Carole McDonnell, was devastated by the loss of her daughter and lobbied on behalf of her daughter tirelessly until the State of New Jersey passed a drowsy driving law [27]. Maggie's Law states that a sleep-deprived driver qualifies as a reckless driver who can be convicted of vehicular homicide. It is an evidentiary rule establishing that proof of driving after 24 hours of sleeplessness "shall give rise to an inference that the defendant was driving recklessly" to convict a defendant for vehicular homicide. The law also states that falling asleep while driving may infer recklessness without regard to sleeplessness. If convicted, punishment may include up to 10 years in prison and a $100,000 fine.

The Arkansas law was proposed by a State Senator in Arkansas, Jason Rapert [28]. He was moved by one of his constituents, who lost his mother in another head-on collision. The driver allegedly was noted to have commented on social media about staying up over 24 hours prior to the crash and fell asleep while driving. Senator Rapert then filed an amendment to the offense of negligent homicide (SB874, Arkansas Senate Bill) which was passed on April 16, 2013 (Act 1296, Arkansas) [29]. In this bill "fatigued driving" is classified as an offense under negligent homicide punishable when the driver involved in a fatal accident has been without sleep for 24 consecutive hours or is in the state of sleep after being without sleep for 24 consecutive hours. If convicted, punishment may include up to 1 year in prison and/or a $2500 fine.

One of the biggest challenges to drowsy driving legislation is being able to define the scope of the problem. There is likely significant underreporting of drowsy driving-related accidents as it is often difficult to determine if a crash is drowsiness related and there is a dearth of drowsiness investigation training and resources devoted to this. A forum (Asleep at the wheel: A Nation of Drowsy Drivers) sponsored by the National Highway Traffic Safety Administration (NHTSA) laid out several future actions that can help improve traffic safety as it applies to drowsy driving [30].

Industry Standards for Safe Driving

Another area of intense interest is the liability of employers who employ drivers of motor vehicles. The legal doctrine, *respondeat superior,* holds that an employer is responsible for the wrongful acts of an employee if such acts occur within the scope of the employment; when this is invoked, typically both the employer and employee are held liable. This doctrine would then include companies such as trucking, bussing, taxi cab, mail delivery, and even ride-sharing services, which could be held liable if their driver falls asleep at the wheel and injures a third party while working on the job; it also implies that employers may be liable for failure to screen for disorders that may impact their employees' ability to drive safely. Trucks and bus accidents have a higher likelihood of multiple injuries because these vehicles are larger, may carry more people or hazardous substances, and may drive long distances. One of the more famous cases of a deadly crash involving a sleepy truck driver occurred in June 2014. A Walmart truck rear-ended a limo-van carrying comedian Tracy Morgan and continued to hit 3 other vehicles before careening to its side on the New Jersey turnpike. Morgan was critically injured but survived; however one of the passengers in his van, James McNair, was killed. The driver was charged with vehicular homicide and 4 counts of aggravated assault. He had driven 12 hours from his home in Georgia to Delaware before starting his shift; therefore he had been awake for 28 hours at the time of the crash. The total settlement is unknown, but Walmart did reach a $10,000,000 settlement with the McNair family.

There has been significant attention devoted to developing standards in the trucking industry for drivers as it relates to both screening for sleep disorders (particularly sleep apnea) and reducing time driving to prevent driver fatigue. Commercial Driver License (CDL) holders are to undergo medical qualification exams every 2 years by a commercial driver medical examiner (CDME) [31]. In the *Code of Federal Regulations*, the most recent recommendation made for CDME guidance regarding OSA was in 1991. CDME certification cannot place work restrictions (limit hours, travel or type of vehicle) and the American Disabilities Act (ADA) does not take precedent over federal medical standards. The CDME's role is: "To detect the presence of physical, mental, or organic conditions of such character and extent as to affect the driver's ability to operate a commercial motor vehicle safely" and indicate the need for further testing and/or require evaluation by a specialist. If the CDME finds the applicant physically qualified to drive a commercial motor vehicle, they complete a certificate and furnish one copy to the applicant and one to the motor carrier that employs him/her. Currently, the *Code of Federal Regulations* (49CFR 391.41 (b)(5)) states the driver: "Has no established medical history or clinical diagnosis of a respiratory dysfunction likely to interfere with his/her ability to control and drive a commercial motor vehicle safely"; and in 1998, the CDME reporting form was addended to: "ask the driver whether he has a sleep disorder, pauses in breathing while asleep, daytime sleepiness or loud snoring". The Federal Motor Carrier Safety Administration (FMCSA) has been working with various groups to re-evaluate this issue for many years; however, Congress has not allowed any substantial changes to occur. In 2013, Congress passed a resolution stating that "no requirements for the trucking industry could be passed without formal rulemaking" and in 2016, the Obama administration passed a federal proposal to examine a requirement for railroad and CDL operators to be screened for obstructive sleep apnea (OSA). However in 2017, the Trump administration reversed the process because it was felt it would be onerous and hurt job growth [32].

In June 2020, FMCSA changed the "hours of service" rules for truck drivers – relaxing some of the restrictions [33]. These rules were initially established to reduce driver fatigue and drowsiness. Drivers carrying property have a 14-hour driving "window" in which they have 14 consecutive hours that they can drive up to 11 hours after being off duty for 10 or more consecutive hours. They are only intended to drive a total of 8 hours without a break, and then a 30-minute break is mandated. Passenger carriers have a 15-hour on-duty limit and 10 hours driving limit. The newer exceptions did not change the hours of service rules, but altered the type of breaks allowed to include that the driver can stay "on-duty" but not drive, as well as be "off-duty" or in the sleeper berth. There were a few other changes to include short-haul drives and adverse driving condition exceptions.

SLEEP DISORDERS THAT CAN AFFECT DRIVING SAFETY

Obstructive Sleep Apnea

OSA is a common sleep disorder among adults [34, 35]. A systematic review and meta-analysis showed that OSA is associated with an increased risk of MVC, with a mean crash-rate ratio falling between 1.21 and 4.89 [36]. An increased associated risk was still present even in those patients who did not report daytime sleepiness [8]. However, some data suggest that patients with OSA who complain of sleepiness are at the highest risk for near miss accidents [37]. Undiagnosed sleep apnea might be a major factor in drowsy driving. In a recent prospective cohort of patients admitted to a level one trauma center as a driver in a MVC, 26% were found to be high risk for OSA based on a STOP-BANG of $\geq$ 5 [38]. Numerous studies have shown improvement in drowsy driving and MVC's in patients with treated OSA. An evidence-based review and meta-analyses commissioned by the FMCSA showed improved crash risk in patients with OSA using CPAP as seen by improvement in sleepiness and simulated driving performance [39]. Therefore, the diagnosis and treatment of OSA in drivers should be a priority in the effort to improve driving safety related to sleepiness.

Once patients are diagnosed and treatment is initiated, close follow up and assurance of adherence is critical. Data from an employer-mandated program in the US trucking industry to screen, diagnose, and monitor OSA treatment adherence illustrates this point. Patients with OSA who were non-adherent to therapy had 5 times the risk of serious preventable crashes compared to matched controls. Comparatively, those with full treatment adherence had crash rates similar to controls [40].

Hypersomnia Disorders

Narcolepsy and other hypersomnia disorders are characterized by problems with sleepiness, sleep state instability, brain fog, and even cataplexy when there is a sudden loss of muscle tone. These issues obviously put patients with these disorders at high risk for sleep related crashes and studies have suggested that it may be threefold compared to those without sleep disorders [41]. Assessing driving risk in these patients is fraught with challenges, and there is little guidance on best practice. If these patients are allowed to drive, methods to mitigate risk are also not well established. A study that specifically examined driving issues in patients with narcolepsy found two-thirds reported falling asleep at the wheel, with almost one third (29%) experiencing cataplexy and 12% having sleep paralysis while driving [42]. A more recent study of patients with a hypersomnia disorder compared to a control population found that those with hypersomnia, with or without treatment, were more likely to have had a driving accident in the prior 5 years [43]. Since 2010, the FMCSA has noted that patients with narcolepsy are ineligible for a CDL, even if medicated [44].

Clinicians are often put in a position to decide whether a patient with a hypersomnia disorder can pursue a motor vehicle license. There are no federal guidelines regarding this, and state laws are variable. Two states (California and Pennsylvania) require mandatory reporting of a narcolepsy diagnosis, however, most states' laws are silent about the issues or expect "self-reporting" on medical issues [45]. It is suggested that health care providers and patients research the laws in their individual state. A variety of tests have been examined to assess driving risk, including the Epworth Sleepiness Scale or similar questionnaires, objective measures of sleepiness like the mean sleep latency test or maintenance of wakefulness test (MWT), simulated driving tests and real driving tests [46]. It has been suggested that if the MWT sleep latency is > 30 minutes, driving may be allowed, but no clear standard has been adopted [47]. The American Academy of Sleep Medicine (AASM) quality measures for narcolepsy, which can probably also be applied to other hypersomnia disorders, recommend that all patients be counselled on safety measures before or at the time of diagnosis. Furthermore, they note that even pharmacotherapy may not return a normal level of daytime alertness and that "road side naps, frequent breaks, intake of caffeinated beverages are useful recommendations" for patients on long-distance trips [48].

Circadian Rhythm Disorders

As noted, circadian rhythm influences sleep and drowsiness. There are a number of circadian rhythm disorders which may affect driving performance. While there are little data on these, patients with these disorders may have reduced driving performance when their internal clock is prompting sleepiness which may be misaligned with the external clock. For instance, a patient with delayed sleep phase disorder syndrome will typically be more alert in the evening hours, but driving in the early morning may be challenging. Alternatively, patients with an advanced sleep phase disorder would likely be more sleepy in the evening, but may be more alert driving in the morning. Similar to hypersomnia disorders, health care providers should discuss these nuances with patients and similar to the recommendations above regarding mitigation strategies, encourage patients to be aware of these risks, particularly with long-distance trips [48].

Many studies have shown an association of increased MVCs with daylight savings time (DST) [49]. A large scale analysis of fatal MVCs across all states in the United States between 1996 and 2017 reported a 6% increase in the risk of fatal MVC in spring DST. Although the risk was increased even in the afternoon hours, despite longer daylight, this risk was most pronounced in the morning hours. This increased risk subsequently decreased the week after the spring DST change [50]. The AASM published an official position statement in 2020, recommending that seasonal time changes should end [51].

CONCLUSION

Drowsiness clearly affects driving safety and performance. Both homeostatic drive and circadian rhythm influence alertness when behind the wheel. Young males are at disproportionate risk due to sleep deprivation, use of alcohol and age-related circadian rhythm delay. Efforts to mitigate drowsy driving accidents include changes made in vehicles to sense the presence of alertness lapses, use of "power naps", caffeine, and avoidance of nocturnal or early morning driving. Drowsy driving laws are in place in only 2 states and are difficult to prosecute. Screening for sleep apnea amongst CDL holders is variable and not consistent in the industry due to reluctance on the federal government to interfere. Employers should be held accountable to screen their drivers for sleep disorders and to assure drivers comply with "hours of service" regulations. Patients with sleep apnea, hypersomnia disorders and circadian rhythm disorders should all be counselled on the risk of driving.

LIST OF ABBREVIATIONS

AAA American Automobile Association

ADA American Disabilities Act

CDC Centers for Disease Control

CDL Commercial driver's license

CDME Commercial driver medical examiner

DD Drowsy driver

FMCSA Federal Motor Carrier Safety Administration

MVC Motor vehicle crash

MWT Maintenance of Wakefulness Test

MSLT Multiple Sleep Latency Test

NHTSA National Highway Traffic Safety Administration

OSA Obstructive sleep apnea

SDLP Standard deviation of lateral position

CONSENT FOR PUBLICATION

Not applicable.

CONFLICT OF INTEREST

The authors declare no conflict of interest, financial or otherwise.

ACKNOWLEDGEMENTS

Declared none.

REFERENCES

[1]   Wheaton AG, Shults RA, Chapman DP, Ford ES, Croft JB. Drowsy driving and risk behaviors - 10 States and Puerto Rico, 2011-2012. MMWR Morb Mortal Wkly Rep 2014; 63(26): 557-62.
[PMID: 24990488]

[2]   Dawson D, Reid K. Fatigue, alcohol and performance impairment. Nature 1997; 388(6639): 235.
[http://dx.doi.org/10.1038/40775] [PMID: 9230429]

[3]   Lowrie J, Brownlow H. The impact of sleep deprivation and alcohol on driving: a comparative study. BMC Public Health 2020; 20(1): 980.
[http://dx.doi.org/10.1186/s12889-020-09095-5] [PMID: 32571274]

[4]   Administration NHTS. Traffic safety facts crash stats: drowsy driving. Washington, DC: US Department of Transportation, National Highway Traffic Safety Administration 2011.

[5]   Tefft BC. Prevalence of Motor Vehicle Crashes Involving Drowsy Drivers, United States 2009-2013 (Technical Report) 2014: Washington, DC.

[6]   Watson NF, Badr MS, Belenky G, *et al.* Recommended Amount of Sleep for a Healthy Adult: A Joint Consensus Statement of the American Academy of Sleep Medicine and Sleep Research Society. Sleep 2015; 38(6): 843-4.
[http://dx.doi.org/10.5665/sleep.4716] [PMID: 26039963]

[7]   Drowsy driving - 19 states and the District of Columbia, 2009-2010. MMWR Morb Mortal Wkly Rep 2013; 61(51-52): 1033-7.
[PMID: 23282860]

[8]   Gottlieb DJ, Ellenbogen JM, Bianchi MT, Czeisler CA. Sleep deficiency and motor vehicle crash risk in the general population: a prospective cohort study. BMC Med 2018; 16(1): 44.
[http://dx.doi.org/10.1186/s12916-018-1025-7] [PMID: 29554902]

[9]   Lim J, Dinges DF. A meta-analysis of the impact of short-term sleep deprivation on cognitive variables. Psychol Bull 2010; 136(3): 375-89.
[http://dx.doi.org/10.1037/a0018883] [PMID: 20438143]

[10]   Vakulin A, Baulk SD, Catcheside PG, *et al.* Effects of moderate sleep deprivation and low-dose alcohol on driving simulator performance and perception in young men. Sleep 2007; 30(10): 1327-33.
[http://dx.doi.org/10.1093/sleep/30.10.1327] [PMID: 17969466]

[11]   Banks S, Van Dongen HP, Maislin G, Dinges DF. Neurobehavioral dynamics following chronic sleep restriction: dose-response effects of one night for recovery. Sleep 2010; 33(8): 1013-26.
[http://dx.doi.org/10.1093/sleep/33.8.1013] [PMID: 20815182]

[12]   Rupp TL, Wesensten NJ, Bliese PD, Balkin TJ. Banking sleep: realization of benefits during subsequent sleep restriction and recovery. Sleep 2009; 32(3): 311-21.
[http://dx.doi.org/10.1093/sleep/32.3.311] [PMID: 19294951]

[13]   Varghese CS. Umesh, National Highway Traffic Safety Administration.NHTSA's National Center for Statistics and Analysis. Washington, DC: National Highway Traffic Safety Administration 2007.

[14]   Zhou X, Ferguson SA, Matthews RW, *et al.* Sleep, wake and phase dependent changes in neurobehavioral function under forced desynchrony. Sleep 2011; 34(7): 931-41.

[PMID: 21731143]

[15]   Owens JA, Dearth-Wesley T, Herman AN, Whitaker RC. Drowsy Driving, Sleep Duration, and Chronotype in Adolescents. J Pediatr 2019; 205: 224-9.
[http://dx.doi.org/10.1016/j.jpeds.2018.09.072] [PMID: 30392873]

[16]   McLellan TM, Caldwell JA, Lieberman HR. A review of caffeine's effects on cognitive, physical and occupational performance. Neurosci Biobehav Rev 2016; 71: 294-312.
[http://dx.doi.org/10.1016/j.neubiorev.2016.09.001] [PMID: 27612937]

[17]   Irwin C, Khalesi S, Desbrow B, McCartney D. Effects of acute caffeine consumption following sleep loss on cognitive, physical, occupational and driving performance: A systematic review and meta-analysis. Neurosci Biobehav Rev 2020; 108: 877-88.
[http://dx.doi.org/10.1016/j.neubiorev.2019.12.008] [PMID: 31837359]

[18]   Philip P, Taillard J, Moore N, *et al.* The effects of coffee and napping on nighttime highway driving: a randomized trial. Ann Intern Med 2006; 144(11): 785-91.
[http://dx.doi.org/10.7326/0003-4819-144-11-200606060-00004] [PMID: 16754920]

[19]   Sagaspe P, Taillard J, Chaumet G, Moore N, Bioulac B, Philip P. Aging and nocturnal driving: better with coffee or a nap? A randomized study. Sleep 2007; 30(12): 1808-13.
[http://dx.doi.org/10.1093/sleep/30.12.1808] [PMID: 18246990]

[20]   Centofanti SA, *et al.* Do night naps impact driving performance and daytime recovery sleep? Accid Anal Prev 2017; 99Pt B : 416-21.

[21]   Dawson D, Searle AK, Paterson JL. Look before you (s)leep: evaluating the use of fatigue detection technologies within a fatigue risk management system for the road transport industry. Sleep Med Rev 2014; 18(2): 141-52.
[http://dx.doi.org/10.1016/j.smrv.2013.03.003] [PMID: 23796506]

[22]   Howard ME, Cori JM, Horrey WJ. Vehicle and Highway Adaptations to Compensate for Sleepy Drivers. Sleep Med Clin 2019; 14(4): 479-89.
[http://dx.doi.org/10.1016/j.jsmc.2019.08.005] [PMID: 31640876]

[23]   Friedrichs F. Y.B. *Drowsiness monitoring by steering and lane data based features under real driving conditions.* 18th European Signal Processing Conference. Aalborg, Denmark. IEEE. 2010.

[24]   Bioulac S, Micoulaud-Franchi JA, Arnaud M, *et al.* Risk of Motor Vehicle Accidents Related to Sleepiness at the Wheel: A Systematic Review and Meta-Analysis. Sleep 2017; 40: 10.
[http://dx.doi.org/10.1093/sleep/zsx134] [PMID: 28958002]

[25]   Tefft B. The Prevalence and Impact of Drowsy Driving. Washington, DC: AAA Foundation for Traffic Safety 2010.

[26]   Inez A Bushnell vs Mark W Bushnell 1925. Supreme Court of Connecticut First Judicial District.

[27]   Maggie's Law: Driving a Vehicle While Fatigued, Maggie's Law: Driving a Vehicle While Fatigued 2003; 11-5.

[28]   Varagur K. Why an Arkansas State Senator pushed to legislate fatgued driving 2017.
https://www.huffpost.com/entry/jason-rapert-fatigued-driv-ng-legislation_n_5756c5ade4b0ca5c7b4ff86e

[29]   An act to amend the offense of negligent homicide: and for other purposes in Arkansas Code 2013; 5: 10-105.

[30]   Higgins JS, Michael J, Austin R, *et al.* Asleep at the wheel-the road to addressing drowsy driving. Sleep 2017; 40: 2.
[http://dx.doi.org/10.1093/sleep/zsx001] [PMID: 28364516]

[31]   Electronic Code of Federal Regulations 2021. https://www.ecfr.gov/cgi-bin/retrieveECFR?gp=1&ty=HTML&h=L&mc=true&=PART&n=pt49.5.391

[32]   Levin A. Trump Administration Drops Rule to Address Truck Driver, Train Engineer Fatigue 2017. https://www.insurancejournal.com/news/national/2017/08/07/460304.htm

[33]   Hours of Service (HOS). Federal Motor Carrier Safety Administration 3/11/2021]; https://www.fmcsa.dot.gov/regulations/hours-of-service

[34]   Peppard PE, Young T, Barnet JH, Palta M, Hagen EW, Hla KM. Increased prevalence of sleep-disordered breathing in adults. Am J Epidemiol 2013; 177(9): 1006-14.
[http://dx.doi.org/10.1093/aje/kws342] [PMID: 23589584]

[35]   Young T, Palta M, Dempsey J, Skatrud J, Weber S, Badr S. The occurrence of sleep-disordered breathing among middle-aged adults. N Engl J Med 1993; 328(17): 1230-5.
[http://dx.doi.org/10.1056/NEJM199304293281704] [PMID: 8464434]

[36]   Tregear S, Reston J, Schoelles K, Phillips B. Obstructive sleep apnea and risk of motor vehicle crash: systematic review and meta-analysis. J Clin Sleep Med 2009; 5(6): 573-81.
[http://dx.doi.org/10.5664/jcsm.27662] [PMID: 20465027]

[37]   Ward KL, Hillman DR, James A, *et al.* Excessive daytime sleepiness increases the risk of motor vehicle crash in obstructive sleep apnea. J Clin Sleep Med 2013; 9(10): 1013-21.
[http://dx.doi.org/10.5664/jcsm.3072] [PMID: 24127145]

[38]   Purtle MW, Renner CH, McCann DA, Mallen JC, Spilman SK, Sahr SM. Driving with undiagnosed obstructive sleep apnea (OSA): High prevalence of OSA risk in drivers who experienced a motor vehicle crash. Traffic Inj Prev 2020; 21(1): 38-41.
[http://dx.doi.org/10.1080/15389588.2019.1709175] [PMID: 31999487]

[39]   Tregear S, Reston J, Schoelles K, Phillips B. Continuous positive airway pressure reduces risk of motor vehicle crash among drivers with obstructive sleep apnea: systematic review and meta-analysis. Sleep 2010; 33(10): 1373-80.
[http://dx.doi.org/10.1093/sleep/33.10.1373] [PMID: 21061860]

[40]   Burks SV, Anderson JE, Bombyk M, *et al.* Nonadherence with employer-mandated sleep apnea treatment and increased risk of serious truck crashes. Sleep 2016; 39(5): 967-75.
[http://dx.doi.org/10.5665/sleep.5734] [PMID: 27070139]

[41]   Philip P, Chaufton C, Taillard J, *et al.* Maintenance of Wakefulness Test scores and driving performance in sleep disorder patients and controls. Int J Psychophysiol 2013; 89(2): 195-202.
[http://dx.doi.org/10.1016/j.ijpsycho.2013.05.013] [PMID: 23727627]

[42]   Broughton R, Ghanem Q, Hishikawa Y, Sugita Y, Nevsimalova S, Roth B. Life effects of narcolepsy in 180 patients from North America, Asia and Europe compared to matched controls. Can J Neurol Sci 1981; 8(4): 299-304.
[http://dx.doi.org/10.1017/S0317167100043419] [PMID: 7326610]

[43]   Pizza F, Jaussent I, Lopez R, *et al.* Car Crashes and Central Disorders of Hypersomnolence: A French Study. PLoS One 2015; 10(6): e0129386.
[http://dx.doi.org/10.1371/journal.pone.0129386] [PMID: 26052938]

[44]   Is Narcolepsy disqualifying? Federal Motor Carrier Safety Administration 4/1/2014;. https://www.fmcsa. dot.gov/faq/narcolepsy-disqualifying

[45]   Narcolepsy and Driving Laws. Narcolepsy Network 2021. http://narcolepsy network.org/narcolepsydrivinglaws/

[46]   McCall CA, Watson NF. Therapeutic Strategies for Mitigating Driving Risk in Patients with Narcolepsy. Ther Clin Risk Manag 2020; 16: 1099-108.
[http://dx.doi.org/10.2147/TCRM.S244714] [PMID: 33209031]

[47]   Ingram DG, Marciarille AM, Ehsan Z, Perry GV, Schneider T, Al-Shawwa B. Assessing readiness to drive in adolescents with narcolepsy: what are providers doing? Sleep Breath 2019; 23(2): 611-7.
[http://dx.doi.org/10.1007/s11325-019-01799-2] [PMID: 30734889]

[48]   Krahn LE, Hershner S, Loeding LD, *et al.* Quality measures for the care of patients with narcolepsy. J Clin Sleep Med 2015; 11(3): 335-55.
[http://dx.doi.org/10.5664/jcsm.4554] [PMID: 25700880]

[49]   Carey RN, Sarma KM. Impact of daylight saving time on road traffic collision risk: a systematic review. BMJ Open 2017; 7(6): e014319.
[http://dx.doi.org/10.1136/bmjopen-2016-014319] [PMID: 28674131]

[50]   Fritz J, VoPham T, Wright KP Jr, Vetter C. A chronobiological evaluation of the acute effects of daylight saving time on traffic accident risk. Curr Biol 2020; 30(4): 729-735.e2.
[http://dx.doi.org/10.1016/j.cub.2019.12.045] [PMID: 32008905]

[51]   Rishi MA, Ahmed O, Barrantes Perez JH, *et al.* Daylight saving time: an American Academy of Sleep Medicine position statement. J Clin Sleep Med 2020; 16(10): 1781-4.
[http://dx.doi.org/10.5664/jcsm.8780] [PMID: 32844740]

CHAPTER 5

Sleep Apnea, Arrhythmias and Sudden Death

Cheryl Augenstein[1] and **Imran H. Iftikhar**[1,*]

[1] *Department of Medicine, Division of Pulmonary, Allergy, Critical Care & Sleep Medicine, Emory University School of Medicine, Atlanta, GA, USA*

Abstract: Converging evidence indicates a link between sleep disordered breathing and arrhythmias. Several OSA-related immediate, intermediate and chronic pathways lead to augmented arrhythmic propensity. The more immediate and intermediate pathways include intermittent hypoxia, autonomic nervous system fluctuations during respiratory events and intrathoracic pressure swings leading to atrial stretch and hypercapnia. Chronic pathways include increased systemic inflammation, oxidative stress, enhanced prothrombotic state and vascular dysfunction. While the more immediate and intermediate pathways are linked to a reduction in the atrial effective refractory period, triggered and abnormal automaticity, the persistence of reentrant arrhythmias and the potential to prolong the QT interval, the more chronic pathways are ultimately linked to cardiac structural and electrical remodeling This paper provides an overview of the main pathophysiologic mechanisms underlying the association between sleep apnea and arrhythmias and discusses the impact of sleep apnea on arrhythmia management.

Keywords: Atrial Fibrillation, Arrhythmia, Obstructive Sleep Apnea.

INTRODUCTION

Obstructive sleep apnea (OSA) is the most common sleep breathing disorder[1]. Cardiac arrhythmias are a common type of heart disease and are associated with significant morbidity and mortality [1]. The association between sleep-disordered breathing and cardiovascular diseases has long been established, especially with hypertension [1], heart failure, atrial fibrillation (AF) and stroke [2]. Several epidemiologic studies have shown that sleep-disordered breathing almost doubles the risk of AF and in patients with OSA and heart failure, the risk is twice to four times higher than those without either condition [3 - 6]. In patients with OSA, apneas and hypopneas are frequently accompanied by oxygen desaturation and microarousals from sleep.

---
* **Corresponding author Imran H. Iftikhar:** Department of Medicine, Division of Pulmonary, Allergy, Critical Care & Sleep Medicine, Emory University School of Medicine, Atlanta, GA, USA; Tel: 803-873-3193; E-mail: Imran.Hasan.Iftikhar@emory.edu

Imran H. Iftikhar and Ali I. Musani (Eds.)

Autonomic imbalances, specifically, cardiac vagal activation during sleep apnea events and predominantly sympathetic activation after the events, could theoretically precipitate arrhythmias [7, 8]. Attempts to breathe against an obstructed upper airway also lead to large intrathoracic pressure swings during sleep apnea events, which could also be a factor in arrhythmogenesis. Repeated acute physiologic insults from intermittent hemodynamic, hypoxemic, and autonomic surges result in cardiac structural and electrical remodeling, creating an altered arrhythmogenic substrate in apnea-induced arrhythmia. Given that OSA is a modifiable risk factor for the development of life-threatening arrhythmias, there is growing interest in understanding the relationship between sleep apnea and arrhythmias in an effort to develop strategies to minimize the risk of deadly arrhythmias. This paper aims to highlight that relationship, review the mechanisms of arrhythmogenesis in the setting of sleep apnea, and suggest a future direction to help mitigate the associated morbidity and mortality.

PATHOPHYSIOLOGIC MECHANISMS

Pathophysiologic mechanisms can be conceptualized by understanding what ensues from sleep-disordered breathing, either immediately or chronically as well as some intermediate-acting mechanisms, as illustrated and discussed in a recent review article and summarized in Fig. (1) [2].

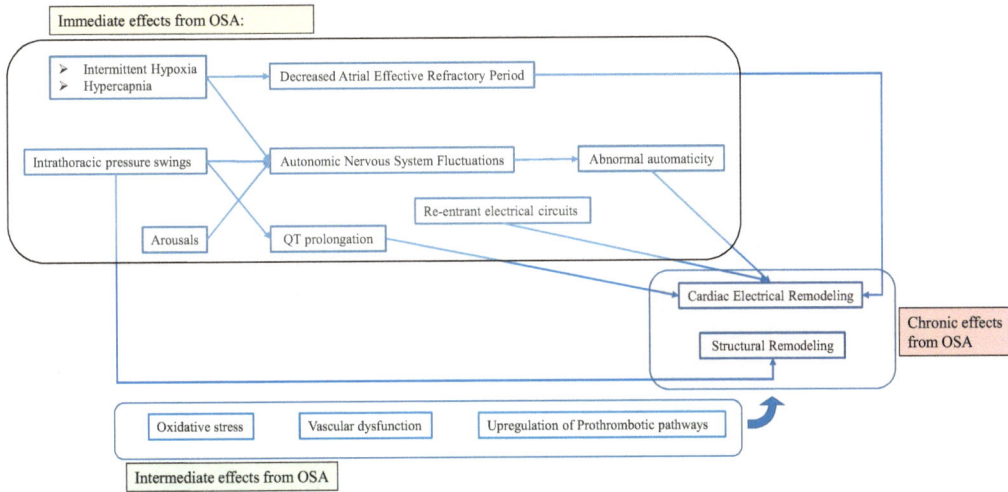

Fig. (1). Mechanistic pathways linking sleep-disordered breathing with arrhythmogenesis.

Immediate Sleep-disordered Breathing Consequences

Autonomic Nervous System Alterations

Sympatho-vagal imbalances during OSA events are primarily responsible for triggering arrhythmogenesis. Specifically, the vagal influences play a direct role in shortening the atrial effective refractory period (ERP), which otherwise would act to prevent arrhythmias. This is because after myocytes produce an action potential, there is a period of time when the activated cells are recovering and unable to produce another action potential, referred to as the ERP. Any disturbance that shortens the atrial ERP, predisposes the heart to arrhythmias. This has been simulated in canine models where OSA with intermittent hypoxia and hypercapnia decreased ERP [9, 10]. After upper airway patency restoration, strong sympathetic responses generated in response to the interacting effects of central respiratory sympathetic coupling, hypoxia, hypercapnia, and absence of sympathoinhibition from normal lung initiation reflexes, further the arrhythmia susceptibility [11].

Observations from animal model studies support the role of autonomic influences in OSA and arrhythmogenesis. In a canine model, ablation of the right ganglionated plexus resulted in inhibition of apnea-induced AF [12]. In a porcine model, simulated tracheal occlusion led to increasing AF inducibility, reduction of the atrial ERP, but these observations were found to be reversed by renal sympathetic denervation and low-level baroreceptor stimulation, which essentially suppressed both sympathetic and parasympathetic activity [13].

Additionally, intermittent hypoxemic episodes (from repetitive OSA events) alone serve to perpetuate recurrent sympathetic discharges triggering atrial activity and abnormal automaticity [14].

Lastly, OSA-induced cardiac structural remodeling (fibrosis and connexin dysregulation) can also lead to conduction slowing, thereby precipitating arrhythmogenesis [15].

Hypoxia

At the end of each OSA event, and following the termination of upper airway obstruction, re-oxygenation in cardiac tissues leads to the formation of hazardous reactive oxygen species (ROS) [16, 17]. Not only is the oxidative stress implicated directly in myocardial hypertrophy, injury, and apoptosis (leading to structural heart changes in mice models) [18, 19], but also ROS has been linked to arrhythmogenesis both in animals and humans, primarily due to alterations in calcium channel activity and microvascular ischemia [20].

Additionally, oxidative stress secondary to hypoxia uncouples endothelial nitric oxide synthase, thereby increasing superoxide generation and decreasing nitric oxide production, and in turn, leads to chronic endothelial dysfunction, which is associated with AF [21]. Oxidative stress also promotes the conversion of myofibroblasts from fibroblasts, leading to perivascular and cardiac interstitial fibrosis that could also slow conduction [22].

Intrathoracic Pressure Changes

Upper airway obstruction (Müller maneuver) generates negative intrathoracic pressure, usually up to -65mmHg, which can lead to increased transmural cardiac pressures, and increased afterload. In turn, this increases atrial distension [23], which in turn leads to acute shortening of atrial ERP *via* vagal activation. The effect of increased venous return in atrial chambers from negative intrathoracic pressures also serves to enhance arrhythmogenicity potential. Simulated obstructive sleep events *via* Müller maneuver in both healthy and AF patients has been shown to lead to premature atrial beats and QTc prolongation [24, 25].

Intermediate Sleep-disordered Breathing Mechanisms

Systemic Inflammation and Oxidative Stress

A number of systemic inflammatory markers have been associated with OSA. These include C-reactive protein (CRP), tumor necrosis factor-α (TNF-α), interleukin (IL)-8, intercellular adhesion molecule, selectin and vascular cellular adhesion molecule. Based on *in-vitro* experiments and animal models, TNF-α can induce gap-junction channel dysfunction through impaired atrial connexin 40 and connexin 43 expression and distribution [26, 27] and these changes occur within a matter of few hours [28]. Levels of IL-6 have been acknowledged to have a strong prognostic value in predicting mortality after an acute cardiac event. Increased levels of IL-6 have been related to acquired long QT-syndrome in patients with systemic inflammation, resulting in higher risks for life-threatening polymorphic ventricular tachycardia [29]. CRP levels are elevated in patients with AF corresponding to the AF burden level and may contribute to AF persistence [30]. Both plasma CRP and IL-6 levels are associated with left atrial dilation and endothelial dysfunction [31, 32].

Prothrombotic State

Emerging evidence suggests a possible bidirectional relationship between hypercoagulability and AF, one causing or leading to the other [33, 34]. In experimental models, hypoxic burden and intermittent hypoxia were found to be associated with platelet activation, fibrinogen, and platelet aggregation and thrombus formation [35, 36]. Additionally, in the participants of the Cleveland Family Study [37], levels of the prothrombotic biomarkers plasminogen activator inhibitor-1 and fibrinogen were found to increase with incremental increases in the apnea-hypopnea index until a plateau was reached at a moderate level of SDB. The relationships persisted after consideration of confounders, including body mass index, medications, and smoking, suggesting that the changes in prothrombotic biomarkers were secondary to mild to moderate levels of sleep-disordered breathing.

Chronic Sleep-disordered Breathing Mechanisms

Cardiac Structural and Electrical Remodeling

It is possible that several months or years of untreated sleep apnea leads to structural changes in the heart, predisposing to arrhythmias. In an observational case-control study assessing atrial electromechanical parameters, interatrial and intra-atrial electromechanical delay and P wave dispersion were found to be prolonged in patients with moderate-to-severe OSA compared to controls, and the specifically interatrial electromechanical delay had a significant correlation with left atrial volume index and left atrial dimension [38]. This study also found a significant correlation between the interatrial electromechanical delay and the lowest nocturnal oxygen saturation and AHI [38]. One study [39] found signs of left atrial remodeling in severe OSA patients when compared with appropriate control participants, and another study [40] showed that moderate/severe OSA was associated with a high prevalence of concentric left ventricular geometry. Overall, these studies indicate that OSA is associated with atrial remodeling and dilation and left ventricular hypertrophy, which are all known predisposing factors for arrhythmogenesis [41].

ROLE OF CARDIAC IMPLANTABLE ELECTRONIC DEVICES IN SLEEP APNEA DETECTION

Some cardiac implantable electronic devices (CIED) have incorporated sleep apnea detection algorithms that can be used as a screening tool for the early detection of sleep apnea in patients with AF. The main advantage seems to be the possibility of prolonged monitoring, allowing an increase in the detection period of respiratory sleep disorders *versus* polysomnography (PSG). The algorithm was previously validated by the manufacturer in the DREAM clinical trial [42]. This trial included unselected patients who had an indication for pacemaker implantation (PM) and the respiratory disturbance index (RDI) obtained from pacemakers correlated with the RDI and AHI obtained from the PSG. An RDI-PM cut-off of ≥20 had 85% specificity and 89% sensitivity for detecting severe sleep apnea. Another study showed a cut-off RDI-PM of 13 for detecting moderate-to-severe sleep apnea with 70% specificity and 100% sensitivity [43]. In another study [44] of 81 patients with OSA RDI-PM showed good diagnostic accuracy for OSAS (area under the curve: 0.767 [95% CI: 0.65–0.88]; $p < 0.001$). At the ideal diagnostic cut-off of 13.3 for RDI, the specificity and sensitivity were both 78% and for detection of moderate-to-severe OSA, a 90% sensitivity. The study also showed a significantly greater AF burden in patients with OSA than in those without OSA. In patients with AF, the RDI-PM cut-off of 13.3 decreased the specificity to 57% compared to the general population [44]. However, in patients without AF the specificity was 100% and sensitivity 77% [44]. This suggests that the presence AF alters the specificity of RDI-PM in the diagnosis of OSAS.

CPAP TREATMENT AND ARRHYTHMIAS

CPAP may have a favorable effect in preventing AF recurrence [45]. A meta-analysis of seven observational studies noted that users of CPAP had a significant reduction in AF recurrence rate compared with nonusers [33.3% *vs.* 58.1%; relative risk: 0.58; 95% confidence intervals (CI): 0.51-0.67; p<0.001] [46]. In a subgroup analysis of 5 studies in which patients underwent pulmonary vein isolation, users of CPAP were found to have a lower risk of AF recurrence in comparison with nonusers (33.3% *vs* 57.6%; relative risk 0.58 [95% CIs: 0.50 to 0.67, p < 0.001] [46]. In another meta-analysis of 8 studies, patients treated with CPAP had a 42% decreased risk of AF (pooled risk ratio, 0.58 ; 95% CIs: 0.47 to 0.70, p <0.001) [47]. Data from these two meta-analyses were primarily based on observational studies. Recently, in a randomized controlled trial [48] of 108 patients with OSA and paroxysmal AF (54 in CPAP and 54 in usual care group), CPAP therapy compared with usual care alone, did not result in a statistically significant reduction in the time in AF and the adherence to CPAP treatment also did not influence this result. However, the study was limited by the small sample size, short duration (5 months) and patients with more severe sleep apnea and subjective daytime sleepiness were excluded from the analysis.

SLEEP APNEA AND SUDDEN CARDIAC DEATH

The link between OSA and sudden cardiac death (SCD) is not clearly understood but possibly related to maladaptive autonomic nervous system changes, altered ion channel expression and hemodynamic shifts. In general, non-REM sleep is characterized by increased baroreceptor gain and vagal tone which can increase the frequency of sinus arrhythmia and bradycardia [49]. Sympathetic nervous activity on the other hand usually predominates phasic REM sleep, but there are usually intermittent bursts of vagal activity, which can also generate bradyarrhythmias.

In a previously published study [50] it was shown that individuals with OSA had an increased risk of SCD from 10 PM to 6 AM and that individuals without OSA had a diurnal pattern of sudden death, peaking between 6 AM and noon, similar to that seen in the general population. In that study, individuals with OSA had a 2.6 fold risk of nocturnal SCD, and the severity of OSA correlated with the magnitude of this risk [50]. In a cohort study of 10,701 adults referred for sleep studies, the presence of OSA predicted incident SCD and this risk was predicted by OSA severity, including the AHI and nocturnal oxygen desaturation [51]. Another controlled, multicenter study showed that during sleep, non-sustained ventricular tachycardia occurred in 5.3% and complex ventricular ectopy occurred in 25% of patients with OSA and central sleep apnea. In that study, after adjustment for comorbidities, patients with sleep apnea had a 3.4-fold risk of such events compared to the 1.7-fold risk in patients with normal sleep [52]. Another controlled longitudinal study of 107 CPAP compliant and 61 non-CPAP users (or discontinued) followed over an average of 7.5 years showed SCD occurring 7% of untreated OSA patients and in 0% of patients treated OSA [53].

Multiple electrocardiographic markers of increased SCD risk are also associated with OSA, and these include premature ventricular contractions, QT interval prolongation, AF, T-wave alternans and atrioventricular block [54]. Those with these ECG abnormalities have an approximately 2-fold increased risk of SCD during sleep [55]. In a cohort of patients with congenital long QT syndrome, increasing severity of OSA was found to be related to the degree of QT interval [56]. Another study showed that the magnitude of QTc was associated with the degree of hypoxia [57]. The MESA study showed that higher AHI was associated with greater odds of abnormal QRS-T angle [58]. It is possible that patients with OSA and ventricular repolarization abnormality such as prolonged QTc or abnormal QRS-T angle represents a higher risk subgroup for SCD. Further evidence on a possible cause-effect relationship between sleep apnea and QT abnormalities was presented in a randomized controlled trial [59] that showed a significant reduction was noted in QTc interval by 11.3 ms with therapeutic CPAP use. This change in QTc interval was most pronounced in patients with baseline QTc >430 ms and during the hours 6 p.m.–12 p.m [59].

CONCLUSION

In closing, this chapter has reviewed the relationship between sleep apnea and arrhythmias. Given that sleep apnea is such a common condition and is considered a modifiable risk factor for arrhythmia development, there has been growing interest in better understanding this condition. Multiple mechanisms for arrhythmia development exist, which means there may be the potential for multiple targets for treatment and early detection. In the future, pacemakers may be used to help detect sleep apnea in patients with previously diagnosed arrhythmias. Blood detection of IL-6 may offer an efficient way to categorize patients with OSA and their risk of developing arrhythmia. Hopefully, future work will allow for widely identifying patients at risk of sleep apnea and arrhythmias, early diagnosis of sleep disordered breathing and effective treatment of both arrhythmias and sleep apnea.

CONSENT FOR PUBLICATION

Not applicable.

CONFLICT OF INTEREST

The author declares no conflict of interest, financial or otherwise.

ACKNOWLEDGEMENTS

Declared none.

REFERENCES

[1]   Marin JM, Agusti A, Villar I, *et al*. Association between treated and untreated obstructive sleep apnea and risk of hypertension. JAMA 2012; 307(20): 2169-76.
        [http://dx.doi.org/10.1001/jama.2012.3418] [PMID: 22618924]

[2]   May AM, Van Wagoner DR, Mehra R. OSA and cardiac arrhythmogenesis: Mechanistic insights. Chest 2017; 151(1): 225-41.
        [http://dx.doi.org/10.1016/j.chest.2016.09.014] [PMID: 27693594]

[3]   Cadby G, McArdle N, Briffa T, *et al*. Severity of OSA is an independent predictor of incident atrial fibrillation hospitalization in a large sleep-clinic cohort. Chest 2015; 148(4): 945-52.
        [http://dx.doi.org/10.1378/chest.15-0229] [PMID: 25927872]

[4]   Gami AS, Hodge DO, Herges RM, *et al*. Obstructive sleep apnea, obesity, and the risk of incident atrial fibrillation. J Am Coll Cardiol 2007; 49(5): 565-71.
        [http://dx.doi.org/10.1016/j.jacc.2006.08.060] [PMID: 17276180]

[5]   Mehra R, Stone KL, Varosy PD, *et al*. Nocturnal Arrhythmias across a spectrum of obstructive and central sleep-disordered breathing in older men: outcomes of sleep disorders in older men (MrOS sleep) study. Arch Intern Med 2009; 169(12): 1147-55.
        [http://dx.doi.org/10.1001/archinternmed.2009.138] [PMID: 19546416]

[6]   Ng CY, Liu T, Shehata M, Stevens S, Chugh SS, Wang X. Meta-analysis of obstructive sleep apnea as predictor of atrial fibrillation recurrence after catheter ablation. Am J Cardiol 2011; 108(1): 47-51.
        [http://dx.doi.org/10.1016/j.amjcard.2011.02.343] [PMID: 21529734]

[7]   Narkiewicz K, Somers VK. The sympathetic nervous system and obstructive sleep apnea: implications for hypertension. J Hypertens 1997; 15(12 Pt 2): 1613-9.
        [http://dx.doi.org/10.1097/00004872-199715120-00062] [PMID: 9488212]

[8]   Narkiewicz K, Somers VK. Sympathetic nerve activity in obstructive sleep apnoea. Acta Physiol Scand 2003; 177(3): 385-90.
        [http://dx.doi.org/10.1046/j.1365-201X.2003.01091.x] [PMID: 12609010]

[9]   Lu Z, Nie L, He B, *et al*. Increase in vulnerability of atrial fibrillation in an acute intermittent hypoxia model: importance of autonomic imbalance. Auton Neurosci 2013; 177(2): 148-53.

[http://dx.doi.org/10.1016/j.autneu.2013.03.014] [PMID: 23622813]

[10] Linz D, Schotten U, Neuberger HR, Böhm M, Wirth K. Combined blockade of early and late activated atrial potassium currents suppresses atrial fibrillation in a pig model of obstructive apnea. Heart Rhythm 2011; 8(12): 1933-9.
[http://dx.doi.org/10.1016/j.hrthm.2011.07.018] [PMID: 21767520]

[11] Leung RS. Sleep-disordered breathing: autonomic mechanisms and arrhythmias. Prog Cardiovasc Dis 2009; 51(4): 324-38.
[http://dx.doi.org/10.1016/j.pcad.2008.06.002] [PMID: 19110134]

[12] Ghias M, Scherlag BJ, Lu Z, *et al.* The role of ganglionated plexi in apnea-related atrial fibrillation. J Am Coll Cardiol 2009; 54(22): 2075-83.
[http://dx.doi.org/10.1016/j.jacc.2009.09.014] [PMID: 19926016]

[13] Linz D, Hohl M, Khoshkish S, *et al.* Low-level but not high-level baroreceptor stimulation inhibits atrial fibrillation in a pig model of sleep apnea. J Cardiovasc Electrophysiol 2016; 27(9): 1086-92.
[http://dx.doi.org/10.1111/jce.13020] [PMID: 27235276]

[14] Volders PG. Novel insights into the role of the sympathetic nervous system in cardiac arrhythmogenesis. Heart Rhythm 2010; 7(12): 1900-6.
[http://dx.doi.org/10.1016/j.hrthm.2010.06.003] [PMID: 20570754]

[15] Iwasaki YK, Kato T, Xiong F, *et al.* Atrial fibrillation promotion with long-term repetitive obstructive sleep apnea in a rat model. J Am Coll Cardiol 2014; 64(19): 2013-23.
[http://dx.doi.org/10.1016/j.jacc.2014.05.077] [PMID: 25440097]

[16] Peng Y, Yuan G, Overholt JL, Kumar GK, Prabhakar NR. Systemic and cellular responses to intermittent hypoxia: evidence for oxidative stress and mitochondrial dysfunction. Adv Exp Med Biol 2003; 536: 559-64.
[http://dx.doi.org/10.1007/978-1-4419-9280-2_71] [PMID: 14635713]

[17] Peng YJ, Yuan G, Ramakrishnan D, *et al.* Heterozygous HIF-1alpha deficiency impairs carotid body-mediated systemic responses and reactive oxygen species generation in mice exposed to intermittent hypoxia. J Physiol 2006; 577(Pt 2): 705-16.
[http://dx.doi.org/10.1113/jphysiol.2006.114033] [PMID: 16973705]

[18] Chen L, Einbinder E, Zhang Q, Hasday J, Balke CW, Scharf SM. Oxidative stress and left ventricular function with chronic intermittent hypoxia in rats. Am J Respir Crit Care Med 2005; 172(7): 915-20.
[http://dx.doi.org/10.1164/rccm.200504-560OC] [PMID: 15976378]

[19] Park AM, Suzuki YJ. Effects of intermittent hypoxia on oxidative stress-induced myocardial damage in mice. J Appl Physiol (1985) 2007; 102(5): 1806-14.
[http://dx.doi.org/10.1152/japplphysiol.01291.2006]

[20] Jeong EM, Liu M, Sturdy M, *et al.* Metabolic stress, reactive oxygen species, and arrhythmia. J Mol Cell Cardiol 2012; 52(2): 454-63.
[http://dx.doi.org/10.1016/j.yjmcc.2011.09.018] [PMID: 21978629]

[21] Khayat R, Patt B, Hayes D Jr. Obstructive sleep apnea: the new cardiovascular disease. Part I: Obstructive sleep apnea and the pathogenesis of vascular disease. Heart Fail Rev 2009; 14(3): 143-53.
[http://dx.doi.org/10.1007/s10741-008-9112-z] [PMID: 18807180]

[22] Gutierrez A, Van Wagoner DR. Oxidant and inflammatory mechanisms and targeted therapy in atrial fibrillation: An update. J Cardiovasc Pharmacol 2015; 66(6): 523-9.
[http://dx.doi.org/10.1097/FJC.0000000000000313] [PMID: 26335221]

[23] Guggisberg AG, Hess CW, Mathis J. The significance of the sympathetic nervous system in the pathophysiology of periodic leg movements in sleep. Sleep 2007; 30(6): 755-66.
[http://dx.doi.org/10.1093/sleep/30.6.755] [PMID: 17580597]

[24] Straus SM, Kors JA, De Bruin ML, *et al.* Prolonged QTc interval and risk of sudden cardiac death in a population of older adults. J Am Coll Cardiol 2006; 47(2): 362-7.

[http://dx.doi.org/10.1016/j.jacc.2005.08.067] [PMID: 16412861]

[25]   Camen G, Clarenbach CF, Stöwhas AC, *et al.* The effects of simulated obstructive apnea and hypopnea on arrhythmic potential in healthy subjects. Eur J Appl Physiol 2013; 113(2): 489-96.
[http://dx.doi.org/10.1007/s00421-012-2457-y] [PMID: 22806087]

[26]   Sawaya SE, Rajawat YS, Rami TG, *et al.* Downregulation of connexin40 and increased prevalence of atrial arrhythmias in transgenic mice with cardiac-restricted overexpression of tumor necrosis factor. Am J Physiol Heart Circ Physiol 2007; 292(3): H1561-7.
[http://dx.doi.org/10.1152/ajpheart.00285.2006] [PMID: 17122196]

[27]   Liew R, Khairunnisa K, Gu Y, *et al.* Role of tumor necrosis factor-α in the pathogenesis of atrial fibrosis and development of an arrhythmogenic substrate. Circ J 2013; 77(5): 1171-9.
[http://dx.doi.org/10.1253/circj.CJ-12-1155] [PMID: 23370453]

[28]   Fernandez-Cobo M, Gingalewski C, Drujan D, De Maio A. Downregulation of connexin 43 gene expression in rat heart during inflammation. The role of tumour necrosis factor. Cytokine 1999; 11(3): 216-24.
[http://dx.doi.org/10.1006/cyto.1998.0422] [PMID: 10209069]

[29]   Mormile R. Obstructive sleep apnea and susceptibility to sudden cardiac death: A single player for both conditions? Cardiovasc Pathol 2020; 47: 107222.
[http://dx.doi.org/10.1016/j.carpath.2020.107222] [PMID: 32375086]

[30]   Chung MK, Martin DO, Sprecher D, *et al.* C-reactive protein elevation in patients with atrial arrhythmias: inflammatory mechanisms and persistence of atrial fibrillation. Circulation 2001; 104(24): 2886-91.
[http://dx.doi.org/10.1161/hc4901.101760] [PMID: 11739301]

[31]   Kaski JC, Arrebola-Moreno AL. Inflammation and thrombosis in atrial fibrillation. Rev Esp Cardiol 2011; 64(7): 551-3.
[http://dx.doi.org/10.1016/j.recesp.2011.03.015] [PMID: 21616576]

[32]   Tousoulis D, Zisimos K, Antoniades C, *et al.* Oxidative stress and inflammatory process in patients with atrial fibrillation: the role of left atrium distension. Int J Cardiol 2009; 136(3): 258-62.
[http://dx.doi.org/10.1016/j.ijcard.2008.04.087] [PMID: 18657327]

[33]   Spronk HM, De Jong AM, Verheule S, *et al.* Hypercoagulability causes atrial fibrosis and promotes atrial fibrillation. Eur Heart J 2017; 38(1): 38-50.
[http://dx.doi.org/10.1093/eurheartj/ehw119] [PMID: 27071821]

[34]   Liak C, Fitzpatrick M. Coagulability in obstructive sleep apnea. Can Respir J 2011; 18(6): 338-48.
[http://dx.doi.org/10.1155/2011/924629] [PMID: 22187690]

[35]   Rahangdale S, Yeh SY, Novack V, *et al.* The influence of intermittent hypoxemia on platelet activation in obese patients with obstructive sleep apnea. J Clin Sleep Med 2011; 7(2): 172-8.
[http://dx.doi.org/10.5664/jcsm.28105] [PMID: 21509332]

[36]   Watson T, Shantsila E, Lip GY. Mechanisms of thrombogenesis in atrial fibrillation: Virchow's triad revisited. Lancet 2009; 373(9658): 155-66.
[http://dx.doi.org/10.1016/S0140-6736(09)60040-4] [PMID: 19135613]

[37]   Mehra R, Xu F, Babineau DC, *et al.* Sleep-disordered breathing and prothrombotic biomarkers: cross-sectional results of the Cleveland Family Study. Am J Respir Crit Care Med 2010; 182(6): 826-33.
[http://dx.doi.org/10.1164/rccm.201001-0020OC] [PMID: 20508215]

[38]   Yagmur J, Yetkin O, Cansel M, *et al.* Assessment of atrial electromechanical delay and influential factors in patients with obstructive sleep apnea. Sleep Breath 2012; 16(1): 83-8.
[http://dx.doi.org/10.1007/s11325-010-0477-6] [PMID: 21221821]

[39]   Drager LF, Bortolotto LA, Figueiredo AC, Silva BC, Krieger EM, Lorenzi-Filho G. Obstructive sleep apnea, hypertension, and their interaction on arterial stiffness and heart remodeling. Chest 2007; 131(5): 1379-86.

[http://dx.doi.org/10.1378/chest.06-2703] [PMID: 17494787]

[40] Cioffi G, Russo TE, Stefenelli C, *et al.* Severe obstructive sleep apnea elicits concentric left ventricular geometry. J Hypertens 2010; 28(5): 1074-82.
[http://dx.doi.org/10.1097/HJH.0b013e328336c90a] [PMID: 20411620]

[41] Chatterjee S, Bavishi C, Sardar P, *et al.* Meta-analysis of left ventricular hypertrophy and sustained arrhythmias. Am J Cardiol 2014; 114(7): 1049-52.
[http://dx.doi.org/10.1016/j.amjcard.2014.07.015] [PMID: 25118122]

[42] Defaye P, de la Cruz I, Martí-Almor J, *et al.* A pacemaker transthoracic impedance sensor with an advanced algorithm to identify severe sleep apnea: the DREAM European study. Heart Rhythm 2014; 11(5): 842-8.
[http://dx.doi.org/10.1016/j.hrthm.2014.02.011] [PMID: 24561163]

[43] Dias M, Gonçalves I, Amann B, *et al.* Utility of new-generation pacemakers in sleep apnea screening. Sleep Med 2017; 37: 27-31.
[http://dx.doi.org/10.1016/j.sleep.2017.06.006] [PMID: 28899536]

[44] Gonçalves IS, Agostinho JR, Silva G, *et al.* Accuracy and utility of a pacemaker respiratory monitoring algorithm for the detection of obstructive sleep apnea in patients with atrial fibrillation. Sleep Med 2019; 61: 88-94.
[http://dx.doi.org/10.1016/j.sleep.2019.01.051] [PMID: 31401011]

[45] Riaz S, Bhatti H, Sampat PJ, Dhamoon A. The Converging Pathologies of Obstructive Sleep Apnea and Atrial Arrhythmias. Cureus 2020; 12(7): e9388.
[http://dx.doi.org/10.7759/cureus.9388] [PMID: 32754415]

[46] Shukla A, Aizer A, Holmes D, *et al.* Effect of Obstructive Sleep Apnea Treatment on Atrial Fibrillation Recurrence: A Meta-Analysis. JACC Clin Electrophysiol 2015; 1(1-2): 41-51.
[http://dx.doi.org/10.1016/j.jacep.2015.02.014] [PMID: 29759338]

[47] Qureshi WT, Nasir UB, Alqalyoobi S, *et al.* Meta-analysis of continuous positive airway pressure as a therapy of atrial fibrillation in obstructive sleep apnea. Am J Cardiol 2015; 116(11): 1767-73.
[http://dx.doi.org/10.1016/j.amjcard.2015.08.046] [PMID: 26482182]

[48] Traaen GM, Aakerøy L, Hunt TE, *et al.* Effect of continuous positive airway pressure on arrhythmia in atrial fibrillation and sleep apnea: a randomized controlled trial. Am J Respir Crit Care Med 2021; 204(5): 573-82.
[http://dx.doi.org/10.1164/rccm.202011-4133OC] [PMID: 33938787]

[49] Somers VK, Dyken ME, Clary MP, Abboud FM. Sympathetic neural mechanisms in obstructive sleep apnea. J Clin Invest 1995; 96(4): 1897-904.
[http://dx.doi.org/10.1172/JCI118235] [PMID: 7560081]

[50] Gami AS, Howard DE, Olson EJ, Somers VK. Day-night pattern of sudden death in obstructive sleep apnea. N Engl J Med 2005; 352(12): 1206-14.
[http://dx.doi.org/10.1056/NEJMoa041832] [PMID: 15788497]

[51] Gami AS, Olson EJ, Shen WK, *et al.* Obstructive sleep apnea and the risk of sudden cardiac death: a longitudinal study of 10,701 adults. J Am Coll Cardiol 2013; 62(7): 610-6.
[http://dx.doi.org/10.1016/j.jacc.2013.04.080] [PMID: 23770166]

[52] Mehra R, Benjamin EJ, Shahar E, *et al.* Association of nocturnal arrhythmias with sleep-disordered breathing: The Sleep Heart Health Study. Am J Respir Crit Care Med 2006; 173(8): 910-6.
[http://dx.doi.org/10.1164/rccm.200509-1442OC] [PMID: 16424443]

[53] Doherty LS, Kiely JL, Swan V, McNicholas WT. Long-term effects of nasal continuous positive airway pressure therapy on cardiovascular outcomes in sleep apnea syndrome. Chest 2005; 127(6): 2076-84.
[http://dx.doi.org/10.1378/chest.127.6.2076] [PMID: 15947323]

[54] Raghuram A, Clay R, Kumbam A, Tereshchenko LG, Khan A. A systematic review of the association

between obstructive sleep apnea and ventricular arrhythmias. J Clin Sleep Med 2014; 10(10): 1155-60.
[http://dx.doi.org/10.5664/jcsm.4126] [PMID: 25317099]

[55]   Schlatzer C, Bratton DJ, Craig SE, Kohler M, Stradling JR. ECG risk markers for atrial fibrillation and sudden cardiac death in minimally symptomatic obstructive sleep apnoea: the MOSAIC randomised trial. BMJ Open 2016; 6(3): e010150.
[http://dx.doi.org/10.1136/bmjopen-2015-010150] [PMID: 26983946]

[56]   Shamsuzzaman AS, Somers VK, Knilans TK, Ackerman MJ, Wang Y, Amin RS. Obstructive Sleep Apnea in Patients with Congenital Long QT Syndrome: Implications for Increased Risk of Sudden Cardiac Death. Sleep 2015; 38(7): 1113-9.
[http://dx.doi.org/10.5665/sleep.4824] [PMID: 26118557]

[57]   Latshang TD, Kaufmann B, Nussbaumer-Ochsner Y, *et al.* Patients with obstructive sleep apnea have cardiac repolarization disturbances when travelling to altitude: randomized, placebo-controlled trial of acetazolamide. Sleep 2016; 39(9): 1631-7.
[http://dx.doi.org/10.5665/sleep.6080] [PMID: 27306264]

[58]   Kwon Y, Misialek JR, Duprez D, *et al.* Sleep-disordered breathing and electrocardiographic QRS-T angle: The MESA study. Ann Noninvasive Electrocardiol 2018; 23(6): e12579.
[http://dx.doi.org/10.1111/anec.12579] [PMID: 29963729]

[59]   Schlatzer C, Bratton DJ, Schwarz EI, *et al.* Effect of continuous positive airway pressure therapy on circadian patterns of cardiac repolarization in patients with obstructive sleep apnoea: data from a randomized trial. J Thorac Dis 2018; 10(8): 4940-8.
[http://dx.doi.org/10.21037/jtd.2018.07.17] [PMID: 30233868]

CHAPTER 6

Transvenous Phrenic Nerve Stimulation for Central Sleep Apnea

William J. Healy[1,*] and **Rami Khayat[2]**

[1] Division of Pulmonary, Critical Care, and Sleep Medicine, The Medical College of Georgia at Augusta University, Augusta, GA 30912, USA

[2] Division of Pulmonary and Critical Care Medicine, University of California-Irvine, Irvine, CA 92868, USA

Abstract: Central sleep apnea (CSA) occurs when there is a recurrent temporary failure of the pontomedullary breathing pacemaker and subsequent cessation of breathing during sleep. The pathophysiological changes of low cardiac output states are the most common causes of CSA. Thus, CSA occurs most frequently in patients with underlying cardiovascular disease and specifically heart failure (HF). However, cessation of inspiratory effort is also observed in other physiologic and pathophysiologic states such as high-altitude induced periodic breathing, narcotic-induced CSA, and idiopathic CSA, along with any processes that may compress the brainstem. CSA is associated with immediate negative consequences, including intermittent hypoxia and sympathetic activation. Several studies have reported an association between CSA and worsened mortality in HF patients. Therefore, the treatment of CSA has been considered part of standard care, especially in patients with HF. In these patients, treatment of CSA can improve sympathetic activation, quality of life and decrease arrhythmias. Previously, the mainstay of treatment for CSA was continuous positive airway pressure (CPAP) therapy and then, as technology evolved, Adaptive Servo Ventilation (ASV). Recent data have suggested increased mortality in patients with HF with reduced ejection fraction (HFrEF) treated with ASV for CSA with EF <45, excluding this otherwise efficacious modality from usage in the majority of patients with CSA. Upon this background, the recent introduction of a novel therapeutic modality, transvenous phrenic nerve stimulation (TPNS), provides a valid treatment option that should be considered in all patients with CSA. In this chapter, we will introduce this treatment modality to the reader and attempt to provide a comprehensive overview of its operation, efficacy data, and application to the treatment of patients with CSA.

* **Corresponding author William J. Healy:** Division of Pulmonary, Critical Care, and Sleep Medicine Medical College of Georgia 1120 15ᵗʰ St, BBR 5513 Augusta, GA 30912, USA; Tel: 706-721-2566; Fax: 706-721-3069; E-mail: wihealy@augusta.edu

Imran H. Iftikhar and Ali I. Musani (Eds.)
All rights reserved-© 2022 Bentham Science Publishers

Keywords: Adaptive Servo, Cardiac Surgery, Central sleep apnea, Cheyne-stokes respiration, CPAP, Heart failure with a preserved ejection fraction, Heart failure with a reduced ejection fraction, Hypersomnia, Perioperative evaluation, Remedē ®, Sleep-disordered breathing, Snoring, Ventilation.

INTRODUCTION

Transvenous phrenic nerve stimulation (TPNS) is a recently introduced treatment modality for central sleep apnea. The only clinically available TPNS is the remedē system® which was approved by the Food and Drug Administration (FDA) in October 2017 for the treatment of moderate to severe central sleep apnea (CSA). This fully implantable system stabilizes breathing by delivering electrical stimulation to the hemidiaphragm. The system includes a stimulation lead placed either in the left pericardiophrenic or right brachiocephalic vein and a sensing lead placed in the Azygos vein. The system is programmed to turn on automatically during the patient's habitual sleep window and turn off prior to their habitual wake time. There are several studies published recently supporting the safety and effectiveness of this system. However, its dissemination and acceptance remain affected by the invasive nature of the therapy and the limited medical insurance coverage. Nevertheless, this modality is currently the only FDA approved therapy for CSA and is likely to gain wider acceptance and coverage as its utilization around the world increases. In this chapter, we will first discuss relevant aspects of the mechanism and consequences of CSA, then proceed to present and discuss in detail the Remede® system and its clinical data and applicability to treatment approaches for CSA.

DEFINITIONS AND CRITERIA FOR CSA

Sleep-disordered breathing (SDB) describes all types of sleep-related breathing disorders, including both obstructive sleep apnea (OSA) and CSA. Diagnosis of SDB depends on the polysomnographic scoring of the type of abnormal respiratory events into apneas and hypopneas. Apnea is an absence of airflow for greater than 10 seconds with a 90% drop in oronasal thermal sensor flow [1]. With hypopneas, a 30% drop in the nasal pressure sensor for greater than 10 seconds with a greater than 4% drop in the oxygen saturation is required [1]. Apneas and hypopneas are further classified into obstructive or central based on whether accompanying respiratory effort is present or absent. A diagnosis of SDB is made if more than 5 abnormal respiratory events (apneas or hypopneas) per hour of sleep were present (Apnea-hypopnea index >5 events/hour) [1]. If more than half of these respiratory events were classified as obstructive, the SDB is classified as OSA(1). The SDB is central sleep apnea if more than half of the events are central (hypopneas and apneas) [1].

A pattern of an oscillatory breathing pattern that includes increased ventilation, followed by decreased ventilation, then a cessation of breathing was described by Hunter, Cheyne, and Stokes in the early to the mid-19th century in patients with obesity, stroke, and heart failure (HF) [2]. This pattern, Hunter-Cheyne-Stokes Respiration (HCSR), features recurrent 60-90 second cycles of slowly increasing ventilation (crescendo), followed by a decrease in ventilation (decrescendo) terminating in a period of apnea [2]. HCSR occurs due to an underlying instability in the respiratory control system [2]. The first polysomnographic description of HCSR was made in 1965 [3]. Occurring during restful wakefulness, exercise, and sleep, HCSR is reported mainly in patients with systolic HF [4, 5].

Diagnosing CSA on a sleep study (polysomnogram) typically is based on the presence of central apnea or hypopnea but does not require the characteristic pattern of HCSR for diagnosis [1]. However, the HCSR pattern will commonly be found on the polysomnograms of patients with HF and CSA. It should be noted that a similar periodic breathing pattern of respiration may be observed in the context of obstructive events or without even meeting the definition of a respiratory event (*i.e.,* no accompanying decrease in oxygen saturation). For this reason, one cannot interchange HCSR and CSA. Patients who demonstrate CSA on their sleep studies may or may not have the same pathophysiology of respiratory control instability that underlies HCSR. The cycle lengths of central apneic periods may be affected by the underlying etiology. The central apneas observed during heart failure often have cycles of 60-90 seconds [6]. High altitude periodic breathing during Non-REM sleep, NREM, is often 10-25 seconds in duration at altitudes above 3000 meters [6]. Similarly, opioid-induced central apneas are also of short duration. Central apneas can also occur immediately prior to obstructive airway closure as part of a mixed apnea. Although patients with central sleep apnea have underlying decreased respiratory motor output, an obstructive component may occur at the end of a central apnea [7]. Finally, a certain patient, especially those with HF, can manifest mixed, central, and obstructive events during a single night since obstruction of the upper airway is part of the mechanism of central apnea [8].

PATHOPHYSIOLOGY OF CENTRAL APNEA DURING SLEEP

A comprehensive discussion of the mechanisms underlying respiratory control and the pathogenesis of CSA is well beyond the scope of this chapter. Recent reviews provide excellent coverage of this topic [6, 9, 10]. We will only briefly cover here the foundational concepts in the pathogenesis of CSA. The sleep state is associated with withdrawal of the wakefulness-related behavioral and metabolic stimuli to the breathing centers. This renders respiration during sleep dependent on $PaCO_2$ [11]. A change in arterial $PaCO_2$ will lead to a corresponding change in ventilation aiming to maintain the prevailing $PaCO_2$ (Eupneic $PaCO_2$) within a narrow physiologic range [12]. Central apnea will occur if the arterial $PaCO_2$ decreases below a reproducible, sensitive hypocapnic apneic threshold [12]. Thus, baseline hypocapneia from hyperventilation, as seen in patients with HF, creates an environment conducive for the CSA in patients with HF [13].

Central hypopneas and apneas occur in a recurrent cyclical pattern during sleep. This results from the negative feedback closed-loop cycle that characterizes the ventilatory control system. This function is often best understood using the concept of the respiratory system "loop gain". In this model, a change in chemical stimuli leads to a corresponding change in ventilation aiming to correct the initial perturbation. A transient increase in minute ventilation induces the opposite of the initial perturbation, causing an increased alveolar PO_2 and decreased PCO_2 [11]. The goal of these control systems is to preserve ventilation and chemical stimuli within a relatively narrow range while responding to changes in sleep state or gas exchange under a variety of physiologic or pathologic conditions. The respiratory system's loop gain combines the response of the ventilatory system to changing $PaCO_2$, (the controller gain), and the lung/chest in lowering $PaCO_2$ in response to hyperventilation (the plant gain) [14]. Changes in either parameter would change the requisite magnitude of hypocapnia to reach central apnea (termed the CO_2 reserve; a lower CO_2 reserve would be associated with an increased tendency to central apnea). Loop gain is a useful concept in understanding control of breathing; however, the applicability of loop gain clinically is limited in part because arousals and upper airway obstruction can abruptly alter the responsiveness of the system to a perturbation in chemical stimuli. TPNS is effective in patients with the predominantly central phenotype of CSA who have minimal upper airway obstruction [15].

CONSEQUENCES OF CSA AND RATIONALE FOR TREATMENT

Both OSA and CSA have cyclical episodes of hypoxia followed by re-oxygenation as hyperventilation follows arousal that ends the respiratory event. Throughout the night, these cycles of cessation of breathing, intermittent hypoxia, and reoxygenation recur in a typical pattern of intermittent nocturnal hypoxia seen in SDB. Nocturnal intermittent hypoxia is a distinct physiologic state associated with a unique profile of respiratory, vascular and neuro-humoral responses [16, 17]. Intermittent hypoxia upregulated the carotid chemoreceptors' output resulting in sustained stimulation in the ventilatory response and destabilizing the respiratory control system in a fashion that propagates SDB [18]. In addition, activation of the chemoreceptors results in sympathetic activation that is sustained throughout the night [16, 19]. The negative impact of increased sympathetic tone is well established in heart failure patients [20]. These perturbations are particularly detrimental to HF patients, although they are linked to other types of cardiovascular disease as well [20]. The consequences of SDB induced sympathetic activation to the failing heart predisposes to tachyarrhythmia and can also contribute to ventricular arrhythmias [21, 22]. Treatment of both CSA and OSA decreases sympathetic activation in HF patients and can reduce myocardial workload [21, 23 - 26].

Given the associated hypoxia and sympathetic activation, it would be expected that CSA, as a comorbidity in HF, would exert its most negative impact during HF hospitalizations. Hospital admissions and readmissions related to heart failure are important health outcomes and have a negative impact on the progression and outcome of HF [27]. The largest study to evaluate the impact of CSA on HF-related post-discharge readmissions enrolled over 800 patients with HF and reduced ejection fraction (HFrEF) who were hospitalized for decompensated HF and underwent in-hospital sleep testing during their admission [28]. In this study, the multivariate modeling of readmission rates adjusted for a set of covariates were found in large HF registries to predict readmissions and mortality [27, 29, 30], provided the novel insight that CSA is an independent predictor of post-discharge HF readmissions [28]. Later, a large prospective study provided the first evidence that SDB has independently associated with post-discharge cardiovascular mortality [31]. This study was a prospective cohort study of over a thousand HFrEF patients who were hospitalized with decompensated HF who had never been evaluated for SDB. These patients underwent in-hospital sleep testing and were followed for a median of 3 years post-discharge. Both CSA and OSA were independently associated with mortality in this cohort. This study was the largest observational study to date evaluating the effect of CSA on HF related mortality [31]. These studies solidify the negative impact of CSA in HF and identify HF decompensation as a critical time in the progression of HF. This is a time in which the patient is most susceptible to the consequences of CSA [31].

It is important to note that there are no adequately powered randomized trials showing a beneficial effect on mortality or readmission for the treatment of CSA at this time. Some authors have suggested that treatment of CSA may not be indicated and that CSA may be a compensatory mechanism in HFrEF and accordingly should not always be treated [32]. This notion is based on the observation that CSR is associated with hyperventilation-related increases in end-expiratory lung volume, intrinsic positive airway pressure, and a possible decrease of work of breathing associated with periodic rest to the respiratory cycle [33]. The recent publication of a negative trial in HFrEF and CSA lead to further support to this hypothesis [33]. However, this notion of CSA as a compensatory mechanism has not been validated or even tested in humans with heart failure, and it stands opposed to numerous studies over the past few decades that demonstrate a negative impact of CSA in HFrEF patients [34]. While the treatment of CSA has not been shown to improve mortality in heart failure patients, the neurohumoral consequences of CSA and their elimination with treatment are well documented [33]. Multiple randomized trials, though limited by a small number of patients, have shown that treatment of CSA decreases sympathetic activity while also decreasing work of breathing and improving respiratory strength [24, 35 - 37]. Several of these compensatory mechanisms of CSA are similarly achieved by the use of positive airway pressure (PAP): CPAP or adaptive servo-ventilation (ASV). PAP stabilizes the airway by improving ventilation-perfusion matching, increasing the end-expiratory pressure, and increasing intra-thoracic volume decreases the work of breathing [38].

Central events produce an identical pattern of cyclical intermittent hypoxia and activation of the sympathetic system to that seen with obstructive events [8, 16, 19] Furthermore, most central events are regularly associated with airway collapse at the end of apnea [7]. The clinical definition of CSA also includes patients that may have a substantial number of obstructive events [39, 40]. OSA and CSA are further associated with periodic breathing that varies from night to night. For these reasons, a decision not to treat a patient with HF and CSA is not justified and would leave this patient exposed to unmitigated hypoxia, airway instability, sympathetic activation, disturbed sleep, and the possibility of arrhythmias.

CURRENT STATE OF TREATMENT OPTIONS FOR CSA

For many years, it was observed that continuous positive airway pressure (CPAP) can at least partially treat CSA [21]. The largest randomized controlled trial (RCT) evaluating continuous PAP (CPAP) for treatment of CSA was done in patients HFrEF [41]. This trial (CANPAP) showed that CPAP did not improve survival in patients with CHF [41]. CPAP was able to decrease the severity of CSA and improve ejection fraction in a subset of patients. Since then, Adaptive Servo Ventilation (ASV) was developed specifically for the treatment of CSA. Early experience with ASV demonstrated superior efficacy in controlling CSA and evidence of improved clinical outcomes in patients with HF [42 - 44]. More recently, SERVE-HF, a multinational, multicenter, RCT evaluated the effects of ASV and optimal medical management compared to medical management alone in symptomatic patients with HFrEF and predominant CSA. This study reported increased mortality in the ASV with optimal medical management group [33]. This resulted in a black box warning for ASV therapy for heart failure patients with an ejection fraction of <45% and left clinicians with a dilemma as to how to manage patients requiring therapy for CSA in heart failure patients.

Other treatments that have been evaluated for CSA include pharmacological agents such as acetazolamide and nocturnal supplemental oxygen [45] These treatments have not been sufficiently studied in adequately powered long-term trials thus far and are not part of the standard approach for the treatment of CSA.

TRANSVENOUS PHRENIC NERVE STIMULATION FOR CENTRAL SLEEP APNEA

Background

Phrenic nerve stimulation (PNS) has been evaluated for a few decades for the treatment of diaphragm paralysis after injuries to the cervical spine [46 - 48]. In the beginning, these devices were surgically implanted in the thoracic cavity and were able to directly stimulate both hemidiaphragms. Subsequent studies showed the phrenic nerve could successfully be stimulated to treat central sleep apnea [15]. This system, the remedē® system (Respicardia, Inc., Minnetonka, Minnesota) is a lead-based device that performs transvenous phrenic nerve stimulation to pace a single hemidiaphragm during periods of central apnea. The procedure is performed by electrophysiologists in the EP suite under conscious sedation to minimize procedural risks as the patients often have prior strokes and advanced heart failure. The device senses respiration *via* transthoracic impedance through a lead placed in the azygous vein.

Validation of TPNS for Treatment of Moderate to Severe CSA

Following its initial conception, a small feasibility study of TPNS was conducted as a proof of concept and to determine safety. The study enrolled a small number of patients (n=16) who underwent implantation of a two-lead, transvenously-inserted PNS device. Participants underwent a two-day polysomnography study comparing one night of control sleep with no phrenic nerve stimulation to a second night with PNS. The investigators observed a significant improvement in the major indices of CSA severity, including AHI, oxygen desaturation index (ODI 4%), central apnea index (CAI), arousal index (AI), and A second short term study was done in China and yielded similar observations [49].

Pivotal Trial for TPNS

The remedē ® system was conclusively evaluated in the pivotal trial completed May 2015, looking at patients with moderate to severe CSA based on a polysomnogram. In the experimental arm the device was turned on after implant and in the control arm the device was inactive for the first three months of the trial. Patients were included if they had CSA diagnosed by PSG within 40 days of implant, AHI greater than 20, Central apnea index (CAI) > 50% with at least 30 central apnea, obstructive apnea index (OAI) <20% of the total AHI and they had to be medically stable prior to the study. Patients were excluded if they had CSA from pain medication, palsy of the phrenic nerve, stroke within 12 months of testing, FEV1/FVC <65% of predicted or FVC < 60% predicted, baseline O_2 saturation <92% while awake, pacemaker dependent subjects, life expectancy <12 months, currently enrolled in a confounding study, or invasive cardiac procedures within 3 months of the procedure [50]. The primary endpoint was a 50% reduction in AHI. Secondary endpoints included sleep architecture, sleep-disordered breathing parameters, ESS and the global patient assessment. Fig. (**1**) describes the percentage improvement in AHI observed in the pivotal trial. Safety measures were tracked throughout the study, including therapy, device, and procedure-related events throughout the study period. 151 patients were divided between treatment, 73, and control, 78. 51% had an AHI reduction of > 50% at 6 months. 11% of the control group had a reduction of AHI of > 50% at 6 months. 91% of patients were free at 12 months of adverse events from the device, procedure, or therapy. After 6 months of the study was completed, the control group had the device turned on and had similar improvements in outcomes to the experimental group. Interestingly, there were improvements in ejection fraction and left ventricular dimension at 12 months compared to baseline (p<0.05). There was an improvement in Minnesota Living with Heart Failure scores in the intervention group (p<0.01) and a trend towards a lower rate of hospitalization in the treatment group at 6 months as compared to control (p=0.065) [51]. Fig. (**1**) shows a decrease in AHI at both 6 and 12 months of therapy during the pivotal trial.

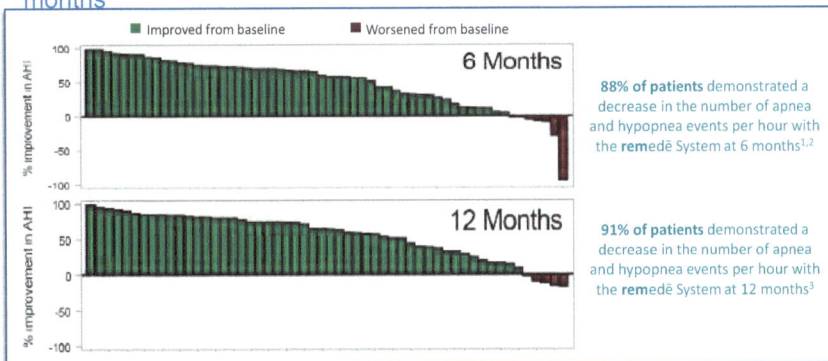

Fig. (1). The percentage of improvement in AHI from baseline is contrasted between 6 and 12 months after implant of the TPNS [50, 53].

Mechanism of Effect

Currently, there are no published studies addressing the mechanism of action of TPNS in CSA. This is partially explained by the novelty of the treatment modality. Such paucity of studies must not be prolonged given that the therapy is relatively invasive and requires a higher burden of the safety of efficacy. The experience with SERVE-HF, evaluating ASV in HFrEF-CSA, is a cautionary tale. The observation of increased mortality in the treatment arm of SERVE-HF remains unexplained, largely due to the limited understanding of the long-term effect of ASV on respiratory control and cardiovascular parameters.

In the absence of mechanistic studies, one can only speculate at this point regarding the mechanism of efficacy of TPNS. As demonstrated in Fig. (2), TPNS paces a unilateral phrenic nerve *via* the wall of an adjacent vein. As such, one hemidiaphragm is "overdriven" or its putative motor output 'overridden" by the system at a set rate and amplitude. It appears that this paced rate and amplitude entrains the other hemidiaphragm, likely *via* a variety of chest wall and lung tissue generated sensory inputs to the central respiratory controller. Fig. (3) contrasts central sleep apnea at baseline and with a patient stabilized breathing once the TPNS device is turned on. The pacing may, in theory, induce a slight hypoventilation or hyperventilation. However, the set stimulation rate and amplitude are often guided by the patient's baseline ventilatory parameters. Nevertheless, studies have not yet reported on the state of $PaCO_2$ or serum bicarbonate in patients who underwent pacing. Published studies and the authors' experience, however, did not include any cases of acid-base disturbance or arrhythmia.

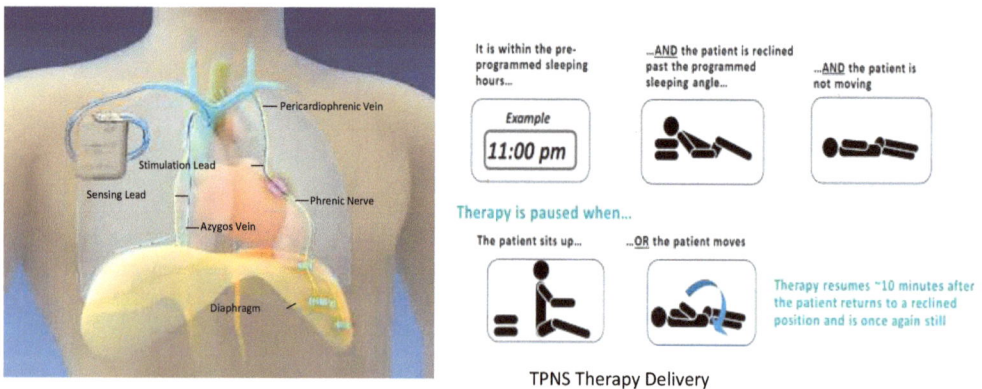

TPNS Therapy Delivery

Fig. (2). The TPNS electrode paces a unilateral phrenic nerve through the adjacent vein to stimulate diaphragmatic contractions during periods of absent inspiratory effort. The TPNS will only start therapy at appropriate times when the patient is reclined and not moving.

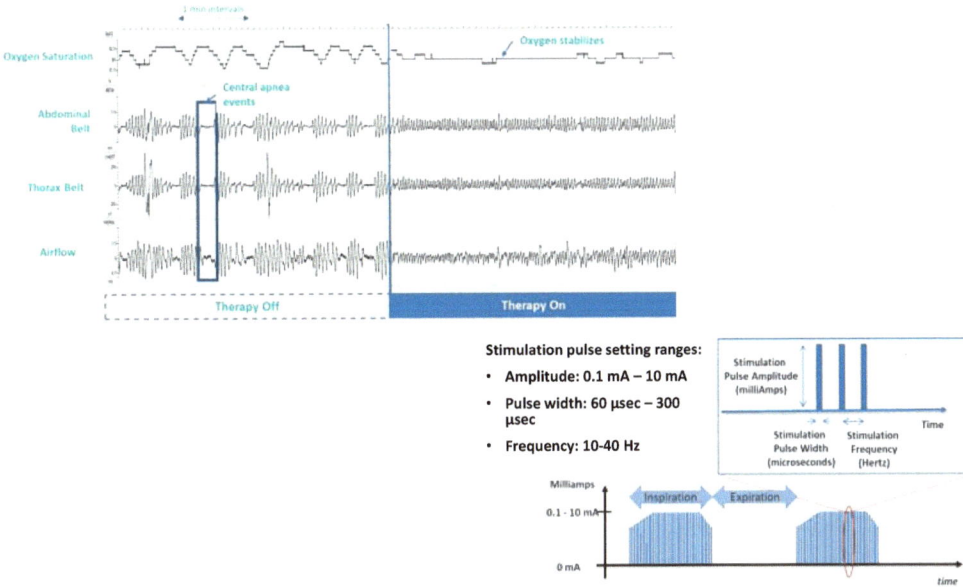

Fig. (3). A representative polysomnogram showing central sleep apnea at baseline and after the TPNS therapy is turned on. Standard stimulation pulse setting ranges are provided for reference.

A hypothetical concern with TPNS is inducing destabilizing pressures on airway patency. Experience with diaphragmatic pacing in children with central alveolar syndrome support this concern [52]. The published pivotal (6 months) and long term follow up (12 and 18 months) studies do not report an increase in the obstructive AHI, as seen in Fig. (**1**) [53]. However, it is clear from the published study that TPNS has no efficacy on obstructive events as its main effect is in reducing the central AHI.

CANDIDATE SELECTION

As an emerging therapy with relatively limited clinical experience in the real world, an important question arises regarding the ideal candidate for receiving the implant. Examining the pivotal trial for TPNS provides two important observations. One is that the modality was effective only for central events and had no positive impact on obstructive events. The second observation is that the inclusion criteria of the trial required patients with the predominantly central disorder (AHI $\geq$ 20; CAI at least 50% of all apneas with at least 30 central apnea events; Obstructive Apnea Index $\leq$ 20% of the total AHI). As such, the ideal candidate would be a patient with predominantly central disorder on the baseline PSG, both etiologically and morphologically. This is in contrast with the general classification of CSA, which allows for patients who have just above 50% of their events defined as centrals to be classified as having CSA.

IMPLANTING AND ACTIVATION

Implantation of the device is an outpatient procedure with moderate sedation to minimize harm to medically fragile patients that would often benefit from the therapy. The device has three components: a sensing lead, a stimulation lead, and an implantable pulse generator [54]. Implantation generally takes 3 to 4 hours to perform and is performed by an electrophysiologist experienced in pacemaker placement. During implant, the stimulation leads can be placed either in the right brachiocephalic vein next to the right phrenic nerve or in the left pericardiophrenic vein next to the left phrenic nerve [50]. The sensing lead is placed in the azygous vein which travels near the diaphragm. These electrodes are connected to the pulse generator which is placed in the right or left pectoral region depending on an available spot. It is confirmed during the implant procedure that the diaphragm moves during stimulation.

The patient returns for follow-up around 4-6 weeks after implant. Since implant, the device has been gathering data on the patient's baseline respiratory rate, sleep pattern, and respiration. The device is programmed to initiate therapy at night during the time window of the patients' habitual sleep time. The amount of stimulation needed for a breath will be determined at this visit. At the next follow-up visit in about 6 more weeks, data will be reviewed and further titration will be performed. Finally, an overnight PSG will be performed, and final programming of the device will be performed at that time. Fig. (**4**) describes the sequence of follow-up visits after implant.

Effective remedē therapy progression – programming follow-up

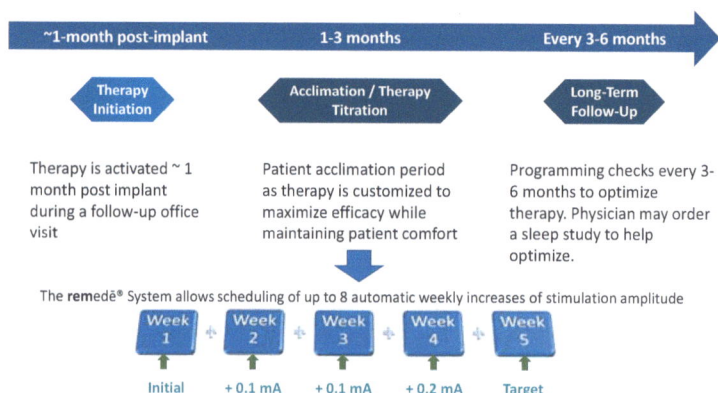

Fig. (4). The follow-up procedures and stimulation amplitude adjustments after TPNS implant are demonstrated at their recommended intervals.

CONCLUSION

TPNS for CSA is an exciting new area of sleep therapeutics with proven patient benefits. The remedē® system has shown itself to be tolerable, safe, and efficacious through multiple studies. Despite the complexity of its intervention, the system can easily be implanted in an outpatient procedure and monitored and adjusted with a few follow-up visits. Candidate selection is critical for success since the technology is effective only for central events.

CONSENT FOR PUBLICATION

Not applicable.

CONFLICT OF INTEREST

The author declares no conflict of interest, financial or otherwise.

ACKNOWLEDGEMENT

Declared none.

REFERENCES

[1]   Berry R, Brooks R, Gamaldo C, Harding S, Lloyd R, Marcus C, *et al.* The AASM Manual for the Scoring of Sleep and Associated Events. 2016.

[2]   Wang Y, Cao J, Feng J, Chen BY. Cheyne-Stokes respiration during sleep: mechanisms and potential interventions. Br J Hosp Med (Lond) 2015; 76(7): 390-6.
        [http://dx.doi.org/10.12968/hmed.2015.76.7.390] [PMID: 26140557]

[3]   Gastaut H, Tassinari CA, Duron B. Polygraphic study of diurnal and nocturnal (hypnic and respiratory) episodal manifestations of Pickwick syndrome. Rev Neurol (Paris) 1965; 112(6): 568-79.
        [PMID: 5856212]

[4]   Poletti R, Passino C, Giannoni A, *et al.* Risk factors and prognostic value of daytime Cheyne-Stokes respiration in chronic heart failure patients. Int J Cardiol 2008.
        [PMID: 18691782]

[5]   Andreas S, Hagenah G, Moller C, Werner GS, Kreuzer H. Cheyne-Stokes respiration and prognosis in congestive heart failure. Am J Cardiol 1996; 78(11): 1260-4.
        [http://dx.doi.org/10.1016/S0002-9149(96)00608-X] [PMID: 8960586]

[6]   Dempsey JA. Central sleep apnea: misunderstood and mistreated! F1000 Res 2019; 8: 8.
        [http://dx.doi.org/10.12688/f1000research.18358.1] [PMID: 31297185]

[7]   Badr MS, Toiber F, Skatrud JB, Dempsey J. Pharyngeal narrowing/occlusion during central sleep apnea. J Appl Physiol 1995; 78(5): 1806-15.
        [http://dx.doi.org/10.1152/jappl.1995.78.5.1806] [PMID: 7649916]

[8]   Javaheri S, Barbe F, Campos-Rodriguez F, *et al.* Sleep apnea: types, mechanisms, and clinical cardiovascular consequences. J Am Coll Cardiol 2017; 69(7): 841-58.
        [http://dx.doi.org/10.1016/j.jacc.2016.11.069] [PMID: 28209226]

[9]   Javaheri S, Brown LK, Khayat RN. Update on Apneas of Heart Failure With Reduced Ejection Fraction: Emphasis on the Physiology of Treatment: Part 2: Central Sleep Apnea. Chest 2020; 157(6):

1637-46.
[http://dx.doi.org/10.1016/j.chest.2019.12.020] [PMID: 31958442]

[10]   Badr MS, Dingell JD, Javaheri S. Central Sleep Apnea: a Brief Review. Curr Pulmonol Rep 2019; 8(1): 14-21.
[http://dx.doi.org/10.1007/s13665-019-0221-z] [PMID: 31788413]

[11]   Costanzo MR, Khayat R, Ponikowski P, *et al.* Mechanisms and clinical consequences of untreated central sleep apnea in heart failure. J Am Coll Cardiol 2015; 65(1): 72-84.
[http://dx.doi.org/10.1016/j.jacc.2014.10.025] [PMID: 25572513]

[12]   Skatrud JB, Dempsey JA. Interaction of sleep state and chemical stimuli in sustaining rhythmic ventilation. J Appl Physiol 1983; 55(3): 813-22.
[http://dx.doi.org/10.1152/jappl.1983.55.3.813] [PMID: 6415011]

[13]   Xie A, Skatrud JB, Puleo DS, Rahko PS, Dempsey JA. Apnea-hypopnea threshold for CO2 in patients with congestive heart failure. Am J Respir Crit Care Med 2002; 165(9): 1245-50.
[http://dx.doi.org/10.1164/rccm.200110-022OC] [PMID: 11991873]

[14]   Dempsey JA, Smith CA, Przybylowski T, *et al.* The ventilatory responsiveness to CO(2) below eupnoea as a determinant of ventilatory stability in sleep. J Physiol 2004; 560(Pt 1): 1-11.
[http://dx.doi.org/10.1113/jphysiol.2004.072371] [PMID: 15284345]

[15]   Ponikowski P, Javaheri S, Michalkiewicz D, *et al.* Transvenous phrenic nerve stimulation for the treatment of central sleep apnoea in heart failure. Eur Heart J 2012; 33(7): 889-94.
[http://dx.doi.org/10.1093/eurheartj/ehr298] [PMID: 21856678]

[16]   Katragadda S, Xie A, Puleo D, Skatrud JB, Morgan BJ. Neural mechanism of the pressor response to obstructive and nonobstructive apnea. J Appl Physiol 1997; 83(6): 2048-54.
[http://dx.doi.org/10.1152/jappl.1997.83.6.2048] [PMID: 9390980]

[17]   Xie A, Skatrud JB, Crabtree DC, Puleo DS, Goodman BM, Morgan BJ. Neurocirculatory consequences of intermittent asphyxia in humans. J Appl Physiol 2000; 89(4): 1333-9.
[http://dx.doi.org/10.1152/jappl.2000.89.4.1333] [PMID: 11007566]

[18]   Peng YJ, Overholt JL, Kline D, Kumar GK, Prabhakar NR. Induction of sensory long-term facilitation in the carotid body by intermittent hypoxia: implications for recurrent apneas. Proc Natl Acad Sci USA 2003; 100(17): 10073-8.
[http://dx.doi.org/10.1073/pnas.1734109100] [PMID: 12907705]

[19]   Morgan BJ, Denahan T, Ebert TJ. Neurocirculatory consequences of negative intrathoracic pressure *vs.* asphyxia during voluntary apnea. J Appl Physiol 1993; 74(6): 2969-75.
[http://dx.doi.org/10.1152/jappl.1993.74.6.2969] [PMID: 8365996]

[20]   Cohn JN, Levine TB, Olivari MT, *et al.* Plasma norepinephrine as a guide to prognosis in patients with chronic congestive heart failure. N Engl J Med 1984; 311(13): 819-23.
[http://dx.doi.org/10.1056/NEJM198409273111303] [PMID: 6382011]

[21]   Javaheri S. Effects of continuous positive airway pressure on sleep apnea and ventricular irritability in patients with heart failure. Circulation 2000; 101(4): 392-7.
[http://dx.doi.org/10.1161/01.CIR.101.4.392] [PMID: 10653830]

[22]   Bitter T, Westerheide N, Prinz C, *et al.* Cheyne-Stokes respiration and obstructive sleep apnoea are independent risk factors for malignant ventricular arrhythmias requiring appropriate cardioverter-defibrillator therapies in patients with congestive heart failure. Eur Heart J 2011; 32(1): 61-74.
[http://dx.doi.org/10.1093/eurheartj/ehq327] [PMID: 20846992]

[23]   Kaye DM, Mansfield D, Aggarwal A, Naughton MT, Esler MD. Acute effects of continuous positive airway pressure on cardiac sympathetic tone in congestive heart failure. Circulation 2001; 103(19): 2336-8.
[http://dx.doi.org/10.1161/01.CIR.103.19.2336] [PMID: 11352880]

[24]   Naughton MT, Benard DC, Liu PP, Rutherford R, Rankin F, Bradley TD. Effects of nasal CPAP on

sympathetic activity in patients with heart failure and central sleep apnea. Am J Respir Crit Care Med 1995; 152(2): 473-9.
[http://dx.doi.org/10.1164/ajrccm.152.2.7633695] [PMID: 7633695]

[25]   Naughton MT, Liu PP, Bernard DC, Goldstein RS, Bradley TD. Treatment of congestive heart failure and Cheyne-Stokes respiration during sleep by continuous positive airway pressure. Am J Respir Crit Care Med 1995; 151(1): 92-7.
[http://dx.doi.org/10.1164/ajrccm.151.1.7812579] [PMID: 7812579]

[26]   Hall AB, Ziadi MC, Leech JA, *et al*. Effects of short-term continuous positive airway pressure on myocardial sympathetic nerve function and energetics in patients with heart failure and obstructive sleep apnea: a randomized study. Circulation 2014; 130(11): 892-901.
[http://dx.doi.org/10.1161/CIRCULATIONAHA.113.005893] [PMID: 24993098]

[27]   Fonarow GC, Stough WG, Abraham WT, *et al*. Characteristics, treatments, and outcomes of patients with preserved systolic function hospitalized for heart failure: a report from the OPTIMIZE-HF Registry. J Am Coll Cardiol 2007; 50(8): 768-77.
[http://dx.doi.org/10.1016/j.jacc.2007.04.064] [PMID: 17707182]

[28]   Khayat R, Abraham W, Patt B, *et al*. Central sleep apnea is a predictor of cardiac readmission in hospitalized patients with systolic heart failure. J Card Fail 2012; 18(7): 534-40.
[http://dx.doi.org/10.1016/j.cardfail.2012.05.003] [PMID: 22748486]

[29]   Abraham WT, Adams KF, Fonarow GC, *et al*. In-hospital mortality in patients with acute decompensated heart failure requiring intravenous vasoactive medications: an analysis from the Acute Decompensated Heart Failure National Registry (ADHERE). J Am Coll Cardiol 2005; 46(1): 57-64.
[http://dx.doi.org/10.1016/j.jacc.2005.03.051] [PMID: 15992636]

[30]   Fonarow GC, Abraham WT, Albert NM, *et al*. Age- and gender-related differences in quality of care and outcomes of patients hospitalized with heart failure (from OPTIMIZE-HF). Am J Cardiol 2009; 104(1): 107-15.
[http://dx.doi.org/10.1016/j.amjcard.2009.02.057] [PMID: 19576329]

[31]   Khayat R, Jarjoura D, Porter K, *et al*. Sleep disordered breathing and post-discharge mortality in patients with acute heart failure. Eur Heart J 2015; 36(23): 1463-9.
[http://dx.doi.org/10.1093/eurheartj/ehu522] [PMID: 25636743]

[32]   Naughton MT. Cheyne-Stokes respiration: friend or foe? Thorax 2012; 67(4): 357-60.
[http://dx.doi.org/10.1136/thoraxjnl-2011-200927] [PMID: 22318163]

[33]   Cowie MR, Woehrle H, Wegscheider K, *et al*. Adaptive Servo-Ventilation for Central Sleep Apnea in Systolic Heart Failure. N Engl J Med 2015; 373(12): 1095-105.
[http://dx.doi.org/10.1056/NEJMoa1506459] [PMID: 26323938]

[34]   Javaheri S, Brown LK, Khayat R. CON: Persistent central sleep apnea/hunter-cheyne-stokes breathing, despite best guideline-based therapy of heart failure with reduced ejection fraction, is not a compensatory mechanism and should be suppressed. J Clin Sleep Med 2018; 14(6): 915-21.
[http://dx.doi.org/10.5664/jcsm.7148] [PMID: 29852913]

[35]   Kasai T, Narui K, Dohi T, *et al*. Efficacy of nasal bi-level positive airway pressure in congestive heart failure patients with cheyne-stokes respiration and central sleep apnea. Circ J 2005; 69(8): 913-21.
[http://dx.doi.org/10.1253/circj.69.913] [PMID: 16041159]

[36]   Sin DD, Logan AG, Fitzgerald FS, Liu PP, Bradley TD. Effects of continuous positive airway pressure on cardiovascular outcomes in heart failure patients with and without Cheyne-Stokes respiration. Circulation 2000; 102(1): 61-6.
[http://dx.doi.org/10.1161/01.CIR.102.1.61] [PMID: 10880416]

[37]   Granton JT, Naughton MT, Benard DC, Liu PP, Goldstein RS, Bradley TD. CPAP improves inspiratory muscle strength in patients with heart failure and central sleep apnea. Am J Respir Crit Care Med 1996; 153(1): 277-82.
[http://dx.doi.org/10.1164/ajrccm.153.1.8542129] [PMID: 8542129]

[38]   Lenique F, Habis M, Lofaso F, Dubois-Randé JL, Harf A, Brochard L. Ventilatory and hemodynamic effects of continuous positive airway pressure in left heart failure. Am J Respir Crit Care Med 1997; 155(2): 500-5.
[http://dx.doi.org/10.1164/ajrccm.155.2.9032185] [PMID: 9032185]

[39]   Berry RB, Budhiraja R, Gottlieb DJ, *et al.* Rules for scoring respiratory events in sleep: update of the 2007 AASM Manual for the Scoring of Sleep and Associated Events. J Clin Sleep Med 2012; 8(5): 597-619.
[http://dx.doi.org/10.5664/jcsm.2172] [PMID: 23066376]

[40]   Ruehland WR, Rochford PD, O'Donoghue FJ, Pierce RJ, Singh P, Thornton AT. The new AASM criteria for scoring hypopneas: impact on the apnea hypopnea index. Sleep 2009; 32(2): 150-7.
[http://dx.doi.org/10.1093/sleep/32.2.150] [PMID: 19238801]

[41]   Bradley TD, Logan AG, Kimoff RJ, *et al.* Continuous Positive Airway Pressure for Central Sleep Apnea and Heart Failure. N Engl J Med 2005; 353(19): 2025-33.
[PMID: 16282177]

[42]   Kasai T, Kasagi S, Maeno K, *et al.* Adaptive servo-ventilation in cardiac function and neurohormonal status in patients with heart failure and central sleep apnea nonresponsive to continuous positive airway pressure. JACC Heart Fail 2013; 1(1): 58-63.
[http://dx.doi.org/10.1016/j.jchf.2012.11.002] [PMID: 24621799]

[43]   Kasai T, Usui Y, Yoshioka T, *et al.* Effect of flow-triggered adaptive servo-ventilation compared with continuous positive airway pressure in patients with chronic heart failure with coexisting obstructive sleep apnea and Cheyne-Stokes respiration. Circ Heart Fail 2010; 3(1): 140-8.
[http://dx.doi.org/10.1161/CIRCHEARTFAILURE.109.868786] [PMID: 19933407]

[44]   Philippe C, Stoïca-Herman M, Drouot X, *et al.* Compliance with and effectiveness of adaptive servoventilation *versus* continuous positive airway pressure in the treatment of Cheyne-Stokes respiration in heart failure over a six month period. Heart 2006; 92(3): 337-42.
[http://dx.doi.org/10.1136/hrt.2005.060038] [PMID: 15964943]

[45]   Eckert DJ, Jordan AS, Merchia P, Malhotra A. Central sleep apnea: Pathophysiology and treatment. Chest 2007; 131(2): 595-607.
[http://dx.doi.org/10.1378/chest.06.2287] [PMID: 17296668]

[46]   Joseph S, Costanzo MR. A novel therapeutic approach for central sleep apnea: Phrenic nerve stimulation by the remedē® System. Int J Cardiol 2016; 206 (Suppl.): S28-34.
[http://dx.doi.org/10.1016/j.ijcard.2016.02.121] [PMID: 26964705]

[47]   Romero FJ, Gambarrutta C, Garcia-Forcada A, *et al.* Long-term evaluation of phrenic nerve pacing for respiratory failure due to high cervical spinal cord injury. Spinal Cord 2012; 50(12): 895-8.
[http://dx.doi.org/10.1038/sc.2012.74] [PMID: 22777487]

[48]   Flageole H, Adolph VR, Davis GM, Laberge JM, Nguyen LT, Guttman FM. Diaphragmatic pacing in children with congenital central alveolar hypoventilation syndrome. Surgery 1995; 118(1): 25-8.
[http://dx.doi.org/10.1016/S0039-6060(05)80005-4] [PMID: 7604375]

[49]   Zhang XL, Ding N, Wang H, *et al.* Transvenous phrenic nerve stimulation in patients with Cheyne-Stokes respiration and congestive heart failure: a safety and proof-of-concept study. Chest 2012; 142(4): 927-34.
[http://dx.doi.org/10.1378/chest.11-1899] [PMID: 22302299]

[50]   Costanzo MR, Ponikowski P, Javaheri S, *et al.* Transvenous neurostimulation for central sleep apnoea: a randomised controlled trial. Lancet 2016; 388(10048): 974-82.
[http://dx.doi.org/10.1016/S0140-6736(16)30961-8] [PMID: 27598679]

[51]   Jagielski D, Ponikowski P, Augostini R, Kolodziej A, Khayat R, Abraham WT. Transvenous stimulation of the phrenic nerve for the treatment of central sleep apnoea: 12 months' experience with the remedē· System. Eur J Heart Fail 2016; 18(11): 1386-93.

[http://dx.doi.org/10.1002/ejhf.593] [PMID: 27373452]

[52]　Chervin RD, Guilleminault C. Diaphragm pacing: review and reassessment. Sleep 1994; 17(2): 176-87.
[http://dx.doi.org/10.1093/sleep/17.2.176] [PMID: 8036373]

[53]　Costanzo MR, Ponikowski P, Javaheri S, *et al.* Sustained 12 Month Benefit of Phrenic Nerve Stimulation for Central Sleep Apnea. Am J Cardiol 2018; 121(11): 1400-8.
[http://dx.doi.org/10.1016/j.amjcard.2018.02.022] [PMID: 29735217]

[54]　Augostini RS, Afzal MR, Costanzo MR, *et al.* How to implant a phrenic nerve stimulator for treatment of central sleep apnea? J Cardiovasc Electrophysiol 2019; 30(5): 792-9.
[http://dx.doi.org/10.1111/jce.13898] [PMID: 30834611]

CHAPTER 7

REM Sleep Behavior Disorder: Diagnosis, Epidemiology & Management

John DuBose[1] and **Emmanuel During**[2,*]

[1] *Atrium Health Sleep Medicine, Charlotte, NC, USA*

[2] *Department of Psychiatry, Division of Sleep Medicine, Department of Neurology, Stanford University, Palo Alto, CA, USA*

Abstract: REM Sleep Behavior Disorder (RBD), often known as injurious dream-enacting behaviors secondary to loss of atonia in REM sleep, was first described in 1986. While in the younger population, RBD can be associated with narcolepsy, posttraumatic stress disorder (PTSD) and antidepressant use, in middle-aged and older adults, RBD is almost always associated with a neurodegenerative disorder of synuclein—primarily Parkinson's disease and dementia with Lewy bodies. For this reason, so-called isolated, or idiopathic RBD (iRBD), is in the great majority of cases a prodromal manifestation of neurodegeneration. Diagnosis of RBD requires video-polysomnography to rule out common mimics. Specific diagnostic procedures and thresholds of electromyography (EMG) activity for the diagnosis of RBD have been developed and show high accuracy. Epidemiological studies have placed the overall prevalence of RBD around 2% across all age groups. Sleep-related injurious behaviors are common in RBD, especially in men, explaining the higher proportion of males diagnosed with RBD. In the management of RBD, safety is therefore paramount. Prognostic counselling is often warranted in iRBD, given the high rate of conversion to overt synucleinopathy. Offending agents, such as serotonergic medications, should be reduced or discontinued as possible as they exacerbate RBD behaviors. Pharmacological management involves primarily melatonin and/or clonazepam, while transdermal rivastigmine and, in select cases, sodium oxybate may be considered in treatment-resistant cases.

Keywords: Antidepressants, Diagnosis, Dream-enacting behavior, Epidemiology, Lewy body dementia, Multiple system atrophy, Management, Narcolepsy, Parasomnia, Parkinson's disease, Prognosis, Posttraumatic stress disorder, PTSD, Polysomnography, PSG, REM sleep behavior disorder, RBD, REM sleep without atonia, RSWA, Sleep-related injury, Synucleinopathy.

* **Corresponding author Emmanuel During:** Department of Psychiatry, Division of Sleep Medicine, Department of Neurology, Stanford University, Palo Alto, CA, USA; Tel: 650-723-6601; Fax: 650-721-3448; E-mail: eduring@stanford.edu

Imran H. Iftikhar and Ali I. Musani (Eds.)

INTRODUCTION

Rapid-eye-movement (REM) sleep behavior disorder (RBD) is due to REM sleep without atonia (RSWA), or loss of normal paralysis during REM sleep, resulting in potentially injurious dream-enacting behaviors (DEB). This parasomnia was first recognized by Schenck in 1986, who reported a series of five patients with a history of injurious dream enactment and loss of skeletal muscle atonia during REM sleep confirmed by video polysomnography (vPSG) [1]. Subsequent case series in adult patients delineated typical clinical features and the male predominance reported by Schenck in the initial report. Patients were often males in the sixth or seventh decade of life presenting with years-long histories of DEB consisting of flailing, punching, kicking, vocalizations, including yelling and screaming. Some patients were either already diagnosed with Parkinson's disease (PD) or had some features of other synucleinopathies such as dementia with Lewy bodies (DLB) or multiple system atrophy (MSA), however, a large proportion of them had no such diagnosis but later developed one of these neurodegenerative diseases. Injuries to the patient and bed partner are common in RBD, including lacerations, ecchymoses, hematomas and fractures, and this incidence is particularly high in men [2 - 4].

Classically, RBD has been subdivided into idiopathic (iRBD) and secondary or symptomatic. Idiopathic RBD has long been recognized as a prodromal feature of neurodegenerative diseases, namely the α-synucleinopathies—Parkinson's disease (PD), Lewy body dementia (DLB), and multisystem atrophy (MSA)—tracing to a cohort study by Schenck published in 1996 [5]. Subsequent studies have shown that the rates of conversion to a clinically manifest neurodegenerative disease exceed 80% [6, 7] and that the underlying pathology is nearly always related to misfolded alpha-synuclein [8]. Because in adult-onset RBD, ultimate conversion is so likely, and the preclinical stage may still represent latent disease, the terms "prodromal RBD" and "cryptogenic RBD" have been suggested [9] in lieu of "idiopathic RBD." A full section in this chapter will be dedicated to iRBD, given its relatively high prevalence in adults and its natural history as a precursor of neurodegeneration.

Secondary or symptomatic RBD is a broader category. The larger group of etiologies includes RBD associated with a clinically manifest synucleinopathy, more often PD and DLB, less commonly MSA. RBD is also common in narcolepsy with cataplexy (30-60%) [10], which is related to loss of hypocretin cells, and closely associated with anti-IgLON-5 disease [11]. Ischemic (strokes), neoplastic, paraneoplastic, autoimmune, inflammatory (neurosarcoidosis), and demyelinating diseases (multiple sclerosis, neuromyelitis optical), as well as a number of neurological diseases (progressive supranuclear palsy, corticobasal syndrome, spinocerebellar ataxias, ALS) affecting the brainstem and/or limbic system, can be associated with RBD [12]. Importantly, RBD can be triggered or exacerbated in the setting of antidepressant use [13, 14]. It may occur in psychiatric disorders such as PTSD and following trauma, even without antidepressant use [15 - 17].

Whereas a probable diagnosis is based on the history of suspicious DEB, vPSG is required for a definitive diagnosis of RBD, demonstrating RSWA, the neurophysiologic hallmark of RBD. Important challenges in the diagnostic procedure of RBD include limited patient awareness of episodes, the frequent lack of an informant, as well as the nuances and specific criteria used to quantify RSWA, which ideally requires the addition of arm electromyography (EMG) leads to the standard vPSG montage.

The management of RBD requires careful consideration of a number of factors. Due to the high risk of sleep-related injuries, safety measures need to be strictly implemented in all patients. Unfortunately, other than clonazepam and melatonin, pharmacological options are relatively limited. Counselling is an essential aspect of the management, especially in iRBD given the high risk of conversion to a neurodegenerative disorder. This chapter will discuss all these aspects of RBD, starting with the diagnosis, followed by the epidemiology and management of RBD.

BOX 1: Clinical Case, part 1

A 62-year-old man with a history of hypertension and morbid obesity presented for loud snoring and unrefreshing sleep after an anesthesiologist had noted long apneas during a recent elective procedure. He denied dream enactment, sleepwalking, or falling out of bed, but he endorsed sleep talking during his initial evaluation. He was scheduled for a diagnostic vPSG which showed severe OSA (AHI 92) with severe oxygen desaturation (O_2 nadir 58%). Less than 25 minutes of highly fragmented REM sleep occurred, but some loss of atonia and limb movements were noted, often associated with arousals. He was advised to return for an overnight PAP titration; however, because RBD was not suspected, arm EMG leads were not placed.

DIAGNOSIS

The diagnosis of RBD can be "probable" or "definite". Probable RBD is based on the clinical history of DEB alone, whereas definite RBD is based on the combination of a history of DEB or evidence of DEB on vPSG, with the neurophysiologic finding of RSWA, which is the electrophysiologic hallmark of RBD.

Clinical Diagnosis

The ICSD-3 criteria for diagnosis of RBD include "repeated episodes of sleep-related vocalization and/or complex motor behaviors", which may have been reported historically or observed during video polysomnography (vPSG). The criteria stipulate that these behaviors be determined by compelling history or vPSG during REM sleep and not be better explained by medications, substances, or other disorders [18].

Often, patients are not aware of their episodes. The largest case series reporting on patient awareness of DEB found that patients could be aware of only 20% of their episodes. Further, until they are diagnosed, almost half of the patients with RBD are unaware of having a disorder causing dream enactment [19]. For these reasons, the history should always include bed partners' and observers' accounts.

There is a wide range of motor manifestations and vocalizations in RBD. As RBD manifestations occur, by definition, only during REM sleep, RBD overall tends to manifest later in the night, as opposed to NREM parasomnias, which almost exclusively occur in the first 3 hours of sleep, dominated by slow wave sleep. Video-PSG studies reviewing visible movements epoch-by-epoch in patients with RBD show that the majority of these movements are short (seconds-long) twitches or jerks predominantly affecting the upper extremities [20 - 22]. These simple, elementary, non-purposeful movements, which could originate in the red nucleus, are more frequent (69%) than complex, purposeful RBD movements enacting dreams, which may originate in the cortex (31%) [23, 24]. The latter, more dramatic behaviors generally prompt patients and families to seek care, delaying the diagnosis by 4-5 years on average. Both extremities are generally involved, and lower extremity movements can be misinterpreted as periodic limb movements during sleep (PLMS), which, by definition, are periodic (every 15-40 seconds) and stereotyped, rarely persist during REM sleep and with some rare exceptions are not associated with violent behaviors or abnormal dreams [25]. The variety of manifestations in the same individual is a characteristic feature of RBD, which contrasts with the stereotyped phenomenology associated with sleep-related hypermotor epilepsy.

Vocalizations in RBD range from gentle, casual, conversational sleep talking, to disruptive screaming, yelling and cursing. Speech is usually intelligible, unlike sleep talking occurring in other, non-REM parasomnias. Illustrating the gender differences in RBD manifestations, profanities are more common in males. Unlike sleep talking occurring during NREM sleep, sleep talking in RBD is often conversational.

Dream contents vary from night to night, between patients as well as RBD phenotypes. However, in RBD associated with an underlying neurodegenerative disorder, either in its prodromal or manifest phase, the nightmares experienced depart from typical dream mentation, as they frequently involve being chased or attacked by people and animals. Those highly unpleasant, action-filled dreams account for the majority of sleep-related injuries. This nighttime aggressiveness, especially observed in male patients, contrasts with their placid daytime personality during wakefulness. When a patient is awakened during an episode, dream recollection is not the rule, as a high proportion of patients may not recall their dreams. In addition, the arousal is rapid and not associated with confusion or sleep inertia. Rather, patients should immediately orient to their surroundings and situation, which contrasts with NREM parasomnias. The only exception to this may be seen in RBD associated with advanced PD, PD dementia and DLB, where RBD can be associated with nocturnal episodes involving hallucinations, sleepwalking and confusion with subsequent amnesia. Such oneiroid states stand at the border of RBD, can be labelled "parasomnia overlap syndrome/disorder", and may be related to more widespread cortical Lewy body pathology.

Since OSA is a common disorder and can occasionally manifest with hypermotor behaviors associated with arousals secondary to obstructive events, it is important to distinguish this condition, also called "pseudo-RBD," from RBD [26]. Since history alone does not suffice to distinguish these two conditions, vPSG should be performed in all patients with suspected RBD to evaluate for any contribution of OSA, and to evaluate for excessive muscle activity during REM sleep, or RSWA, as detailed in the next section.

Polysomnographic Diagnosis (RSWA)

RBD is the only parasomnia that requires video-polysomnography for a definitive diagnosis [18]. The electrophysiologic hallmark of RBD is the loss of normal atonia during REM sleep, also called RSWA. Various degrees of increased EMG activity can be observed in other circumstances than RBD, as well as in the general population, supporting the notion of a continuum between normal and pathological states [27]. Further, in individuals with isolated RSWA without dream-enactment episodes, the RSWA severity (RSWA index) tends to increase over time until behaviors eventually emerge [28]. It is therefore likely that in adult-onset RBD related to synucleinopathy, years before progressing to clinically manifest RBD and vPSG-defined RSWA, patients display subtle findings or low-grade abnormalities that may represent a prodromal, preclinical phase of the disease.

Although several other methods have been tested, the current consensus method scoring RSWA uses SINBAR criteria [29]. Periods of sustained tonic activity (elevation of EMG tone above lowest baseline seen in NREM sleep) were observed in the chin (mentalis) muscle and/or excessive phasic activity (transient elevations, at least 4 times above background lasting at least 0.1 sec) in chin or limb muscles need to be observed during REM sleep. RSWA is said to occur in any 30-sec epoch of REM sleep if the abnormal tonic activity is observed in the chin for 50% of the epoch, or if out of this 30-sec epoch, phasic activity occurs in the chin and/or limbs in at least 50% of 3-sec mini-epochs, i.e., in at least 5 mini-epochs (Fig. **1**). Once all REM sleep epochs for that night have been reviewed and scored for RSWA, an RSWA index (%) can be calculated as the percentage of REM sleep 30-sec epochs in which RSWA was observed.

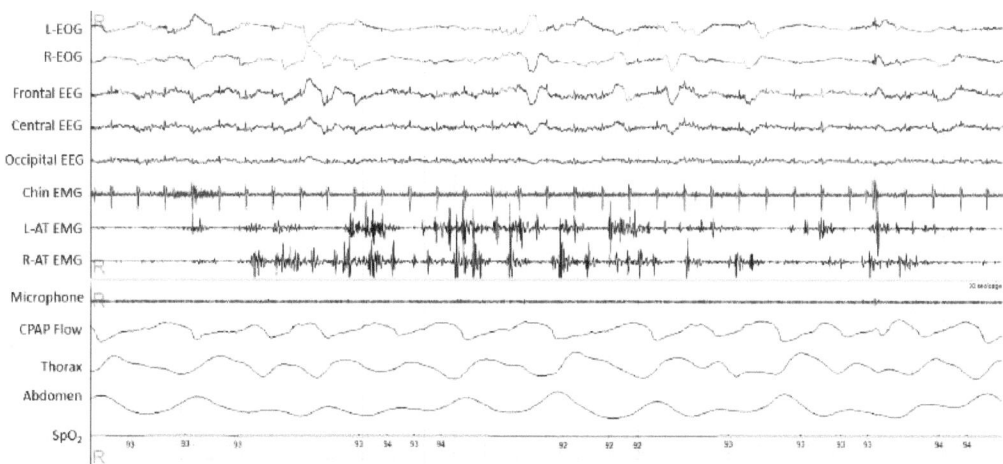

Fig. (1). A 30-second epoch of REM sleep demarcated into 3-second mini-epochs for our case example. Excessive phasic activity in the anterior tibialis leads (L-AT and R-AT EMG) occurs in 9 out of 10 mini-epochs, so this epoch is demonstrating RSWA. Phasic activity in the mentalis EMG is seen in the second 3 sec-mini-epoch as well. Note that ECG artifact is seen throughout the chin EMG tracing.

RSWA cutoffs cited by the current classification and referred to in most studies as the gold standard diagnostic criteria are derived from a series of investigations by the Sleep Innsbruck Barcelona (SINBAR) Group. The SINBAR studies showed that the highest rates of EMG augmentation in patients with RBD were observed in the mentalis, flexor digitorum superficialis, and extensor digitorum brevis muscles of the upper extremities [30], which comports with the observation that the majority of RBD movements are distal [22]. A 2012 landmark study established that the following cutoffs have the highest accuracy (100% specificity and areas under the curve ≥ 0.99) for the diagnosis of RBD [29]:

- Using any mentalis EMG activity alone: 14% of REM sleep considered in 30-second epochs (or 18% in 3-second mini-epochs)
- Using a combination of any mentalis EMG activity and phasic flexor digitorum superficialis activity: 27% of REM sleep considered in 30-second epochs (or 32% in 3-second mini-epochs)
- Using a combination of any mentalis EMG activity and anterior tibialis phasic activity: 45% of REM sleep considered in 30-second epochs (or 46% in 3-second mini-epochs)

Although the last combination of the chin and lower extremity EMG is the most widely used—being part of the standard vPSG montage, it is also more susceptible to artefacts and misinterpretations than a combination of chin and upper extremity EMG. It should also be noted that although cut offs for 3-sec mini-epochs method are provided as a reference, as they could improve sensitivity, such an approach is generally not used in clinical practice.

Table 1. Diagnostic RSWA thresholds for selected EMG combinations using 30-second epochs.

Muscles	Rate with 100% specificity
Mentalis "any"	14.5
Ment tonic	8.7
Ment "any" + FDS	27.2
FDS L + R	7.7
AT L + R	30.6
Ment "any" + AT	45.5

FDS: flexor digitorum superficialis, AT: anterior tibialis, adapted from Frauscher, 2012 [29].

In practice, the mentalis-FDS montage for RBD, is thus recommended as the diagnostic standard, but conventions and capabilities vary between sleep centers, and when RBD is an incidental finding (as in the provided case example), FDS leads may not have been requested. In these situations, chin alone or the combination of the chin and lower extremity EMG can be used.

There are a number of challenges and barriers to the implementation of the SINBAR method using conventional manual scoring in general clinical practice. This procedure is time and resource-intensive and requires a high level of expertise. In addition, it has limited interrater reliability [31]. The most common error that leads to missing the diagnosis of RSWA and RBD is due to underestimating the amount of REM sleep and staging an epoch as REM sleep only if it meets the standard definition of normal REM sleep, i.e., when muscle atonia occurs. This common mistake can be avoided by carefully reviewing the context and any behaviors displayed by the patient that would have been recorded with video and/or audio. This approach will help to identify periods showing important muscle activation and abnormal behaviors. Another common pitfall is related to EMG augmentation accompanying arousals due to breathing events in OSA. Such events are common, especially in the supine position. Again, the broader context and the sequence, timing and appearance of EMG augmentation about reduced airflow and/or snoring can help distinguish OSA-related increased EMG tone during REM sleep from true RSWA.

Automated methods have been developed to complement or replace human scoring of RSWA using mentalis EMG [32, 33] and the SINBAR montage [34]. Researchers have reported the high reliability of these methods compared with visual scoring approaches. More recently, machine learning approaches using EMG and other signals have shown high performance in differentiating individuals with RBD vs controls. It is conceivable that, in the near future, such approaches will be used in the clinical setting [35].

BOX 2: Case Example, part 2

Our patient underwent a full-night PAP titration in which high pressures were required. His disordered breathing was well-controlled with bilevel PAP. He achieved over 80 minutes of stable REM sleep after his breathing was controlled. During this time, he was observed to gesture in an animated fashion, pointing assertively and barking out orders to an imagined subordinate. He was noted to have excessive muscle activity during REM. His RSWA-index was 51% for a combination of "any" mentalis EMG activity or phasic EMG activity in the anterior tibialis leads (see Table 1 for SINBAR thresholds and Figure 1 for an example of a positive epoch). Based on this finding along with clear dream enactment captured on vPSG, he was diagnosed with RBD and given prognostic counseling. Upon further interview, the patient endorsed recent onset of constipation, increased urinary frequency and some longstanding loss of smell, however he showed no overt signs of parkinsonism on physical exam. The patient inquired about the significance of his condition, as he learned online that RBD is often a precursor of Parkinson's disease. He was educated on the prognosis and at his request, referred to a neurologist for further evaluation and care. This case illustrates the value of high-specificity diagnostic thresholds when the history is not compelling, RBD is discovered incidentally, and confidence in making the diagnosis is not high. It also shows the utility of having thresholds available for multiple EMG combinations. It also illustrates the complex ethical and medical questions related to the care and prognosis of patients with idiopathic RBD.

THE SPECIFIC CASE OF IDIOPATHIC RBD: PRESENTATION AND NATURAL HISTORY

As discussed in the introduction, the so-called idiopathic form of RBD has a very high predictive value for future progression to a neurodegenerative disorder. This fact, together with a relatively high prevalence of RBD in the adult population (estimated around 1%), has been the subject of a significant amount of literature and longitudinal studies in the last two decades describing the phenotype and progression of iRBD, as well as the associated features that allow risk stratification of patients in terms of neurodegenerative risk.

Clinical Features

The largest study of clinical features conducted in Spain on 203 consecutive iRBD patients referred to a sleep center found a 4:1 male: female ratio, median age of 63 at symptom onset and 68 at diagnosis, and a minimum age at diagnosis of 50. While the majority had been referred for dream-enacting behaviors (DEB), 11% had been referred for other reasons, and 44% of the patients would have been unaware of their behaviors had they not been informed by their bed partner. A large majority (93%) of these patients recalled negative dream content, most frequently being attacked, argued with, or chased. A majority (77%) had fallen out of bed, often more than once. Notably, 24% left the bed to stand, 9% walked, among which some left the room and even the house. Clinicians should be aware that while these behaviors are more classically associated with NREM parasomnias, they do not preclude RBD, as only one of these patients had a known history of sleepwalking. On the other hand, these behaviors tended to be rare compared to the context of more frequent DEB in these patients, and the possibility of comorbid disorders of arousal/NREM parasomnias could not be excluded. Injuries were common, had affected a majority of patients (59%) and a fraction of bed partners (21%). Women were less likely to have assaulted their bed partners (5% vs. 27% of men), though their bed partners were similarly likely to be incidentally injured. Women were more likely to dream that their children were in life-threatening situations (32% vs 8%) [19].

Conversion to Synucleinopathy

That idiopathic RBD is a harbinger of neurodegenerative disorder has been well-established through several cohort studies. Schenck first reported in 1996 that 38% of 29 male patients aged 50 and older with vPSG-confirmed iRBD developed a parkinsonian disorder after a mean interval of 3.7 years following diagnosis and 12.7 years after symptom onset [5]. A subsequent report was published in 2013, at which time 81% of the cohort (excluding 3 lost to follow-up) had converted to parkinsonism or dementia with a mean interval from RBD onset to the conversion of 14.2 years (range 5-29 years). Of the 26 patients in the report, 13 (50%) had developed PD, 3 DLB, 2 MSA, 2 Alzheimer's disease, and one unspecified dementia. The two cases of Alzheimer's dementia were classified as having comorbid limbic-predominant Lewy body disease following postmortem neuropathological examination. Notably, the only living patient yet to convert in the cohort had a 53-year history of iRBD and parasomnia overlap disorder [6].

Iranzo and colleagues followed a Spanish cohort of 44 patients with iRBD, first reporting the development of a parkinsonian disorder in 16 and MCI in 4 after 3.8 years from polysomnographic iRBD diagnosis [36]. In a subsequent report [7], of the 42 patients still part of the cohort, 82% had developed PD, DLB or MCI. Notably, 3 of the patients diagnosed with MCI in the initial report had developed DLB, 4 patients remained undiagnosed and 2 died with iRBD. All 4 of the patients who remained disease-free showed at least one biomarker of short-term Lewy body conversion. The median interval from RBD symptom onset to conversion was 12 years. Importantly, this Spanish cohort was expanded upon to include 130 patients diagnosed subsequently, and while they couldn't be followed up for an equivalent period, they were included in the estimated risk of conversion analysis to yield close to 33% at 5 years, 75% at 10 years, and 91% at 14 years from RBD onset [37].

A large, multi-center prospective study from 24 centers in the International RBD Study Group (IRBD-SG) was recently published, which included 1,280 patients (mean age 66.3, 82.5% male). The mean interval to conversion in this group was 4.6 years and the annual conversion rate was 8%. Phenoconversion risk was reported to be 31.3% after 5 years, 60.2% after 10 years, and 73.5% after 12 years. The ratio of parkinsonism to dementia was 5:4, and only 4.5% of those with parkinsonism had probable MSA [38].

Taking these data together, we can say that risks of conversion to clinical alpha-synucleinopathy exceed 80% at 14 years, that the majority of patients will develop PD or DLB in roughly equal proportions, a minority isolated cognitive impairment, and less than 5% will develop MSA. A recent meta-analysis of studies through 2017 reported that the conversion rate to any neurodegenerative disease (to include Alzheimer's Dementia) at 14 years was 96.6% [39]. Although conversion within a decade-plus is more common than not, there are individuals whose progression spans more than one or two decades. The Mayo Clinic reported on a group of 27 late converters showing a median time to conversion of 25 years [40]. The Barcelona group also reported on long-standing (10+ years) iRBD patients and found a high incidence of prodromal neurodegenerative features [41]. Individual genetic and environmental protective factors may explain the differences observed in the rate of disease progression.

Predicting Conversion and Subtype

A separate prognostic question is to which neurodegenerative disease a patient will convert among PD, DLB and MSA. The task of predicting between phenotypes at conversion can be challenging given the similarities and frequent intermediary phenotypes between PD and DLB associated with prodromal RBD.

A number of additional predictors of neurodegenerative disease were identified by Postuma and the IRBDSG in patients with RBD, including abnormal motor testing, abnormal olfaction, erectile dysfunction, MCI, constipation, and older age [38]. Only abnormal cognitive performance and color vision testing were predictive of DLB rather than PD. In contrast to prodromal PD and DLB where reduced olfaction and MCI are often present, preserved olfaction and cognition combined with early bladder dysfunction is strongly predictive of future progression to MSA [42].

Regarding vPSG findings, Postuma found that a higher degree of loss of atonia (as measured by tonic chin activity) was associated with conversion to PD rather than dementia in a small study [43]. A recent study by the Mayo group, found a higher amount of tonic chin elevation associated with MSA compared to other phenotypes, however, it is unknown whether this feature is present before phenoconversion [44].

EPIDEMIOLOGY

As RBD is more common in older adults, most prevalence studies have been conducted in this population group. The data is more limited to younger adults and children.

Adult General Population

The best evidence places the prevalence of definite RBD in the adult population at approximately 1%, though estimates have ranged widely. Early estimates were based on survey findings of violent behavior and injury occurring during sleep and ranged from 0.5 to 0.8 percent [45, 46]. Since only a fraction of patients with RBD experience violent or injurious behaviors, these are likely to be underestimated. Studies utilizing RBD screening questionnaires are designed for high sensitivity and cast a wider net as they are meant to diagnose probable RBD. Validated questionnaires include the Innsbruck RBD-Inventory (RBD-I), the RBD Screening Questionnaire (RBDSQ), and the Mayo Screening Questionnaire (MSQ), which were applied to large elderly populations in two studies, finding probable RBD in 4.6% to 7.7% [47, 48]. However, two large multi-stage investigations wherein patients who screened positive on the questionnaire were subjected to vPSG have reported a predictive value of no greater than 0.25 [49, 50]. Two large population-based studies utilizing vPSG on all patients to determine the incidence of RBD have been published [51], including the HypnoLaus Sleep Cohort study, performed in Lausanne, Switzerland, which reported an estimated prevalence of 1.06% [52].

Adult Clinic Population

While the prevalence in the general population may be approximately 1%, it is certainly higher among patients referred to sleep clinics. In 2010, Frauscher published a report on a series of 703 consecutive referrals to the Sleep Disorders Unit at Innsbruck Medical University that was studied to determine the prevalence of RBD in a sleep laboratory population. Thirty-four of the patients (4.8%, 27 men and 7 women) were diagnosed with vPSG-confirmed RBD, including 32% of those with Parkinsonian syndromes. Notably, only 6 of these 34 were referred for dream enactment [53].

α-Synucleinopathies

In PD, the prevalence of RBD ranges from about 20% to as high as 70%, depending on the methods used and disease stage. A 2017 meta-analysis of 8 case-control studies on patients with PD found a prevalence of 23.6% in PD *vs.* 3.4% in controls [54]. The studies reviewed, however, tended to employ RBD screening questionnaires which can underestimate the prevalence in the PD population due to lack of awareness and lead to overestimates in the control population due to the presence of mimics. Adler and colleagues reported RBD prevalence as high as 69% in PD, regardless of RBD preceding PD diagnosis or emerging later in the course of the disease [55].

In DLB, the prevalence of RBD is generally higher. In a clinical population in which almost all had reported dream-enactment, the prevalence of vPSG-confirmed RBD was 83% [56]. This estimation is consistent with findings from a large longitudinal study conducted at Mayo in which 76% of autopsy-confirmed DLB patients had RBD, and 84% had evidence of RSWA on vPSG [57].

RBD is present in almost all patients with MSA. A multicenter cross-sectional study found that over 80% of patients with MSA reported symptoms of RBD, and 81% had vPSG-confirmed RBD. A meta-analysis performed by the same authors found RBD symptoms in 73% of patients with MSA, and a pooled sample of 217 subjects found a vPSG-confirmed prevalence of 88% [58].

Psychiatric Population: PTSD and Antidepressants

While RBD occurring in the setting of antidepressant use has often been assumed to be iatrogenic, cases where RBD persisted long after discontinuation was recognized as early as 1992 [59] and have been described since [19, 60].

RBD associated with psychiatric disease has been proposed as a distinct phenotype, one younger and more predominantly female compared to the male predominant idiopathic RBD. Studies on this population have been small, and the rate of antidepressant use among the patients is so high that it is difficult to determine whether mood or psychotic disorders can cause RBD independently of psychotropic use [15, 61]. A study from Mayo suggests, however that antidepressant use rather than depression mediates RSWA [62].

The existence of DEB in patients with PTSD has been well-documented [63, 64], and a novel category of parasomnia termed "trauma-associated sleep disorder" (TSD) was proposed to describe the combination of trauma-associated nightmares autonomic hyperarousal, and DEB [65]. A recent study estimated the prevalence of DEB and vPSG-confirmed RBD in 394 veteran sleep clinic patients (mean age 54) to be 9% in the entire sample, in addition to 7% for isolated RSWA [17]. Of note, the group included 19% of patients with PTSD, 9% with TBI, and 10% with both PTSD and TBI. Interestingly, those with PTSD had a high (15%) prevalence of RBD, while the combination of PTSD and TBI was associated with the highest (21%) prevalence of RBD.

Narcolepsy

The nature of RBD in narcolepsy is different than that of iRBD, with episodes occurring less frequently and with less violent behaviors [66]. Estimates for the occurrence of RBD in narcolepsy vary widely due to disparate criteria and methodologies. An initial report by Schenck in 1992 found that 7% of 142 patients met the criteria for RBD [67], but subsequent studies have reported RBD symptoms in up to 63% [68 - 72]. The largest PSG study of patients with type 1 narcolepsy reported that in a subset of 295 patients, RBD incidence was 46% in males and 54% in females [72]. RBD also occurs in type 2 narcolepsy but less frequently [69, 71]. Generally, there is more global sleep motor dysregulation in patients with narcolepsy, broadly affecting NREM stages as well [66]. RSWA in children with narcolepsy is so specific to that condition that it has been proposed a diagnostic biomarker with a 96% specificity and 53% sensitivity above a mentalis RSWA index of 8% [73].

Gender Differences

Case series have consistently reported a male predominance with a ratio of about 3:1 [2, 6]. On the one hand, this may reflect differential susceptibility to the neurodegenerative process, as a male predominance, albeit less pronounced, has also been observed in Parkinson's disease [74]. On the other hand, the largest population vPSG study on RBD did not find a disparity [52], though due to the low base-rate of RBD, this large study may not have been powered to detect a gender disparity. Gender prevalence approaches equality in younger RBD populations, where a higher incidence of narcolepsy, trauma-related disorders, and antidepressant use is found [75, 76].

It has been speculated that the gender disparity in older populations is illusory, perhaps due to a referral bias owing to more violent DEB in men [77]. It is possible that men with RBD have more dream-related movements and are more likely to fall out of bed [78]. Although a recent study found that women with RBD had higher phasic activity during REM sleep [79], most studies support the notion that men with RBD have a more pronounced loss of atonia. A recent vPSG study of RBD patients found that males with RBD have a higher degree of phasic muscular activity with a higher burden of myoclonic jerks and truncal motor events [80], consistent with prior findings of a higher loss of atonia, particularly in the lower limbs [81] in iRBD, and RBD associated with PD [82].

MANAGEMENT

The management of RBD is complex. This complexity is due to the nature of RBD itself—since the severity and occurrence of DEB are unpredictable—but also due to the limited number of drug options, and in the case of adult-onset idiopathic RBD, the future risk of neurodegeneration. For all these reasons, a good understanding of the disorder and its implications and an up-to-date knowledge of the ever-growing literature is necessary for appropriate counselling and treating patients.

Safety Measures

The immediate concern with a new diagnosis of RBD is a risk of injury to the patient and bed partner. While leaving the bed and sustaining injuries may not frequently occur for a given patient with RBD, the majority of patients and over 20% of bed partners sustain injuries [4, 19]. The burden on the bed partner can be important and may often be underrecognized. Bed partners suffer, if not from directly injurious behaviors, from frequently disrupted sleep due to loud vocalizations and cursing during DEB. They may develop insomnia and frequently report anxiety and depression. The quality of marital relationships frequently suffers [4]. Safety measures are recommended as the highest level-A recommendation per AASM guidelines [83], which is higher than any pharmacotherapy. This should include a diligent evaluation of the patient's sleep environment and the implementation of strict measures to protect patients and their partners in case of injurious DEB. Those measures may include placing the mattress on the floor, dressing windows with heavy drapes, removing heavy objects and padding sharp corners, and of course, removing guns or weapons. While patients occasionally improvise protective measures for themselves and their bed partners, restraints might be dangerous given the unpredictability of behaviors. The bed partner may be advised to sleep in separate quarters until the behaviors are controlled.

Pharmacotherapy

A number of drugs have been tried to reduce symptoms in RBD, but the two most widely used drugs remain melatonin and clonazepam. The quality of the evidence for these two drugs, as for most drugs used in RBD, is low.

Melatonin

The evidence on the efficacy of melatonin stems mostly from open label studies, case series, and anecdotal reports. The utility of melatonin in RBD was first reported in a 1997 case report [84], followed by an open-label pilot study by the same group on six patients reporting a dramatic benefit [85]. A subsequent small cross-over placebo-controlled RCT in 8 patients showed improvements in CGI and RSWA compared to placebo. Notably, this RSWA effect seemed to persist in the patients who crossed over from treatment to placebo [86]. Kunz has proposed that this durability in efficacy is due to a persistent circadian benefit and, for this reason, recommended consistently timed dosing [87]. In the last two decades, multiple open-label prospective and retrospective studies have supported the efficacy of melatonin in RBD at doses in the range of 3-12 mg [88 - 91]. Given the ease of prescription and the rare side effects, melatonin is usually considered or recommended as first-line treatment. Melatonin may also be preferable in cases in which comorbid OSA is untreated or undertreated due to a lower potential to exacerbate obstructive sleep apnea [92]. However, the true efficacy of melatonin has been challenged by two recent RCTs, testing various doses of prolonged-release melatonin in iRBD and RBD associated with PD, which both failed to show superiority against placebo. In conclusion, although melatonin appears to be a promising and safe drug treatment for RBD, which may possibly have neuroprotective effects [87], future studies need to determine its true efficacy against placebo [93, 94]. The appropriate dose and formulation (instant versus prolonged release) continue to be a matter of debate. Notably, it has not been shown that a higher dose is more effective than a low dose.

Clonazepam

Clonazepam was reported to be effective in 4 of 4 patients in the first case series [1]. It has since become the most widely prescribed drug in RBD and is often considered to be the most effective first-line drug. Several large case series have shown at least partial response in more than 80% of patients and complete response in at least half of them with doses ranging 0.125–2 mg and above [2, 95 - 98]. Unlike melatonin, the efficacy of clonazepam is dose-dependent, with higher doses observed to be more effective than lower doses. Although usually effective, tolerability varies. Common side effects include early morning sedation, cognitive slowing, and impaired balance. Although no falls were reported in a large case series that included a majority of patients with PD and MSA [2], these side effects warrant cautious use in the elderly and in those with manifest neurodegenerative disease.

The mechanism of clonazepam in improving RBD is not fully understood but could be related to an improvement in the patients' dreaming experience, more specifically, a reduction of more violent vivid dreams and nightmares. Although Lapierre and Montplaisir reported a reduction in phasic EMG activity with clonazepam in a small study in five RBD patients [99], this was not observed in a larger, more recent study [100].

Although clonazepam is generally considered to be the most effective available drug, its efficacy was recently challenged when a first double-blind RCT comparing 0.5mg clonazepam dose against placebo in patients with PD failed to show more than a trend toward improvement in CGI-I score [101]. As expected, the treatment group reported a higher incidence of daytime sleepiness, dizziness, and postural instability. Though this study was negative, there are a few caveats. The patients enrolled had no vPSG confirmation of RBD, which raises the possibility that some RBD mimics could have been enrolled in the study. Importantly, clonazepam was used at a low dose, lower than what is generally observed to be effective in clinical practice, and many of the patients enrolled were using dopaminergic drugs, which may partially treat RBD [93].

Transdermal Rivastigmine

The agent with the best quality evidence for treatment-resistant RBD is the cholinergic agent rivastigmine, an acetylcholinesterase inhibitor (AChEi). Two small crossover RCTs, one in 12 patients with PD, the other in 25 patients with MCI, have evaluated the 4.6mg rivastigmine patch for the treatment of vPSG-confirmed RBD in patients who had failed melatonin and clonazepam [102, 103].

The two studies demonstrated a consistent large effect size of 50% reduction in DEB frequency vs 8-15% under placebo. Although rivastigmine is not known to commonly cause sedation, 40% of patients with RBD and MCI reported such a side effect [103]. Larger studies are needed to replicate these findings as rivastigmine would constitute an interesting alternative in the treatment of iRBD and RBD associated with PD or DLB, since cholinergic deficit has been described in these patients [104, 105]. Although transdermal rivastigmine appears to be effective in some individuals with RBD, the efficacy of AChEi as a class is inconsistent. Specifically, donepezil does not show the same consistent results [106, 107], and oral rivastigmine may even induce RBD in some patients with Alzheimer's Disease [108, 109].

Pramipexole

Many other agents have been trialled in case reports, case series, and open-label studies. The most studied is pramipexole. In the largest retrospective study testing pramipexole, in which 81 patients with iRBD were titrated, as tolerated, up to 1.5 mg, 62% of patients reported at least 50% symptom reduction [110]. However, in this study, the patients were not randomized to pramipexole but chose the drug after discussing with their physician the risks and benefits of pramipexole and clonazepam, the alternative treatment offered. The authors attempted to find traits that may predict pramipexole response and found a higher RSWA-index to be predictive. Taken together, the quality of the data on pramipexole for iRBD and secondary RBD is low and does not strongly support its use unless other therapies have been tried and failed [111].

Sodium Oxybate

Sodium oxybate deserves mention despite its limited evidence due to the stark results reported in 7 previously refractory adult cases of iRBD or RBD associated with PD [112 - 114]. The drug, taken in one single dose or two nightly doses ranging 3–9g provided, in most patients, rapid, complete and sustained benefit without significant side effects. The mechanism of action of sodium oxybate in RBD is unclear but could involve REM suppression and regulation of sleep/wake motor control. Although sodium oxybate is generally used in narcolepsy to reduce symptoms of sleepiness and cataplexy, it has shown to also reduce sleepiness in patients with PD [115]. Sodium oxybate reduces symptoms of RBD, which are often present in narcolepsy, and this effect could be mediated by a normalization of REM-related atonia [116]. A recent open-label investigation in children and adolescents (mean age 12.5) with narcolepsy showed statistically significant improvement in RBD episodes and the REM atonia index [117]. Most common side effects included transient nausea during the first weeks of titration, confusional episodes with subsequent amnesia (NREM parasomnias), enuresis, and anxiety. The potential to reduce other symptoms commonly associated with RBD, such as insomnia and daytime sleepiness, could make sodium oxybate a particularly helpful pharmacological intervention for RBD, however, considerations such as high sodium load in the older preparation and limited availability limit its use. In most countries, sodium oxybate is not available outside the strict indication of narcolepsy. Sodium oxybate is currently being compared against a placebo in a double-blind randomized clinical trial for treatment-resistant RBD (NCT04006925).

Other Agents

All other agents for the treatment of RBD are not supported by sufficient evidence or have shown no benefit. These include memantine [118], levodopa, donepezil, temazepam, ramelteon, carbamazepine, ropinirole, gabapentin, pregabalin, zopiclone, and Yi-Gan San [119].

Prognosis and Counselling

A large proportion of adult patients with a diagnosis of RBD present other subtle signs or symptoms of prodromal synucleinopathy—anosmia, constipation, orthostasis, cognitive impairment, and depression—as all of these symptoms are commonly seen in the preclinical phase of PD and DLB [41]. When indicated, a careful neurological examination may reveal impairment in executive and visuospatial functions and motor symptoms of hypomimia, bradykinesia with finger or foot tapping, reduced arm swing during casual gait, and a kinetic (finger-to-nose) more often than resting tremor [12]. Referral to a neurologist may be considered if any of these deficits are detected.

Whether patients should be counselled on prognosis remains an open debate since conversion to neurodegenerative disease for a specific individual may neither be imminent nor certain [120]. However, a recent study showed that today, the wide majority of practitioners (93%) do counsel their patients on this eventuality [121]. Although disclosing the long-term risk of neurodegeneration associated with RBD can generate anxiety and pose an ethical issue since no neuroprotection or disease-modifying drugs are yet available [122], other factors merit consideration. First, an increasing proportion of patients can now access an abundant source of information about RBD on the internet, and as a result, learn about the association with synucleinopathy before they even discuss this with their doctor. Second, it is conceivable that, as drugs are being developed, a number of patients diagnosed with iRBD today may soon become eligible to participate in neuroprotection trials against synucleinopathies (NCT03623672). In sum, rather than a rigid approach to counselling and disclosing the available data about disease progression, we advocate for an individualized, center-based approach that takes into account factors such as individual resilience, support systems, goals, combined with medical aspects, including the perceived stages of progression toward a neurodegenerative disorder.

With regards to RBD in patients taking antidepressants, the risk of synucleinopathy is less clear. Postuma conducted a prospective cohort study in 100 patients with RBD, including 27 antidepressant users (similarly aged, no specific temporal relationship to RBD), compared with 45 age and sex-matched controls followed annually up to 8 years. Patients with RBD taking antidepressants converted to synucleinopathy at a lower rate (5-year risk: 22% vs. 59%), but they had a similar incidence of prodromal markers, including constipation, MCI, and deficits in olfaction, color vision, and motor testing. The authors concluded that antidepressants could unmask a latent neurodegenerative process rather than independently cause RBD in these patients [14]. A caveat regarding this study finding is that the population of patients with RBD taking antidepressants were older than the psychiatric populations reported earlier. We might conclude that antidepressant use is somewhat reassuring that conversion is less imminent. More research is needed on younger patients, especially those with trauma, to determine whether they are at risk for synucleinopathy. In all cases, reduction, and ideally discontinuation and replacement of exacerbating medications (including antidepressants) should be considered, as feasible. Bupropion might be substituted for serotonergic medications where an antidepressant is needed [60].

Follow-up should occur at least semi-annually to assess for RBD symptom control and insidious or overt signs of disease progression. Specifically, patients and bedpartners should be encouraged to keep a journal of their symptoms. Control of comorbid sleep disorders, particularly OSA [26] and PLMD [25], is important in reducing the frequency of disruptive behaviors.

CONCLUSION

Since its first polysomnographic description in humans more than three decades ago, RBD has been a matter of intense research and important discoveries. Most child and adolescent cases are associated with narcolepsy and mild severity. With the possible exception of RBD associated with PTSD or TBI, adult-onset RBD is, until proven otherwise, a prodrome of neurodegenerative disease, namely PD or DLB. Although behaviors during dreams can be complex and vigorous, many patients with RBD are not aware of their episodes, and most will consult with a physician only after they or their bed partners are injured. Observer reports are therefore paramount for the diagnosis and monitoring of RBD symptoms. When

RBD is clinically suspected, vPSG is necessary not only to confirm the loss of REM sleep atonia but to rule out common mimics such as OSA-related hypermotor arousals and severe PLMs. While considering a reduction of alcohol use and any offending drug such as serotonergic antidepressants, the first and most effective intervention for patients and their bed partners is to implement some strict safety measures. Although melatonin and clonazepam are still the most widely used treatments to reduce RBD symptoms, other pharmacological agents, including transdermal rivastigmine and dopamine agonists, may be effective and available in clinical practice. The timing and modality of the discussion of prognosis in adult patients with high suspicion of prodromal RBD, should be decided on a case-by-case rather than one-size-fits-all basis and may require the involvement of a neurologist familiar with this particular condition.

Although much insight has been gained about the pathophysiology and implications of RBD, more research is needed for impactful changes in the care of our patients. A few unmet needs include the study of protective mechanisms against the progression of neurodegenerative disease, more effective symptomatic treatments and disease-modifying therapies. Additionally, while the current standard diagnostic procedure is the in-lab vPSG, automated methods, including ambulatory procedures for diagnosing RBD in the clinic and the general population, are being developed. This approach could result in a larger recognition of this serious condition and allow many more patients to be diagnosed and receive counselling and treatment earlier in their disease course.

CONSENT FOR PUBLICATION

Not applicable.

CONFLICT OF INTEREST

The author declares no conflict of interest, financial or otherwise.

ACKNOWLEDGEMENTS

Declared none.

REFERENCES

[1]   Schenck CH, Bundlie SR, Ettinger MG, Mahowald MW. Chronic behavioral disorders of human REM sleep: a new category of parasomnia. Sleep 1986; 9(2): 293-308.
        [http://dx.doi.org/10.1093/sleep/9.2.293] [PMID: 3505730]

[2]   Olson EJ, Boeve BF, Silber MH. Rapid eye movement sleep behaviour disorder: demographic, clinical and laboratory findings in 93 cases. Brain 2000; 123(Pt 2): 331-9.
        [http://dx.doi.org/10.1093/brain/123.2.331] [PMID: 10648440]

[3]   Schenck CH, Mahowald MW. REM sleep behavior disorder: clinical, developmental, and

neuroscience perspectives 16 years after its formal identification in SLEEP. Sleep 2002; 25(2): 120-38.
[http://dx.doi.org/10.1093/sleep/25.2.120] [PMID: 11902423]

[4]   Lam SP, Wong CC, Li SX, *et al.* Caring burden of REM sleep behavior disorder - spouses' health and marital relationship. Sleep Med 2016; 24: 40-3.
[http://dx.doi.org/10.1016/j.sleep.2016.08.004] [PMID: 27810184]

[5]   Schenck CH, Bundlie SR, Mahowald MW. Delayed emergence of a parkinsonian disorder in 38% of 29 older men initially diagnosed with idiopathic rapid eye movement sleep behaviour disorder. Neurology 1996; 46(2): 388-93.
[http://dx.doi.org/10.1212/WNL.46.2.388] [PMID: 8614500]

[6]   Schenck CH, Boeve BF, Mahowald MW. Delayed emergence of a parkinsonian disorder or dementia in 81% of older men initially diagnosed with idiopathic rapid eye movement sleep behavior disorder: a 16-year update on a previously reported series. Sleep Med 2013; 14(8): 744-8.
[http://dx.doi.org/10.1016/j.sleep.2012.10.009] [PMID: 23347909]

[7]   Iranzo A, Tolosa E, Gelpi E, *et al.* Neurodegenerative disease status and post-mortem pathology in idiopathic rapid-eye-movement sleep behaviour disorder: an observational cohort study. Lancet Neurol 2013; 12(5): 443-53.
[http://dx.doi.org/10.1016/S1474-4422(13)70056-5] [PMID: 23562390]

[8]   Boeve BF, Silber MH, Ferman TJ, *et al.* Clinicopathologic correlations in 172 cases of rapid eye movement sleep behavior disorder with or without a coexisting neurologic disorder. Sleep Med 2013; 14(8): 754-62.
[http://dx.doi.org/10.1016/j.sleep.2012.10.015] [PMID: 23474058]

[9]   Dauvilliers Y, Schenck CH, Postuma RB, *et al.* REM sleep behaviour disorder. Nat Rev Dis Primers 2018; 4(1): 19.
[http://dx.doi.org/10.1038/s41572-018-0016-5] [PMID: 30166532]

[10] Antelmi E, Pizza F, Franceschini C, Ferri R, Plazzi G. REM sleep behavior disorder in narcolepsy: A secondary form or an intrinsic feature? Sleep Med Rev 2020; 50: 101254.
[http://dx.doi.org/10.1016/j.smrv.2019.101254] [PMID: 31931470]

[11] Sabater L, Gaig C, Gelpi E, *et al.* A novel non-rapid-eye movement and rapid-eye-movement parasomnia with sleep breathing disorder associated with antibodies to IgLON5: a case series, characterisation of the antigen, and post-mortem study. Lancet Neurol 2014; 13(6): 575-86.
[http://dx.doi.org/10.1016/S1474-4422(14)70051-1] [PMID: 24703753]

[12] Högl B, Iranzo A. Rapid Eye Movement Sleep Behavior Disorder and Other Rapid Eye Movement Sleep Parasomnias. Continuum (Minneap Minn) 2017 Aug;23(4, Sleep Neurology): 2017; 1017-34.

[13] Winkelman JW, James L. Serotonergic antidepressants are associated with REM sleep without atonia. Sleep 2004; 27(2): 317-21.
[http://dx.doi.org/10.1093/sleep/27.2.317] [PMID: 15124729]

[14] Postuma RB, Gagnon JF, Tuineaig M, *et al.* Antidepressants and REM sleep behavior disorder: isolated side effect or neurodegenerative signal? Sleep 2013; 36(11): 1579-85.
[http://dx.doi.org/10.5665/sleep.3102] [PMID: 24179289]

[15] Lam SP, Li SX, Chan JW, *et al.* Does rapid eye movement sleep behavior disorder exist in psychiatric populations? A clinical and polysomnographic case-control study. Sleep Med 2013; 14(8): 788-94.
[http://dx.doi.org/10.1016/j.sleep.2012.05.016] [PMID: 22841026]

[16] Mysliwiec V, O'Reilly B, Polchinski J, Kwon HP, Germain A, Roth BJ. Trauma associated sleep disorder: a proposed parasomnia encompassing disruptive nocturnal behaviors, nightmares, and REM without atonia in trauma survivors. J Clin Sleep Med 2014; 10(10): 1143-8.
[http://dx.doi.org/10.5664/jcsm.4120] [PMID: 25317096]

[17] Elliott JE, Opel RA, Pleshakov D, *et al.* Posttraumatic stress disorder increases the odds of REM sleep

behavior disorder and other parasomnias in Veterans with and without comorbid traumatic brain injury. Sleep 2020; 43(3): zsz237.
[http://dx.doi.org/10.1093/sleep/zsz237] [PMID: 31587047]

[18]   The International Classification of Sleep Disorders: Diagnostic and Coding Manual (Revised and Extended). 3rd ed., American Academy of Sleep Medicine 2014.

[19]   Fernández-Arcos A, Iranzo A, Serradell M, Gaig C, Santamaria J. The Clinical Phenotype of Idiopathic Rapid Eye Movement Sleep Behavior Disorder at Presentation: A Study in 203 Consecutive Patients. Sleep 2016; 39(1): 121-32.
[http://dx.doi.org/10.5665/sleep.5332] [PMID: 26940460]

[20]   Sixel-Döring F, Schweitzer M, Mollenhauer B, Trenkwalder C. Intraindividual variability of REM sleep behavior disorder in Parkinson's disease: a comparative assessment using a new REM sleep behavior disorder severity scale (RBDSS) for clinical routine. J Clin Sleep Med 2011; 7(1): 75-80.
[http://dx.doi.org/10.5664/jcsm.28044] [PMID: 21344049]

[21]   Bugalho P, Lampreia T, Miguel R, Mendonça M, Caetano A, Barbosa R. Characterization of motor events in REM sleep behavior disorder. J Neural Transm (Vienna) 2017; 124(10): 1183-6.
[http://dx.doi.org/10.1007/s00702-017-1759-y] [PMID: 28721577]

[22]   Frauscher B, Gschliesser V, Brandauer E, et al. Video analysis of motor events in REM sleep behavior disorder. Mov Disord 2007; 22(10): 1464-70.
[http://dx.doi.org/10.1002/mds.21561] [PMID: 17516467]

[23]   Iranzo A. The REM sleep circuit and how its impairment leads to REM sleep behavior disorder. Cell Tissue Res 2018; 373(1): 245-66.
[http://dx.doi.org/10.1007/s00441-018-2852-8] [PMID: 29846796]

[24]   Manni R, Terzaghi M, Glorioso M. Motor-behavioral episodes in REM sleep behavior disorder and phasic events during REM sleep. Sleep 2009; 32(2): 241-5.
[http://dx.doi.org/10.1093/sleep/32.2.241] [PMID: 19238811]

[25]   Gaig C, Iranzo A, Pujol M, Perez H, Santamaria J. Periodic Limb Movements During Sleep Mimicking REM Sleep Behavior Disorder: A New Form of Periodic Limb Movement Disorder. Sleep 2017; 40: 3.
[http://dx.doi.org/10.1093/sleep/zsw063] [PMID: 28364416]

[26]   Iranzo A, Santamaría J. Severe obstructive sleep apnea/hypopnea mimicking REM sleep behavior disorder. Sleep 2005; 28(2): 203-6.
[http://dx.doi.org/10.1093/sleep/28.2.203] [PMID: 16171244]

[27]   Feemster JC, Jung Y, Timm PC, et al. Normative and isolated rapid eye movement sleep without atonia in adults without REM sleep behavior disorder. Sleep 2019; 42(10): zsz124.
[http://dx.doi.org/10.1093/sleep/zsz124] [PMID: 31587043]

[28]   Stefani A, Gabelia D, Högl B, et al. Long-Term Follow-up Investigation of Isolated Rapid Eye Movement Sleep Without Atonia Without Rapid Eye Movement Sleep Behavior Disorder: A Pilot Study. J Clin Sleep Med 2015; 11(11): 1273-9.
[http://dx.doi.org/10.5664/jcsm.5184] [PMID: 26156949]

[29]   Frauscher B, Iranzo A, Gaig C, et al. Normative EMG values during REM sleep for the diagnosis of REM sleep behavior disorder. Sleep 2012; 35(6): 835-47.
[http://dx.doi.org/10.5665/sleep.1886] [PMID: 22654203]

[30]   Frauscher B, Iranzo A, Högl B, et al. Quantification of electromyographic activity during REM sleep in multiple muscles in REM sleep behavior disorder. Sleep 2008; 31(5): 724-31.
[http://dx.doi.org/10.1093/sleep/31.5.724] [PMID: 18517042]

[31]   Bliwise DL, Fairley J, Hoff S, et al. Inter-rater agreement for visual discrimination of phasic and tonic electromyographic activity in sleep. Sleep 2018; 41: 7.
[http://dx.doi.org/10.1093/sleep/zsy080] [PMID: 29722892]

[32]   Ferri R, Gagnon JF, Postuma RB, Rundo F, Montplaisir JY. Comparison between an automatic and a visual scoring method of the chin muscle tone during rapid eye movement sleep. Sleep Med 2014; 15(6): 661-5.
[http://dx.doi.org/10.1016/j.sleep.2013.12.022] [PMID: 24831249]

[33]   Frandsen R, Nikolic M, Zoetmulder M, Kempfner L, Jennum P. Analysis of automated quantification of motor activity in REM sleep behaviour disorder. J Sleep Res 2015; 24(5): 583-90.
[http://dx.doi.org/10.1111/jsr.12304] [PMID: 25923472]

[34]   Frauscher B, Gabelia D, Biermayr M, *et al.* Validation of an integrated software for the detection of rapid eye movement sleep behavior disorder. Sleep 2014; 37(10): 1663-71.
[http://dx.doi.org/10.5665/sleep.4076] [PMID: 25197814]

[35]   Cesari M, Christensen JAE, Muntean ML, *et al.* A data-driven system to identify REM sleep behavior disorder and to predict its progression from the prodromal stage in Parkinson's disease. Sleep Med 2021; 77: 238-48.
[http://dx.doi.org/10.1016/j.sleep.2020.04.010] [PMID: 32798136]

[36]   Iranzo A, Molinuevo JL, Santamaría J, *et al.* Rapid-eye-movement sleep behaviour disorder as an early marker for a neurodegenerative disorder: a descriptive study. Lancet Neurol 2006; 5(7): 572-7.
[http://dx.doi.org/10.1016/S1474-4422(06)70476-8] [PMID: 16781987]

[37]   Iranzo A, Fernández-Arcos A, Tolosa E, *et al.* Neurodegenerative disorder risk in idiopathic REM sleep behavior disorder: study in 174 patients. PLoS One 2014; 9(2): e89741.
[http://dx.doi.org/10.1371/journal.pone.0089741] [PMID: 24587002]

[38]   Postuma RB, Iranzo A, Hu M, *et al.* Risk and predictors of dementia and parkinsonism in idiopathic REM sleep behaviour disorder: a multicentre study. Brain 2019; 142(3): 744-59.
[http://dx.doi.org/10.1093/brain/awz030] [PMID: 30789229]

[39]   Galbiati A, Verga L, Giora E, Zucconi M, Ferini-Strambi L. The risk of neurodegeneration in REM sleep behavior disorder: A systematic review and meta-analysis of longitudinal studies. Sleep Med Rev 2019; 43: 37-46.
[http://dx.doi.org/10.1016/j.smrv.2018.09.008] [PMID: 30503716]

[40]   Claassen DO, Josephs KA, Ahlskog JE, Silber MH, Tippmann-Peikert M, Boeve BF. REM sleep behavior disorder preceding other aspects of synucleinopathies by up to half a century. Neurology 2010; 75(6): 494-9.
[http://dx.doi.org/10.1212/WNL.0b013e3181ec7fac] [PMID: 20668263]

[41]   Iranzo A, Stefani A, Serradell M, *et al.* Characterization of patients with longstanding idiopathic REM sleep behavior disorder. Neurology 2017; 89(3): 242-8.
[http://dx.doi.org/10.1212/WNL.0000000000004121] [PMID: 28615430]

[42]   Kaufmann H, Norcliffe-Kaufmann L, Palma JA, *et al.* Natural history of pure autonomic failure: A United States prospective cohort. Ann Neurol 2017; 81(2): 287-97.
[http://dx.doi.org/10.1002/ana.24877] [PMID: 28093795]

[43]   Postuma RB, Gagnon JF, Rompré S, Montplaisir JY. Severity of REM atonia loss in idiopathic REM sleep behavior disorder predicts Parkinson disease. Neurology 2010; 74(3): 239-44.
[http://dx.doi.org/10.1212/WNL.0b013e3181ca0166] [PMID: 20083800]

[44]   McCarter SJ, Feemster JC, Tabatabai GM, *et al.* Submentalis Rapid Eye Movement Sleep Muscle Activity: A Potential Biomarker for Synucleinopathy. Ann Neurol 2019; 86(6): 969-74.
[http://dx.doi.org/10.1002/ana.25622] [PMID: 31621939]

[45]   Ohayon MM, Caulet M, Priest RG. Violent behavior during sleep. J Clin Psychiatry 1997; 58(8): 369-76.
[http://dx.doi.org/10.4088/JCP.v58n0808] [PMID: 9515980]

[46]   Chiu HF, Wing YK, Lam LC, *et al.* Sleep-related injury in the elderly--an epidemiological study in Hong Kong. Sleep 2000; 23(4): 513-7.

[http://dx.doi.org/10.1093/sleep/23.4.1e] [PMID: 10875558]

[47]   Boot BP, Boeve BF, Roberts RO, *et al.* Probable rapid eye movement sleep behavior disorder increases risk for mild cognitive impairment and Parkinson disease: a population-based study. Ann Neurol 2012; 71(1): 49-56.
[http://dx.doi.org/10.1002/ana.22655] [PMID: 22275251]

[48]   Mahlknecht P, Seppi K, Frauscher B, *et al.* Probable RBD and association with neurodegenerative disease markers: A population-based study. Mov Disord 2015; 30(10): 1417-21.
[http://dx.doi.org/10.1002/mds.26350] [PMID: 26208108]

[49]   Pujol M, Pujol J, Alonso T, *et al.* Idiopathic REM sleep behavior disorder in the elderly Spanish community: a primary care center study with a two-stage design using video-polysomnography. Sleep Med 2017; 40: 116-21.
[http://dx.doi.org/10.1016/j.sleep.2017.07.021] [PMID: 29042180]

[50]   Sasai-Sakuma T, Takeuchi N, Asai Y, Inoue Y, Inoue Y. Prevalence and clinical characteristics of REM sleep behavior disorder in Japanese elderly people. Sleep 2020; 12;43(8) zsaa024.
[http://dx.doi.org/10.1093/sleep/zsaa024]

[51]   Kang SH, Yoon IY, Lee SD, Han JW, Kim TH, Kim KW. REM sleep behavior disorder in the Korean elderly population: prevalence and clinical characteristics. Sleep 2013; 36(8): 1147-52.
[http://dx.doi.org/10.5665/sleep.2874] [PMID: 23904674]

[52]   Haba-Rubio J, Frauscher B, Marques-Vidal P, *et al.* Prevalence and determinants of rapid eye movement sleep behavior disorder in the general population. Sleep 2018; 41(2): zsx197.
[http://dx.doi.org/10.1093/sleep/zsx197] [PMID: 29216391]

[53]   Frauscher B, Gschliesser V, Brandauer E, *et al.* REM sleep behavior disorder in 703 sleep-disorder patients: the importance of eliciting a comprehensive sleep history. Sleep Med 2010; 11(2): 167-71.
[http://dx.doi.org/10.1016/j.sleep.2009.03.011] [PMID: 20022299]

[54]   Zhang J, Xu CY, Liu J. Meta-analysis on the prevalence of REM sleep behavior disorder symptoms in Parkinson's disease. BMC Neurol 2017; 17(1): 23.
[http://dx.doi.org/10.1186/s12883-017-0795-4] [PMID: 28160778]

[55]   Adler CH, Hentz JG, Shill HA, *et al.* Probable RBD is increased in Parkinson's disease but not in essential tremor or restless legs syndrome. Parkinsonism Relat Disord 2011; 17(6): 456-8.
[http://dx.doi.org/10.1016/j.parkreldis.2011.03.007] [PMID: 21482171]

[56]   Pao WC, Boeve BF, Ferman TJ, *et al.* Polysomnographic findings in dementia with Lewy bodies. Neurologist 2013; 19(1): 1-6.
[http://dx.doi.org/10.1097/NRL.0b013e31827c6bdd] [PMID: 23269098]

[57]   Ferman TJ, Boeve BF, Smith GE, *et al.* Inclusion of RBD improves the diagnostic classification of dementia with Lewy bodies. Neurology 2011; 77(9): 875-82.
[http://dx.doi.org/10.1212/WNL.0b013e31822c9148] [PMID: 21849645]

[58]   Palma JA, Fernandez-Cordon C, Coon EA, *et al.* Prevalence of REM sleep behavior disorder in multiple system atrophy: a multicenter study and meta-analysis. Clin Auton Res 2015; 25(1): 69-75.
[http://dx.doi.org/10.1007/s10286-015-0279-9] [PMID: 25739474]

[59]   Schenck CH, Mahowald MW, Kim SW, O'Connor KA, Hurwitz TD. Prominent eye movements during NREM sleep and REM sleep behavior disorder associated with fluoxetine treatment of depression and obsessive-compulsive disorder. Sleep 1992; 15(3): 226-35.
[http://dx.doi.org/10.1093/sleep/15.3.226] [PMID: 1621023]

[60]   Lam SP, Zhang J, Tsoh J, *et al.* REM sleep behavior disorder in psychiatric populations. J Clin Psychiatry 2010; 71(8): 1101-3.
[http://dx.doi.org/10.4088/JCP.l05877gry] [PMID: 20797385]

[61]   Teman PT, Tippmann-Peikert M, Silber MH, Slocumb NL, Auger RR. Idiopathic rapid-eye-movement sleep disorder: associations with antidepressants, psychiatric diagnoses, and other factors, in relation to

age of onset. Sleep Med 2009; 10(1): 60-5.
[http://dx.doi.org/10.1016/j.sleep.2007.11.019] [PMID: 18226952]

[62]   McCarter SJ, St Louis EK, Sandness DJ, *et al.* Antidepressants Increase REM Sleep Muscle Tone in Patients with and without REM Sleep Behavior Disorder. Sleep 2015; 38(6): 907-17.
[PMID: 25325487]

[63]   Ross RJ, Ball WA, Dinges DF, *et al.* Motor dysfunction during sleep in posttraumatic stress disorder. Sleep 1994; 17(8): 723-32.
[http://dx.doi.org/10.1093/sleep/17.8.723] [PMID: 7701184]

[64]   Husain AM, Miller PP, Carwile ST. Rem sleep behavior disorder: potential relationship to post-traumatic stress disorder. J Clin Neurophysiol 2001; 18(2): 148-57.
[http://dx.doi.org/10.1097/00004691-200103000-00005] [PMID: 11435805]

[65]   Mysliwiec V, Brock MS, Creamer JL, O'Reilly BM, Germain A, Roth BJ. Trauma associated sleep disorder: A parasomnia induced by trauma. Sleep Med Rev 2018; 37: 94-104.
[http://dx.doi.org/10.1016/j.smrv.2017.01.004] [PMID: 28363448]

[66]   Antelmi E, Pizza F, Donadio V, *et al.* Biomarkers for REM sleep behavior disorder in idiopathic and narcoleptic patients. Ann Clin Transl Neurol 2019; 6(9): 1872-6.
[http://dx.doi.org/10.1002/acn3.50833] [PMID: 31386270]

[67]   Schenck CH, Mahowald MW. Motor dyscontrol in narcolepsy: rapid-eye-movement (REM) sleep without atonia and REM sleep behavior disorder. Ann Neurol 1992; 32(1): 3-10.
[http://dx.doi.org/10.1002/ana.410320103] [PMID: 1642469]

[68]   Mayer G, Meier-Ewert K. Motor dyscontrol in sleep of narcoleptic patients (a lifelong development?). J Sleep Res 1993; 2(3): 143-8.
[http://dx.doi.org/10.1111/j.1365-2869.1993.tb00078.x] [PMID: 10607086]

[69]   Nightingale S, Orgill JC, Ebrahim IO, de Lacy SF, Agrawal S, Williams AJ. The association between narcolepsy and REM behavior disorder (RBD). Sleep Med 2005; 6(3): 253-8.
[http://dx.doi.org/10.1016/j.sleep.2004.11.007] [PMID: 15854856]

[70]   Dauvilliers Y, Rompré S, Gagnon JF, Vendette M, Petit D, Montplaisir J. REM sleep characteristics in narcolepsy and REM sleep behavior disorder. Sleep 2007; 30(7): 844-9.
[http://dx.doi.org/10.1093/sleep/30.7.844] [PMID: 17682654]

[71]   Knudsen S, Gammeltoft S, Jennum PJ. Rapid eye movement sleep behaviour disorder in patients with narcolepsy is associated with hypocretin-1 deficiency. Brain 2010; 133(Pt 2): 568-79.
[http://dx.doi.org/10.1093/brain/awp320] [PMID: 20129934]

[72]   Luca G, Haba-Rubio J, Dauvilliers Y, *et al.* Clinical, polysomnographic and genome-wide association analyses of narcolepsy with cataplexy: a European Narcolepsy Network study. J Sleep Res 2013; 22(5): 482-95.
[http://dx.doi.org/10.1111/jsr.12044] [PMID: 23496005]

[73]   Bin-Hasan S, Videnovic A, Maski K. Nocturnal REM Sleep Without Atonia Is a Diagnostic Biomarker of Pediatric Narcolepsy. J Clin Sleep Med 2018; 14(2): 245-52.
[http://dx.doi.org/10.5664/jcsm.6944] [PMID: 29351827]

[74]   Haaxma CA, Bloem BR, Borm GF, *et al.* Gender differences in Parkinson's disease. J Neurol Neurosurg Psychiatry 2007; 78(8): 819-24.
[http://dx.doi.org/10.1136/jnnp.2006.103788] [PMID: 17098842]

[75]   Bonakis A, Howard RS, Ebrahim IO, Merritt S, Williams A. REM sleep behaviour disorder (RBD) and its associations in young patients. Sleep Med 2009; 10(6): 641-5.
[http://dx.doi.org/10.1016/j.sleep.2008.07.008] [PMID: 19109063]

[76]   Ju YE, Larson-Prior L, Duntley S. Changing demographics in REM sleep behavior disorder: possible effect of autoimmunity and antidepressants. Sleep Med 2011; 12(3): 278-83.
[http://dx.doi.org/10.1016/j.sleep.2010.07.022] [PMID: 21317035]

[77]   Bodkin CL, Schenck CH. Rapid eye movement sleep behavior disorder in women: relevance to general and specialty medical practice. J Womens Health (Larchmt) 2009; 18(12): 1955-63.
[http://dx.doi.org/10.1089/jwh.2008.1348] [PMID: 20044857]

[78]   Zhou J, Zhang J, Li Y, *et al.* Gender differences in REM sleep behavior disorder: a clinical and polysomnographic study in China. Sleep Med 2015; 16(3): 414-8.
[http://dx.doi.org/10.1016/j.sleep.2014.10.020] [PMID: 25660814]

[79]   Takeuchi N, Sasai-Sakuma T, Inoue Y. Gender differences in clinical findings and α-synucleiopath--related markers in patients with idiopathic REM sleep behavior disorder. Sleep Med 2020; 66: 216-9.
[http://dx.doi.org/10.1016/j.sleep.2019.11.1261] [PMID: 31978865]

[80]   Bugalho P, Salavisa M. Factors Influencing the Presentation of REM Sleep Behavior Disorder: The Relative Importance of Sex, Associated Neurological Disorder, and Context of Referral to Polysomnography. J Clin Sleep Med 2019; 15(12): 1789-98.
[http://dx.doi.org/10.5664/jcsm.8086] [PMID: 31855164]

[81]   McCarter SJ, St Louis EK, Boeve BF, Sandness DJ, Silber MH. Greatest rapid eye movement sleep atonia loss in men and older age. Ann Clin Transl Neurol 2014; 1(9): 733-8.
[http://dx.doi.org/10.1002/acn3.93] [PMID: 25493286]

[82]   Bliwise DL, Trotti LM, Greer SA, Juncos JJ, Rye DB. Phasic muscle activity in sleep and clinical features of Parkinson disease. Ann Neurol 2010; 68(3): 353-9.
[http://dx.doi.org/10.1002/ana.22076] [PMID: 20626046]

[83]   Aurora RN, Zak RS, Maganti RK, *et al.* Best practice guide for the treatment of REM sleep behavior disorder (RBD). J Clin Sleep Med 2010; 6(1): 85-95.
[http://dx.doi.org/10.5664/jcsm.27717] [PMID: 20191945]

[84]   Kunz D, Bes F. Melatonin effects in a patient with severe REM sleep behavior disorder: case report and theoretical considerations. Neuropsychobiology 1997; 36(4): 211-4.
[http://dx.doi.org/10.1159/000119383] [PMID: 9396020]

[85]   Kunz D, Bes F. Melatonin as a therapy in REM sleep behavior disorder patients: an open-labeled pilot study on the possible influence of melatonin on REM-sleep regulation. Mov Disord 1999; 14(3): 507-11.
[http://dx.doi.org/10.1002/1531-8257(199905)14:3<507::AID-MDS1021>3.0.CO;2-8]   [PMID: 10348479]

[86]   Kunz D, Mahlberg R. A two-part, double-blind, placebo-controlled trial of exogenous melatonin in REM sleep behaviour disorder. J Sleep Res 2010; 19(4): 591-6.
[http://dx.doi.org/10.1111/j.1365-2869.2010.00848.x] [PMID: 20561180]

[87]   Kunz D, Bes F. Twenty years after: Another case report of melatonin effects on rem sleep behavior disorder, using serial dopamine transporter imaging. Neuropsychobiology 2017; 76(2): 100-4.
[http://dx.doi.org/10.1159/000488893] [PMID: 29860260]

[88]   Takeuchi N, Uchimura N, Hashizume Y, *et al.* Melatonin therapy for REM sleep behavior disorder. Psychiatry Clin Neurosci 2001; 55(3): 267-9.
[http://dx.doi.org/10.1046/j.1440-1819.2001.00854.x] [PMID: 11422870]

[89]   Boeve BF, Silber MH, Ferman TJ. Melatonin for treatment of REM sleep behavior disorder in neurologic disorders: results in 14 patients. Sleep Med 2003; 4(4): 281-4.
[http://dx.doi.org/10.1016/S1389-9457(03)00072-8] [PMID: 14592300]

[90]   Lin C-M, Chiu H-Y, Guilleminault C. Melatonin and REM behavior disorder. J Sleep Disord Ther 2013; 2(3): 1-9.
[http://dx.doi.org/10.4172/2167-0277.1000118]

[91]   McCarter SJ, Boswell CL, St Louis EK, *et al.* Treatment outcomes in REM sleep behavior disorder. Sleep Med 2013; 14(3): 237-42.
[http://dx.doi.org/10.1016/j.sleep.2012.09.018] [PMID: 23352028]

[92]   Schaefer C, Kunz D, Bes F. Melatonin effects in REM sleep behavior disorder associated with obstructive sleep apnea syndrome: A case series. Curr Alzheimer Res 2017; 14(10): 1084-9.
[http://dx.doi.org/10.2174/1567205014666170523094938] [PMID: 28545360]

[93]   During EH, Miglis MG. Clinical trials in REM sleep behavior disorder: an urgent need for better evidence. Sleep Med 2019; 63: 1-2.
[http://dx.doi.org/10.1016/j.sleep.2019.06.001] [PMID: 31600655]

[94]   During EH, Schenck CH. Factors hampering the discovery of new therapeutics for rapid eye movement sleep behavior disorder. JAMA Neurol 2019; 76(10): 1137-8.
[http://dx.doi.org/10.1001/jamaneurol.2019.2062] [PMID: 31329218]

[95]   Schenck CH, Hurwitz TD, Mahowald MW. Symposium: Normal and abnormal REM sleep regulation: REM sleep behaviour disorder: an update on a series of 96 patients and a review of the world literature. J Sleep Res 1993; 2(4): 224-31.
[http://dx.doi.org/10.1111/j.1365-2869.1993.tb00093.x] [PMID: 10607098]

[96]   Iranzo A, Santamaría J, Rye DB, et al. Characteristics of idiopathic REM sleep behavior disorder and that associated with MSA and PD. Neurology 2005; 65(2): 247-52.
[http://dx.doi.org/10.1212/01.wnl.0000168864.97813.e0] [PMID: 16043794]

[97]   Li SX, Lam SP, Zhang J, et al. A prospective, naturalistic follow-up study of treatment outcomes with clonazepam in rapid eye movement sleep behavior disorder. Sleep Med 2016; 21: 114-20.
[http://dx.doi.org/10.1016/j.sleep.2015.12.020] [PMID: 27448481]

[98]   Lee HJ, Choi H, Yoon IY. Age of Diagnosis and Comorbid PLMD Predict Poor Response of REM Behavior Disorder to Clonazepam. J Geriatr Psychiatry Neurol 2021; 34(2): 142-9.
[http://dx.doi.org/10.1177/0891988720915517] [PMID: 32233817]

[99]   Lapierre O, Montplaisir J. Polysomnographic features of REM sleep behavior disorder: development of a scoring method. Neurology 1992; 42(7): 1371-4.
[http://dx.doi.org/10.1212/WNL.42.7.1371] [PMID: 1620348]

[100] Ferri R, Marelli S, Ferini-Strambi L, et al. An observational clinical and video-polysomnographic study of the effects of clonazepam in REM sleep behavior disorder. Sleep Med 2013; 14(1): 24-9.
[http://dx.doi.org/10.1016/j.sleep.2012.09.009] [PMID: 23098778]

[101] Shin C, Park H, Lee WW, Kim HJ, Kim HJ, Jeon B. Clonazepam for probable REM sleep behavior disorder in Parkinson's disease: A randomized placebo-controlled trial. J Neurol Sci 2019; 401: 81-6.
[http://dx.doi.org/10.1016/j.jns.2019.04.029] [PMID: 31035190]

[102] Di Giacopo R, Fasano A, Quaranta D, Della Marca G, Bove F, Bentivoglio AR. Rivastigmine as alternative treatment for refractory REM behavior disorder in Parkinson's disease. Mov Disord 2012; 27(4): 559-61.
[http://dx.doi.org/10.1002/mds.24909] [PMID: 22290743]

[103] Brunetti V, Losurdo A, Testani E, et al. Rivastigmine for refractory REM behavior disorder in mild cognitive impairment. Curr Alzheimer Res 2014; 11(3): 267-73.
[http://dx.doi.org/10.2174/1567205011666140302195648] [PMID: 24597506]

[104] Kotagal V, Albin RL, Müller ML, et al. Symptoms of rapid eye movement sleep behavior disorder are associated with cholinergic denervation in Parkinson disease. Ann Neurol 2012; 71(4): 560-8.
[http://dx.doi.org/10.1002/ana.22691] [PMID: 22522445]

[105] Bedard MA, Aghourian M, Legault-Denis C, et al. Brain cholinergic alterations in idiopathic REM sleep behaviour disorder: a PET imaging study with ^{18}F-FEOBV. Sleep Med 2019; 58: 35-41.
[http://dx.doi.org/10.1016/j.sleep.2018.12.020] [PMID: 31078078]

[106] Ringman JM, Simmons JH. Treatment of REM sleep behavior disorder with donepezil: a report of three cases. Neurology 2000; 55(6): 870-1.
[http://dx.doi.org/10.1212/WNL.55.6.870] [PMID: 10994012]

[107]   Kazui H, Adachi H, Kanemoto H, *et al.* Effects of donepezil on sleep disturbances in patients with dementia with Lewy bodies: An open-label study with actigraphy. Psychiatry Res 2017; 251: 312-8.
[http://dx.doi.org/10.1016/j.psychres.2017.02.039] [PMID: 28236784]

[108]   Yeh SB, Yeh PY, Schenck CH. Rivastigmine-induced REM sleep behavior disorder (RBD) in a 88-year-old man with Alzheimer's disease. J Clin Sleep Med 2010; 6(2): 192-5.
[http://dx.doi.org/10.5664/jcsm.27771] [PMID: 20411699]

[109]   Carlander B, Touchon J, Ondze B, Billiard M. REM sleep behavior disorder induced by cholinergic treatment in Alzheimer's disease. J Sleep Res 1996; 5 (Suppl. 1): 28.

[110]   Sasai T, Matsuura M, Inoue Y. Factors associated with the effect of pramipexole on symptoms of idiopathic REM sleep behavior disorder. Parkinsonism Relat Disord 2013; 19(2): 153-7.
[http://dx.doi.org/10.1016/j.parkreldis.2012.08.010] [PMID: 22989561]

[111]   Tan SM, Wan YM. Pramipexole in the treatment of REM sleep behaviour disorder: A critical review. Psychiatry Res 2016; 243: 365-72.
[http://dx.doi.org/10.1016/j.psychres.2016.06.055] [PMID: 27449005]

[112]   Shneerson JM. Successful treatment of REM sleep behavior disorder with sodium oxybate. Clin Neuropharmacol 2009; 32(3): 158-9.
[http://dx.doi.org/10.1097/WNF.0b013e318193e394] [PMID: 19483483]

[113]   Liebenthal J, Valerio J, Ruoff C, Mahowald M. A Case of Rapid Eye Movement Sleep Behavior Disorder in Parkinson Disease Treated With Sodium Oxybate. JAMA Neurol 2016; 73(1): 126-7.
[http://dx.doi.org/10.1001/jamaneurol.2015.2904] [PMID: 26595534]

[114]   Antelmi E, Plazzi G. Rapid eye movement sleep behavior disorder and sodium oxybate: efficacy and viewpoint Sleep 2020; 12;43(11) zsaa149.
[http://dx.doi.org/10.1093/sleep/zsaa149]

[115]   Büchele F, Hackius M, Schreglmann SR, *et al.* Sodium Oxybate for Excessive Daytime Sleepiness and Sleep Disturbance in Parkinson Disease: A Randomized Clinical Trial. JAMA Neurol 2018; 75(1): 114-8.
[http://dx.doi.org/10.1001/jamaneurol.2017.3171] [PMID: 29114733]

[116]   Mayer G, Rodenbeck A, Kesper K. Sodium oxybate treatment in narcolepsy and its effect on muscle tone. Sleep Med 2017; 35: 1-6.
[http://dx.doi.org/10.1016/j.sleep.2017.03.023] [PMID: 28619175]

[117]   Antelmi E, Filardi M, Pizza F, *et al.* REM Sleep Behavior Disorder in Children With Type 1 Narcolepsy Treated With Sodium Oxybate. Neurology 2021; 96(2): e250-4.
[PMID: 33177222]

[118]   Larsson V, Aarsland D, Ballard C, Minthon L, Londos E. The effect of memantine on sleep behaviour in dementia with Lewy bodies and Parkinson's disease dementia. Int J Geriatr Psychiatry 2010; 25(10): 1030-8.
[http://dx.doi.org/10.1002/gps.2506] [PMID: 20872929]

[119]   Gilat M, Marshall NS, Testelmans D, Buyse B, Lewis SJG. A critical review of the pharmacological treatment of REM sleep behavior disorder in adults: time for more and larger randomized placebo. J Neurol 2022; 269(1): 125-48.
[http://dx.doi.org/10.1007/s00415-020-10353-0]

[120]   Sixel-Döring F. Prognostic counseling for patients with idiopathic/isolated rapid eye movement sleep behavior disorder: Should we tell them what's coming? No. Mov Disord Clin Pract (Hoboken) 2019; 6(8): 669-71.
[http://dx.doi.org/10.1002/mdc3.12813] [PMID: 31745476]

[121]   Teigen LN, Sharp RR, Hirsch JR, *et al.* Specialist approaches to prognostic counseling in isolated REM sleep behavior disorder. Sleep Med 2021; 79: 107-12.
[http://dx.doi.org/10.1016/j.sleep.2020.12.014] [PMID: 33486257]

[122] Arnaldi D, Antelmi E, St Louis EK, Postuma RB, Arnulf I. Idiopathic REM sleep behavior disorder and neurodegenerative risk: To tell or not to tell to the patient? How to minimize the risk? Sleep Med Rev 2017; 36: 82-95.
[http://dx.doi.org/10.1016/j.smrv.2016.11.002] [PMID: 28082168]

CHAPTER 8

Surgical Treatment Options for Obstructive Sleep Apnea

Sneha Giri[1]**, Robson Capasso**[2]**, Stanley YC Liu**[2] **and Michael Awad**[1,2,*]

[1] *Department of Otolaryngology / Head & Neck Surgery, Northwestern University, Chicago, Illinois, USA*

[2] *Department of Otolaryngology-Head and Neck Surgery, Division of Sleep Surgery, Stanford Hospital and Clinics, Stanford, California, USA*

Abstract: Advances in upper airway evaluation, along with the improved understanding of OSA phenotypes and evolving approaches to surgical techniques, have enabled targeted multi-level interventions for obstructive sleep apnea (OSA). A variety of surgical techniques to address the nasal cavity, palate, oropharynx, hypopharynx, tongue, epiglottis and facial skeleton exist. Surgery has proven to be an effective treatment modality that reduces objective and subjective OSA measures as well as associated neurocognitive and cardiovascular morbidities.

Keywords: Drug-induced sleep endoscopy (DISE), Genioglossus Advancement (GGA), Lingual Tonsillectomy, Maxillomandibular Advancement (MMA), Palatine Tonsillectomy, Palatopharyngoplasty (PPP), Septoplasty, Turbinate Reduction, Upper Airway Stimulation (UAS).

INTRODUCTION

Modern techniques in sleep surgery offer solutions for obstructive sleep apnea (OSA) patients with symptoms refractory to non-surgical measures, including positive airway pressure, behavioral management positional therapy and oral appliances (mandibular advancement, tongue stabilizing devices).

Several surgical options for OSA exist and the choice of technique should be tailored to an individual's anatomy. Evaluation of the OSA patient for surgical management entails a thorough clinical assessment including a complete head and neck examination with specific evaluation of the following factors: BMI, neck cir-

---

[*] **Corresponding author Michael Awad:** Department of Otolaryngology / Head & Neck Surgery, Northwestern University, Chicago, Illinois, USA and Department of Otolaryngology-Head and Neck Surgery, Division of Sleep Surgery, Stanford Hospital and Clinics, Stanford, California, USA; E-mail: michael.awad@nm.org

Imran H. Iftikhar and Ali I. Musani (Eds.)

cumference, nasal cavity, occlusion, retrognathia/micrognathia, palatal transverse dimension, tongue size/position, tonsil size, and palate position. Awake flexible endoscopy should also be performed to evaluate lingual tonsil size, tongue position, epiglottis position, and lateral wall laxity. If no clear cause of obstruction is identified on awake physical examination or flexible endoscopy, drug-induced sleep endoscopy (DISE) can be used for a dynamic airway evaluation. Surgical intervention is subsequently tailored towards the specific site(s) of obstruction identified on an exam. When multiple levels of obstruction are observed, surgery may be performed on the same day ("multi-level approach") or staged.

Drug-Induced Sleep Endoscopy (DISE)

A. A technique developed by Croft and Pringle in the UK in 1991, drug-induced sleep endoscopy (DISE) has since been adopted worldwide [1]. The goal of DISE is to reproduce patterns of OSA seen during natural sleep. During this procedure, an anaesthetist titrates sedation, typically propofol or dexmedetomidine (Precedex), until the patient transitions to loss of consciousness. Flexible endoscopy is subsequently performed, and subsites within the airway are scored in terms of magnitude and direction of obstruction [2]. DISE offers the advantage of a dynamic assessment that allows for direct visualization of the location of the obstruction. Various positions (supine, lateral, patient's natural sleep position) and maneuvers (jaw thrust, mouth closure) can be trialled during DISE to assess their impact on airway obstruction. The validity of DISE has been demonstrated in several studies [3, 4]. DISE has also been shown to have moderate to good test-retest and inter-rater reliability [5, 6].

  A. Scoring- The most widely accepted scoring system is the VOTE classification (Fig. 1) [7]. This scoring system classifies DISE findings by anatomical level (Velum, Oropharynx, Tongue base, and Epiglottis) and direction (anteroposterior, lateral, and concentric). The magnitude of obstruction in each domain is graded on a 0-2 scale in which 0 indicates no obstruction (<50%; no vibration), 1 partial obstruction (50-75%; vibration), and 2 complete obstructions (>75%; collapse). This scoring system allows for standardization and comparison of findings across centers.

  B. Limitations- Controversy exists as to whether the drug-induced state is reflective of natural sleep. Sedatives decrease muscle tone and diminish the respiratory drive and therefore may artificially worsen OSA and alter the pattern of collapse. Propofol-induced sleep is known to alter sleep architecture and is unable to reproduce rapid eye movement (REM) sleep, a stage in which AHI is frequently increased.

VOTE classification system			
		Direction	
Level	A-P	Lateral	Concentric
Velum			
Oropharynx	■		■
Tongue base		■	
Epiglottis			■

Fig. (1). VOTE Classification system. Established by Kezirian and colleagues in 2011. This scoring system classifies DISE findings by level (Velum, Oropharynx, Tongue base, and Epiglottis) and direction (anteroposterior, lateral, and concentric). Magnitude of obstruction in each domain is graded on a 0-2 scale: 0, no obstruction (<50%, no vibration); 1, partial obstruction (50-75%, vibration), and 2 indicates complete obstruction (>75%, collapse). Figure adapted from [7].

Surgical Treatment Options

Surgical intervention should be targeted toward the specific site(s) of obstruction identified on physical exam, awake flexible endoscopy, and/or DISE (Fig. **2**). A multilevel approach can be used when multiple levels of obstruction are identified.

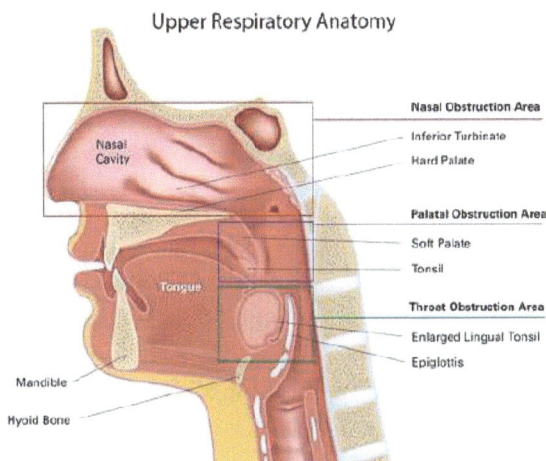

Fig. (2). Upper airway anatomy. The site of obstruction in OSA can be localized to one of several subsites within the upper airway including the velum/palate, oropharynx, tongue, and epiglottis. Surgical interventions can be targeted toward each of these subsites.

Nasal Cavity

a. Septoplasty, turbinate reduction: Nasal obstruction may impair airflow and resultantly impact CPAP compliance and adherence. The most common anatomical issues to cause nasal obstruction are nasal septal deviation, inferior turbinate hypertrophy, nasal valve collapse, nasal polyps, or edematous mucosa. Surgery can be considered in patients who have failed medical management, including nasal saline irrigations and topical/oral steroids/antihistamines. The most common surgeries used to address nasal obstruction are septoplasty and turbinate reduction. Septoplasty is used to correct the nasal septal deviation and can be performed endoscopically, externally, or *via* an open approach in combination with rhinoplasty when correction of the nasal valve is desired. Inferior turbinate hypertrophy can be addressed *via* submucous resection or ablation. Nasal surgery alone should not be directed to treat OSA but can improve subjective sleep quality, sleep architecture and symptoms of daytime sleepiness while reducing disruptive snoring. Moreover, nasal surgery is associated with significant improvements in CPAP tolerance and adherence [8].

b. Distraction Osteogenesis Maxillary Expansion (DOME): Patients with persistent nasal obstruction following nasal surgery are often found to exhibit a narrow, high-arched hard palate creating increased resistance at the level of the nasal floor [9]. Patients exhibiting this phenotype may benefit from DOME to achieve maxillary expansion [10]. Modern adaptations to the DOME Procedure involve an endoscopically assisted technique (MINE-DOME), reducing peri-operative recovery and morbidity.

Palatal/Pharyngeal Procedures

a. Palatopharyngoplasty (PPP): Patients with circumferential narrowing or redundant pharyngeal tissue with low tongue position and relative normoglossia are ideal candidates for PPP. Described by Fujita and colleagues in 1981, uvulopalatopharyngoplasty (UPPP) was amongst the first surgical options available for OSA and remained the most commonly performed surgery for OSA worldwide [11]. The aim of PPP is to expand the potential airspace in the oropharynx *via* excision/rearrangement of tissue of the soft palate, uvula, tonsillar pillar, and tonsils. Friedman and colleagues described predictors of success in patients undergoing UPPP in 2002: Patients grouped into the Stage I category (palate position 1 or 2, tonsil size 3 or 4) were found to have the greatest success with UPPP, and conversely, patients with small tonsils (1 or 2), a large tongue (3 or 4), or elevated BMI (>40) were found to have the least success [12]. The short and long-term sequelae of UPPP include foreign body sensation, dry throat, voice changes, velopharyngeal insufficiency (VPI), and swallow dysfunction [13]. UPPP has historically been and continues to be the most common pharyngeal surgery performed for OSA. Several technical variations for more conservative PPP have since been developed with promising results, including expansion sphincter pharyngoplasty (ESP), tissue-preserving palatopharyngoplasty, and barbed pharyngoplasty [14, 15]. Studies have shown these techniques to effectively address lateral wall collapse without the associated complications of traditional UPPP [16].

b. Palatine tonsillectomy: Palatine tonsil hypertrophy is a common source of upper airway obstruction. The relationship between palatine tonsil size and degree of OSA severity has been well described [17]. Tonsillectomy involves separating the tonsil from the anterior and posterior tonsillar pillars as well as the superior pharyngeal constrictor laterally. Several techniques exist for tonsillectomy, including Bovie electrocautery, coblation, and cold steel, among others. A 2016 meta-analysis of 17 studies (216 patients) found that, on average, patients undergoing palatine tonsillectomy have significant improvement in AHI (Mean Reduction 40.5 to 14), minimum O_2 saturation (78% to 86%), and Epworth Sleepiness Scale (ESS) scores [18].

c. Partial epiglottectomy: Epiglottis collapse is estimated to exist in approximately 12% of adults with OSA [19]. Much remains to be understood regarding the role of the epiglottis in adult OSA. While CPAP may be ineffective for these patients and may actually accentuate collapse, lateral positional therapy can be helpful. Surgical techniques to address epiglottis collapse include partial epiglottectomy or coblation of the lingual surface of the epiglottis. However, data are limited on the efficacy of these approaches [20].

Tongue

a. Upper airway stimulation (UAS): Approved in 2014, the Inspire® hypoglossal nerve stimulator is currently the only FDA-approved device for upper airway stimulation (Fig. 3). This technology uses stimulation of the hypoglossal nerve to increase muscle tone and reduce upper airway collapsibility during inspiration. Candidates must meet the following criteria to qualify for UAS implantation: AHI 15-65, age >22, absence of complete concentric palate collapse on DISE, and <25% central apneas [21]. The device consists of three components: a respiratory sensor implanted between the 4th-6th rib spaces, a battery/pulse generator implanted in the chest, and a stimulation cuff placed in the neck around the hypoglossal nerve. The stimulation cuff is placed to include hypoglossal nerve branches that innervate muscles of tongue protrusion and exclude branches innervating muscles involved in tongue retraction (hyoglossus, styloglossus). The device is typically activated one month after placement, with patients gradually titrated to their final optimal voltage, configuration and polarity settings. This device has been shown to have a multilevel impact, including tongue base, palate, lateral pharyngeal wall, and epiglottis.

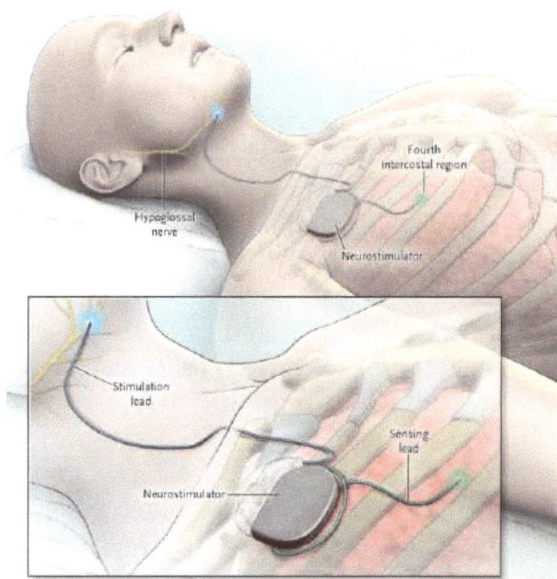

Fig. (3). Upper airway stimulation. The Inspire® hypoglossal nerve stimulator is currently the only FDA approved device for upper airway stimulation. Stimulation of the hypoglossal nerve increases muscle tone and reduces upper airway collapsibility during inspiration. The device consists of three components: a respiratory sensor implanted in axilla, battery/pulse generator implanted in chest, and a stimulation lead placed in the neck around the hypoglossal nerve.

The 2014 STAR trial, a multicenter prospective cohort study, found UAS to be safe and effective in treating moderate-severe OSA with significant improvement in both subjective and objective measurements of the severity of OSA [22]. Five-year outcomes from the STAR trial published in 2018 have shown lasting improvements with an AHI response rate (AHI <20 events/hour and >50% reduction) of 75% and a low rate of serious device-related events (6%) [23]. The ADHERE registry, the largest cohort of patients with UAS enrolling over 1,000 patients to date, has similarly found high patient satisfaction, good therapy adherence, and significant improvement in subjective and objective OSA measures [24, 25]. Limitations of this iteration of the device include MRI incompatibility, a ~10 year battery life, and patient intolerance. Recent studies aimed at identifying responders have found that lower CPAP pressure, lower BMI, female sex, and older age may be factors associated with improved outcomes [25, 26]. In patients who are found to have concentric collapse on DISE, palatopharyngoplasty can be used to resolve concentric collapse and render previously ineligible candidates eligible [27]. Further research must be done to understand factors that predict success and/or failure to allow for optimal patient selection.

a. Lingual tonsillectomy/tongue base reduction: Lingual tonsil hypertrophy refers to the overgrowth of lymphatic tissue at the tongue base. Techniques used to perform lingual tonsillectomy include transoral robotic surgery (TORS) and coblation [28]. Several studies have compared the efficacy of lingual tonsillectomy *via* TORS *versus* coblation and found no significant difference in outcomes [29, 30].
b. Genioglossus advancement (GGA)/genioplasty: The genioglossus acts as the primary pharyngeal dilator muscle of the upper airway during sleep. Its role in OSA has been established, given that airway collapse can occur secondary to failure of the dilator muscle to maintain tension/patency during respiration [31, 32]. In GGA, the genial tubercle and associated muscles are advanced *via* an osteotomy within the anterior aspect of the mandible. In contrast, genioplasty advances the genial tubercle *via* a horizontal sliding osteotomy. Typically, this type of surgery is performed in a multilevel approach, either in combination with soft tissue procedures or maxillomandibular advancement. Rarely, GGA is performed in isolation for patients exhibiting exclusive tongue base collapse.

Facial Skeleton

a. Maxillomandibular advancement (MMA): MMA is the most effective multilevel procedure available for treatment of OSA, resulting in expansion at multiple airway levels from the nasopharynx to the hypopharynx. In 2015, Liu and colleagues studied 16 patients undergoing MMA with pre- and post-op DISE and found that post-MMA DISE showed the most significant improvement at the level of the lateral pharyngeal wall, with obstruction decreasing from 100% (87% complete collapse) to 13% with partial collapse (no complete collapse) [33]. The technique of MMA advances both the maxilla and mandible antero-superiorly relative to the airway, which results in dilation of the airway secondary to increased tension of the attached suprahyoid muscles. Incorporation of counter clockwise rotation of the maxilla around the nasolabial complex confers improved the ability to achieve large scale advancements while balancing facial cosmesis. The surgical success and cure rates of MMA have been shown to be of 85.5% and 38.5%, respectively [34]. The degree of maxillary advancement is correlated to the efficacy of MMA, but large maxillary advancements are known to cause profound change to the nasolabial region. Recent adaptations to the technique of MMA, such as concurrent septoplasty and inferior turbinate reduction at the time of maxillary osteotomy, have helped to reduce morbidity by reducing the frequency of corrective nasal surgery following MMA [35, 36].

FUTURE DIRECTIONS

Study in sleep apnea surgery continues to be directed towards clinically relevant outcomes, with recent literature identifying that sleep apnea surgery can reduce systemic (neurologic, cardiovascular and endocrine) complications of OSA [37].

Understanding predictors of success for each type of surgery is essential for optimizing patient selection.

Current efforts are also aimed at improving the assessment of the airway in a natural sleep state rather than a drug-induced state. And while the Inspire® hypoglossal nerve stimulator is currently the only FDA-approved device for upper airway stimulation, other devices such as the LivaNova Imthera (a device that offers constant upper airway stimulation) and the Nyxoah Genio system (a device that offers bilateral stimulation with a minimally invasive surgical approach and external battery) are currently under investigation. The Bilateral Hypoglossal Nerve Stimulation for Treatment of OSA (BLAST) trial in Europe has shown promising results for the safety and efficacy of Nyxoah in patients with moderate-to-severe OSA [38]. In June 2020, Nyxoah's Genio system received IDE exemption approval by the FDA for its DREAM study in the US.

CONCLUSION

Surgical interventions for OSA should be offered to all patients who have failed behavioral and medical treatments and can be considered in patients presenting with significant anatomical anomalies on physical examination and upper airway endoscopy. Modern surgical techniques are tailored toward individual clinical phenotypes. Tools such as DISE enable dynamic airway evaluation, which enables targeted interventions. Surgical techniques to address the nasal cavity, palate, oropharynx, hypopharynx, tongue, and epiglottis exist. Optimal patient selection is key to the success of these procedures.

CONSENT FOR PUBLICATION

Not applicable.

CONFLICT OF INTEREST

The authors declare no conflict of interest, financial or otherwise.

ACKNOWLEDGEMENTS

Declared none.

REFERENCES

[1]   Croft CB, Pringle M. Sleep nasendoscopy: a technique of assessment in snoring and obstructive sleep apnoea. Clin Otolaryngol Allied Sci 1991; 16(5): 504-9.
[http://dx.doi.org/10.1111/j.1365-2273.1991.tb01050.x] [PMID: 1742903]

[2]   Awad M, Okland TS, Nekhendzy V. Drug-Induced Sleep Endoscopy. Atlas Oral Maxillofac Surg Clin North Am 2019; 27(1): 7-10.
[http://dx.doi.org/10.1016/j.cxom.2018.11.010] [PMID: 30717927]

[3]   Steinhart H, Kuhn-Lohmann J, Gewalt K, Constantinidis J, Mertzlufft F, Iro H. Upper airway collapsibility in habitual snorers and sleep apneics: evaluation with drug-induced sleep endoscopy. Acta Otolaryngol 2000; 120(8): 990-4.
[http://dx.doi.org/10.1080/000164800750218753] [PMID: 11200597]

[4]   Berry S, Roblin G, Williams A, Watkins A, Whittet HB. Validity of sleep nasendoscopy in the investigation of sleep related breathing disorders. Laryngoscope 2005; 115(3): 538-40.
[http://dx.doi.org/10.1097/01.mlg.0000157849.16649.6e] [PMID: 15744173]

[5]   Rodriguez-Bruno K, Goldberg AN, McCulloch CE, Kezirian EJ. Test-retest reliability of drug-induced sleep endoscopy. Otolaryngol Head Neck Surg 2009; 140(5): 646-51.
[http://dx.doi.org/10.1016/j.otohns.2009.01.012] [PMID: 19393404]

[6]   Kezirian EJ, White DP, Malhotra A, Ma W, McCulloch CE, Goldberg AN. Interrater reliability of drug-induced sleep endoscopy. Arch Otolaryngol Head Neck Surg 2010; 136(4): 393-7.
[http://dx.doi.org/10.1001/archoto.2010.26] [PMID: 20403857]

[7]   Kezirian EJ, Hohenhorst W, de Vries N. Drug-induced sleep endoscopy: the VOTE classification. Eur Arch Otorhinolaryngol 2011; 268(8): 1233-6.
[http://dx.doi.org/10.1007/s00405-011-1633-8] [PMID: 21614467]

[8]   Ishii L, Roxbury C, Godoy A, Ishman S, Ishii M. Does Nasal Surgery Improve OSA in Patients with Nasal Obstruction and OSA? A Meta-analysis. Otolaryngol Head Neck Surg 2015; 153(3): 326-33.
[http://dx.doi.org/10.1177/0194599815594374] [PMID: 26183522]

[9]   Awad M, Capasso R. Skeletal Surgery for Obstructive Sleep Apnea. Otolaryngol Clin North Am 2020; 53(3): 459-68.
[http://dx.doi.org/10.1016/j.otc.2020.02.008] [PMID: 32334864]

[10]   Abdelwahab M, Yoon A, Okland T, Poomkonsarn S, Gouveia C, Liu SY. Impact of Distraction Osteogenesis Maxillary Expansion on the Internal Nasal Valve in Obstructive Sleep Apnea. Otolaryngol Head Neck Surg 2019; 161(2): 362-7.
[http://dx.doi.org/10.1177/0194599819842808] [PMID: 31084256]

[11]   Fujita S, Conway W, Zorick F, Roth T. Surgical correction of anatomic azbnormalities in obstructive sleep apnea syndrome: uvulopalatopharyngoplasty. Otolaryngol Head Neck Surg 1981; 89(6): 923-34.
[http://dx.doi.org/10.1177/019459988108900609] [PMID: 6801592]

[12]   Friedman M, Ibrahim H, Bass L. Clinical staging for sleep-disordered breathing. Otolaryngol Head Neck Surg 2002; 127(1): 13-21.
[http://dx.doi.org/10.1067/mhn.2002.126477] [PMID: 12161725]

[13]   Tang JA, Salapatas AM, Bonzelaar LB, Friedman M. Long-Term Incidence of Velopharyngeal Insufficiency and Other Sequelae following Uvulopalatopharyngoplasty. Otolaryngol Head Neck Surg 2017; 156(4): 606-10.
[http://dx.doi.org/10.1177/0194599816688646] [PMID: 28116979]

[14]   Pang KP, Woodson BT. Expansion sphincter pharyngoplasty: a new technique for the treatment of obstructive sleep apnea. Otolaryngol Head Neck Surg 2007; 137(1): 110-4.
[http://dx.doi.org/10.1016/j.otohns.2007.03.014] [PMID: 17599576]

[15]   Awad M, Gouveia C, Capasso R, Liu SY. Tonsillectomy and Pharyngoplasty: Tissue-Preserving Techniques. Atlas Oral Maxillofac Surg Clin North Am 2019; 27(1): 17-22.

[http://dx.doi.org/10.1016/j.cxom.2018.11.005] [PMID: 30717919]

[16]   Hong SN, Kim HG, Han SY, *et al.* Indications for and outcomes of expansion sphincter pharyngoplasty to treat lateral pharyngeal collapse in patients with obstructive sleep apnea. JAMA Otolaryngol Head Neck Surg 2019; 145(5): 405-12.
[http://dx.doi.org/10.1001/jamaoto.2019.0006] [PMID: 30844019]

[17]   Jara SM, Weaver EM. Association of palatine tonsil size and obstructive sleep apnea in adults. Laryngoscope 2018; 128(4): 1002-6.
[http://dx.doi.org/10.1002/lary.26928] [PMID: 29205391]

[18]   Camacho M, Li D, Kawai M, *et al.* Tonsillectomy for adult obstructive sleep apnea: A systematic review and meta-analysis. Laryngoscope 2016; 126(9): 2176-86.
[http://dx.doi.org/10.1002/lary.25931] [PMID: 27005314]

[19]   Catalfumo FJ, Golz A, Westerman ST, Gilbert LM, Joachims HZ, Goldenberg D. The epiglottis and obstructive sleep apnoea syndrome. J Laryngol Otol 1998; 112(10): 940-3.
[http://dx.doi.org/10.1017/S0022215100142136] [PMID: 10211216]

[20]   Torre C, Camacho M, Liu SY-C, Huon L-K, Capasso R. Epiglottis collapse in adult obstructive sleep apnea: A systematic review. Laryngoscope 2016; 126(2): 515-23.
[http://dx.doi.org/10.1002/lary.25589] [PMID: 26371602]

[21]   Baptista PM, Costantino A, Moffa A, Rinaldi V, Casale M. Hypoglossal Nerve Stimulation in the Treatment of Obstructive Sleep Apnea: Patient Selection and New Perspectives. Nat Sci Sleep 2020; 12: 151-9.
[http://dx.doi.org/10.2147/NSS.S221542] [PMID: 32104122]

[22]   Strollo PJ Jr, Soose RJ, Maurer JT, *et al.* Upper-airway stimulation for obstructive sleep apnea. N Engl J Med 2014; 370(2): 139-49.
[http://dx.doi.org/10.1056/NEJMoa1308659] [PMID: 24401051]

[23]   Woodson BT, Strohl KP, Soose RJ, *et al.* Upper Airway Stimulation for Obstructive Sleep Apnea: 5-Year Outcomes. Otolaryngol Head Neck Surg 2018; 159(1): 194-202.
[http://dx.doi.org/10.1177/0194599818762383] [PMID: 29582703]

[24]   Boon M, Huntley C, Steffen A, *et al.* Upper Airway Stimulation for Obstructive Sleep Apnea: Results from the ADHERE Registry. Otolaryngol Head Neck Surg 2018; 159(2): 379-85.
[http://dx.doi.org/10.1177/0194599818764896] [PMID: 29557280]

[25]   Thaler E, Schwab R, Maurer J, *et al.* Results of the ADHERE upper airway stimulation registry and predictors of therapy efficacy. Laryngoscope 2020; 130(5): 1333-8.
[http://dx.doi.org/10.1002/lary.28286] [PMID: 31520484]

[26]   Heiser C, Steffen A, Boon M, *et al.* Post-approval upper airway stimulation predictors of treatment effectiveness in the ADHERE registry. Eur Respir J 2019; 53(1): 1801405.
[http://dx.doi.org/10.1183/13993003.01405-2018] [PMID: 30487205]

[27]   Liu SY-C, Hutz MJ, Poomkonsarn S, Chang CP, Awad M, Capasso R. Palatopharyngoplasty Resolves Concentric Collapse in Patients Ineligible for Upper Airway Stimulation. Laryngoscope 2020; 130(12): E958-62.
[http://dx.doi.org/10.1002/lary.28595] [PMID: 32109324]

[28]   Miller SC, Nguyen SA, Ong AA, Gillespie MB. Transoral robotic base of tongue reduction for obstructive sleep apnea: A systematic review and meta-analysis. Laryngoscope 2017; 127(1): 258-65.
[http://dx.doi.org/10.1002/lary.26060] [PMID: 27346300]

[29]   Hwang CS, Kim JW, Kim JW, *et al.* Comparison of robotic and coblation tongue base resection for obstructive sleep apnoea. Clin Otolaryngol 2018; 43(1): 249-55.
[http://dx.doi.org/10.1111/coa.12951] [PMID: 28800204]

[30]   Tsou Y-A, Chang W-D. Comparison of transoral robotic surgery with other surgeries for obstructive sleep apnea. Sci Rep 2020; 10(1): 18163.

[http://dx.doi.org/10.1038/s41598-020-75215-1] [PMID: 33097783]

[31]   Mezzanotte WS, Tangel DJ, White DP. Waking genioglossal electromyogram in sleep apnea patients *versus* normal controls (a neuromuscular compensatory mechanism). J Clin Invest 1992; 89(5): 1571-9.
         [http://dx.doi.org/10.1172/JCI115751] [PMID: 1569196]

[32]   Eckert DJ, Malhotra A. Pathophysiology of adult obstructive sleep apnea. Proc Am Thorac Soc 2008; 5(2): 144-53.
         [http://dx.doi.org/10.1513/pats.200707-114MG] [PMID: 18250206]

[33]   Liu SY, Huon LK, Iwasaki T, *et al.* Efficacy of Maxillomandibular Advancement Examined with Drug-Induced Sleep Endoscopy and Computational Fluid Dynamics Airflow Modeling. Otolaryngol Head Neck Surg 2016; 154(1): 189-95.
         [http://dx.doi.org/10.1177/0194599815611603] [PMID: 26740522]

[34]   Zaghi S, Holty J-EC, Certal V, *et al.* Maxillomandibular Advancement for Treatment of Obstructive Sleep Apnea: A Meta-analysis. JAMA Otolaryngol Head Neck Surg 2016; 142(1): 58-66.
         [http://dx.doi.org/10.1001/jamaoto.2015.2678] [PMID: 26606321]

[35]   Liu SY, Lee PJ, Awad M, Riley RW, Zaghi S. Corrective Nasal Surgery after Maxillomandibular Advancement for Obstructive Sleep Apnea: Experience from 379 Cases. Otolaryngol Head Neck Surg 2017; 157(1): 156-9.
         [http://dx.doi.org/10.1177/0194599817695807] [PMID: 28417661]

[36]   Liu SY, Awad M, Riley RW. Maxillomandibular advancement: Contemporary approach at stanford. Atlas Oral Maxillofac Surg Clin North Am 2019; 27(1): 29-36.
         [http://dx.doi.org/10.1016/j.cxom.2018.11.011] [PMID: 30717921]

[37]   Ibrahim B, de Freitas Mendonca MI, Gombar S, Callahan A, Jung K, Capasso R. Association of systemic diseases with surgical treatment for obstructive sleep apnea compared with continuous positive airway pressure. JAMA Otolaryngol Head Neck Surg 2021; 147(4): 329-35.
         [http://dx.doi.org/10.1001/jamaoto.2020.5179] [PMID: 33475682]

[38]   Eastwood PR, Barnes M, MacKay SG, *et al.* Bilateral hypoglossal nerve stimulation for treatment of adult obstructive sleep apnoea. Eur Respir J 2020; 55(1): 1901320.
         [http://dx.doi.org/10.1183/13993003.01320-2019] [PMID: 31601716]

CHAPTER 9

Cognitive Behavioral Therapy for Insomnia

Jennifer M. Mundt[1,*] and **Alicia J. Roth**[2]

¹ Department of Neurology, Center for Circadian and Sleep Medicine, Northwestern University Feinberg School of Medicine, Chicago, IL 60611, USA

² Sleep Disorders Center, Neurological Institute, Cleveland Clinic, Cleveland, OH 44124, USA

Abstract: Cognitive behavioral therapy for insomnia (CBT-I) is a multi-component treatment that typically combines sleep education, sleep hygiene instructions, stimulus control therapy, sleep restriction therapy, cognitive therapy, and relaxation training. CBT-I is considered the first line treatment for chronic insomnia due to evidence of its efficacy, including sustained improvement in insomnia over the long term. Compared to pharmacological treatment, CBT-I has similar short-term efficacy but better long-term durability. CBT-I improves subjective measures of time spent awake at night, resulting in improved sleep continuity. CBT-I is typically delivered in 4-8 face to face individual sessions, though the efficacy of different formats has also been demonstrated, including group therapy, telehealth, and digital therapeutics. Individuals with chronic insomnia frequently have medical and psychiatric comorbidities, and the efficacy of CBT-I has been demonstrated in numerous comorbid populations.

Keywords: Cognitive behavior therapy, Counter control, Cognitive therapy, Insomnia, Relaxation, Sleep hygiene, Stimulus control, Sleep restriction, Sleep compression.

INTRODUCTION

Cognitive behavioral therapy for insomnia (CBT-I) is an effective, time-limited treatment that is considered the first line treatment for adult and pediatric patients with chronic insomnia [1 - 6]. Multicomponent CBT-I includes sleep education, cognitive therapy, stimulus control, and sleep restriction [2]. It also frequently includes sleep hygiene and relaxation training. This chapter provides an overview of CBT-I, including a discussion of each of these components (summarized in Table **1**).

* **Corresponding author Jennifer M. Mundt:** Department of Neurology, Center for Circadian and Sleep Medicine, Northwestern University Feinberg School of Medicine, Chicago, IL 60611, USA; Tel: 312-695-7950; Fax: 312-92--4771; fax:312-926-4771; E-mail: jennifer.mundt@nm.org

Imran H. Iftikhar and Ali I. Musani (Eds.)

We will also discuss the efficacy of CBT-I with various populations, the efficacy of various delivery methods, and important considerations for assessment when delivering CBT-I.

Table 1. Components of Cognitive Behavioral Therapy for Insomnia (CBT-I).

Component	Rationale	Description	Notes and Contraindications
Sleep education	Corrects misconceptions about sleep/insomnia and provides a rationale for subsequent recommendations.	Topics addressed include why we sleep, the two-process model, sleep stages, normal sleep, age-related changes in sleep, and the 3-P model of chronic insomnia.	Education should be tailored to the individual to provide information most relevant to them. Clinicians should also consider what and how much information to provide based on factors such as a patient's age and cognitive function.
Sleep hygiene	Poor sleep hygiene will interfere with the success of subsequent CBT-I components.	Sleep hygiene recommendations vary widely but often include: • Avoid caffeine in the afternoon/evening. • Exercise regularly. • Keep regular bed and wake times. • Avoid or limit naps. • Keep electronics such as TV and computers out of the bedroom. • Keep the bedroom cool, dark, and quiet. • Avoid nicotine, exercise, alcohol, and heavy meals close to bedtime.	Sleep hygiene recommendations alone are typically insufficient to treat chronic insomnia. Most patients presenting with chronic insomnia are aware of these recommendations and have excellent (perhaps even overzealous) adherence to sleep hygiene. Recommendations regarding the details of implementation vary widely. For example, some sources recommend avoiding caffeine or nicotine entirely, while others advise moderation and attention to timing (*e.g.*, no caffeine after lunch, no alcohol within 3 hours of bed).
Stimulus control	Reduces unhelpful conditioned responses of the bed/bedroom with wakefulness and negative emotions. Strengthens the association of the bed with sleep so that the bed becomes a cue for sleep.	• Go to bed only when sleepy. • Use the bed for sleep and intimacy only. • If unable to sleep, get up and go to another room. Repeat this as often as necessary. • Wake up at the same time every day regardless of the prior night's sleep. • Avoid napping or dozing.	Patients at risk of falls should remain in bed when unable to sleep. They can practice counter control as an alternative. This involves sitting up in bed and engaging in a calming activity. This strategy may also be necessary for individuals unable to leave the bed because of space limitations, such as when in a hotel or dorm room. Naps are encouraged if needed for safety.

(Table 1) cont.....

Component	Rationale	Description	Notes and Contraindications
Sleep restriction	Consolidates sleep by regulating the homeostatic sleep drive. Reducing time in bed increases sleep pressure, thereby reducing time awake (sleep onset latency and wake after sleep onset).	• Time in bed is restricted based on total sleep time (TST; average from prior 1-2 weeks sleep diaries). • The sleep window (prescribed time in bed) is typically equal to TST (total sleep time) or TST + 30 minutes. • Sleep window is adjusted at subsequent sessions based on sleep efficiency. • Setting and adjusting the sleep window is a collaborative process that takes into account sleep diary data, subjective daytime function, and patient preferences. • Avoid napping or dozing, as this will reduce the sleep drive.	Sleep restriction is an iterative process and patients should be aware that sleep may initially temporarily worsen, resulting in increased daytime tiredness and sleepiness. The sleep window will continue to be adjusted until sleep is consolidated and of adequate duration, as evidenced by patient's subjective daytime function. A gradual approach (sleep compression) should be used with individuals for whom increased sleepiness would potentially be hazardous.
Relaxation training	Reduces cognitive and physiological arousal.	• Patients are recommended to practice during the day (to build skills) as well as at bedtime. • Types of relaxation include diaphragmatic breathing, guided imagery, autogenic relaxation, progressive muscle relaxation.	A small number of people have a paradoxical reaction of increased anxiety when practising relaxation.

(Table 1) cont.....

Component	Rationale	Description	Notes and Contraindications
Cognitive therapy	Reduces thoughts and emotions which interfere with sleep.	• Provide education on the cognitive behavioral model. • Identify maladaptive daytime and nighttime thoughts related to sleep and encourage self-monitoring to increase awareness of these thoughts. • Cognitive restructuring: unhelpful thoughts are challenged using Socratic questioning and the patient is encouraged to consider alternative perspectives.	Cognitive therapy can be approached in a formal manner through the use of thought records and cognitive restructuring worksheets. It may also be done informally *via* discussions throughout the course of treatment.

INSOMNIA

Insomnia symptoms and insomnia disorder are highly prevalent across the lifespan, though estimates of prevalence vary depending on how insomnia is defined and measured. Insomnia symptoms are present in approximately one-third of adults [7] and children [8]. The prevalence of adults with daytime dysfunction related to insomnia is 10-15%, and 6-10% meet the criteria for insomnia disorder based on DSM or ICSD criteria [7]. Chronic insomnia disorder is defined as difficulty falling or staying asleep at least three times per week for a duration of at least three months, along with accompanying distress or impairment in functioning (*e.g.*, mood, attention, fatigue, occupational/school performance) resulting from the sleep disturbance [9, 10]. In children, insomnia may manifest as resisting going to bed, difficulty sleeping without caregiver reassurance, or requiring objects or activities associated with sleep onset [5].

The likelihood of insomnia increases with age, a finding attributed to multiple factors, including increases in chronic medical conditions, polypharmacy, and sleep disorders such as sleep apnea and restless legs syndrome, which may contribute to insomnia [11, 12]. Decreasing physical function and psychosocial factors such as grief also contribute to insomnia in older adults [12]. Women are approximately 1.5 times as likely as men to experience insomnia and more likely to experience persistent insomnia [13]. Moreover, the relative risk of insomnia for women compared to men increases with age, rising from 1.28 at ages 15-30 to 1.73 by age 65 [14]. The experience of discrimination has been linked to higher rates of insomnia for members of marginalized racial/ethnic groups [15, 16]. Similarly, discrimination and stigma contribute to an increased incidence of sleep problems (insomnia disorder per se has yet to be investigated) among sexual and gender minorities [17, 18].

Medical and/or psychiatric comorbidities are present in most individuals with insomnia [19]. Among adults, medical comorbidities include cancer [20], chronic pain [21], neurological disorders [22, 23], traumatic brain injury [24], cardiovascular disorders [25], and diabetes [26]. Similarly, pediatric insomnia is associated with numerous medical conditions such as chronic pain, gastrointestinal disorders, type 1 diabetes, cystic fibrosis, Down syndrome, headaches, and traumatic brain injury [27]. The likelihood of insomnia increases in tandem with the number of medical comorbidities [28]. Psychiatric comorbidities common among adults with insomnia include depressive, bipolar, anxiety, trauma-related, and substance use disorders [19]. Children and adolescents with anxiety, depressive, and autism spectrum disorders have higher rates of insomnia [8, 27]. The co-occurrence of depression with insomnia is particularly high; among individuals with depression, 90% have insomnia symptoms and 40.5% meet criteria for insomnia disorder [29, 30]. Insomnia is also associated with an increased risk for suicidal ideation and suicidal behaviors [31].

The onset of insomnia can be precipitated by medical or psychiatric symptoms or any other type of life change or stressors, such as those related to work, school, relationships, sociopolitical events, or natural disasters. Regardless of the initial cause, when insomnia becomes chronic, it typically takes on a life of its own and is maintained primarily by the development of additional factors—referred to as perpetuating factors—distinct from those which caused the initial onset. For this reason, chronic insomnia which developed in the context of a medical or psychiatric condition is typically considered an independent (rather than secondary) disorder that requires separate treatment. Insomnia is one of the most common residual symptoms of depression [32] and PTSD [33], persisting even after other symptoms have abated with treatment.

The progression and confluence of factors contributing to chronic insomnia are described by Spielman's "3-P" model of chronic insomnia, which identifies the role of predisposing, precipitating, and perpetuating factors implicated in insomnia [34]. It provides a framework for understanding the role of CBT-I in ameliorating insomnia symptoms and is clinically useful for identifying relevant treatment targets for patients [35]. In this model, predisposing factors represent genetic, physiological, or psychological factors that confer risk for developing insomnia (*e.g.*, family history, neuroticism) [35, 36]. Precipitating factors are the aforementioned life changes/stressors which contribute to the initial onset of insomnia. While precipitating factors often resolve over time, maladaptive cognitive and behavioral changes (perpetuating factors) which occur in reaction to insomnia serve to maintain insomnia over the long-term. Perpetuating factors include sleep-related anxiety or frustration, increased time in bed, conditioned arousal, and increased effort and focus directed toward sleep (*e.g.*, reading about sleep, purchasing products for the purpose of improving sleep, tracking one's sleep, frequently thinking about sleep during the daytime). CBT-I targets these perpetuating factors with systematic changes to behaviors and thought patterns known to maintain chronic insomnia.

GUIDELINES, EVIDENCE, AND OUTCOMES

Multicomponent CBT-I is recommended as the first-line treatment for chronic insomnia in adults according to guidelines from the American Academy of Sleep Medicine [1, 2], American College of Physicians [4], and the European Sleep Research Society [3]. Researchers have also recommended CBT-I as the first line treatment for pediatric insomnia [5, 6]. Compared to medication, CBT-I has similar short-term efficacy but better durability and lower risk for adverse effects. Insomnia remits for approximately half of individuals who receive CBT-I, and a majority (70-80%) experienced improvement in insomnia symptoms [37].

While the efficacy of individual face-to-face treatment has been well-established, evidence also indicates that CBT-I can be successfully delivered *via* telemedicine [38], in groups [39], or *via* digital therapeutics [40, 41]. Furthermore, the efficacy of CBT-I has been demonstrated with individuals who have medical and psychiatric comorbidities [42 - 45], an important finding given the high prevalence of such comorbidities as discussed above. CBT-I may even result in improvement in comorbidities such as depression, anxiety, PTSD, bipolar disorder, and chronic pain [46 - 51].

CBT-I consistently results in improvements in subjective measures of sleep, though improvements demonstrated *via* actigraphy are less consistent and changes in polysomnography are not consistently found [52]. According to meta-analytic reviews, CBT-I improves scores on the Insomnia Severity Index [53] and Pittsburgh Sleep Quality Index [54] as well as on sleep diary-derived measures of sleep continuity, including sleep onset latency, wake time after sleep onset, and sleep efficiency [55, 56]. Moreover, a meta-analysis demonstrated that these improvements are maintained for a year following treatment [57]. Of note, improvement in sleep duration is a less consistent finding.

ASSESSMENT CONSIDERATIONS

Insomnia is diagnosed on the basis of a patient's (and/or caregiver's) subjective report of sleep. Caregiver interviews are vital for the assessment of pediatric insomnia [8]. Objective measures of sleep such as actigraphy, polysomnography, and multiple sleep latency test (MSLT) are not indicated in the routine evaluation of insomnia [1]. Actigraphy is indicated for the assessment of possible circadian rhythm sleep-wake disorders, and polysomnography is needed only if there is suspicion for an underlying sleep disorder such as sleep-related breathing disorder, movement disorder, or violent/injurious parasomnia. Polysomnography may also be recommended if insomnia does not remit with treatment.

The American Academy of Sleep Medicine (AASM) guideline for the evaluation and management of chronic insomnia in adults [1] recommends obtaining a thorough sleep history including insomnia symptoms, pre-sleep conditions, sleep-wake patterns, other sleep-related symptoms, daytime consequences of sleep concerns, and a measure of daytime sleepiness such as the Epworth Sleepiness Scale [58]. AASM further notes the importance of obtaining medical, substance, and psychiatric history. For pediatric insomnia, an interview with both caregiver and child is advised [8].

Two weeks of sleep diaries are recommended to provide data supporting the formal diagnosis of insomnia disorder [1, 8], and sleep diaries are used throughout CBT-I to assess symptom changes, inform recommendations, and monitor adherence to recommendations. Various versions of sleep diaries exist for use in clinical practice. The Consensus Sleep Diary has been developed by an expert panel [59] in order to facilitate the comparison of data across research studies, though this diary may also be used in routine clinical practice. The Consensus Sleep Diary includes a Core diary as well as alternate versions with additional items. The Core diary collects the following variables: bed time, time the patient tried to sleep, sleep onset latency (SOL), number of awakenings, wake time after sleep onset (WASO), final wake time, and sleep quality. From these variables, clinicians can calculate variables used during sleep restriction therapy: total sleep time (TST), total time in bed (TIB), and sleep efficiency (SE, the percent of the time in bed spent sleeping). Additional items in other versions of the Consensus Sleep Diary include time spent napping/dozing, sleep medications, alcohol, and caffeine.

Visual analog sleep diaries represent an alternative to diaries such as the Consensus Sleep Diary. Visual analog diaries such as that created by the American Academy of Sleep Medicine [60] record sleep/wake patterns in a visual format similar to that provided by actigraphy. This format is typically preferred for patients presenting with possible circadian disorders because it allows for rapid visual assessment of sleep timing patterns. In patients with insomnia, visual analog sleep diaries may be preferred if circadian issues are suspected or if sleep is highly irregular or fragmented across the 24-hour day. Visual analog diaries may also be used because of patient or clinician preference, including when this format is deemed easier to comprehend or complete because of a patient's writing abilities or cognitive function.

Differential Diagnosis

Patients with a variety of sleep disorders may report a primary concern of difficulty falling or staying asleep, which is initially suggestive of insomnia. Differential diagnoses to be considered include sleep apnea, restless legs syndrome, and circadian rhythm sleep-wake disorders. The ICSD-3 [9] also notes the potential for insomnia to arise from sleep-disruptive environmental circumstances such as noise, light, movement of a bed partner, or an unsafe environment. However, in these instances, insomnia disorder would not be diagnosed because these factors would disturb the sleep of most individuals. Insomnia disorder is diagnosed only when an individual has difficulty sleeping in the context of a sleep-conducive environment.

For a diagnosis of insomnia disorder, sufficient sleep opportunity must also be present. Insomnia must therefore be distinguished from insufficient sleep syndrome (ISS), a disorder of hypersomnolence characterized by excessive daytime sleepiness (EDS) resulting from insufficient sleep opportunity rather than difficulty sleeping [9]. Individuals with ISS will demonstrate a high sleep efficiency compared to those with insomnia. For example, an individual with insomnia may report spending 9 hours in bed but sleeping only a total of 6 hours because of lengthy sleep onset latency and/or time awake after sleep onset. In contrast, an individual with ISS might report spending only 6 hours in bed but sleeping virtually the entire time. Additionally, they will have daytime periods of irrepressible need to sleep or lapses into sleep. In ISS, the extension of total sleep time resolves daytime sleepiness.

While daytime tiredness or fatigue is a common concern of individuals with insomnia, EDS is not typically present. In fact, some studies have demonstrated that individuals with insomnia have longer sleep latency on the MSLT [61]. Individuals with insomnia will characteristically describe feeling "tired but wired" and report being unable to nap. Thus when EDS is present, a careful assessment must be undertaken to determine whether the patient's sleep complaints are better accounted for by another sleep disorder or whether the patient has insomnia comorbid with another sleep disorder associated with EDS, such as sleep apnea or narcolepsy. Based on a meta-analysis, COMISA (comorbid insomnia and sleep apnea) is fairly common; 35% of individuals with insomnia have comorbid sleep apnea, and 38% of individuals with OSA also have insomnia [62].

GENERAL ASPECTS OF TREATMENT

Individual or group CBT-I is typically provided over the course of 4 to 8 sessions, with sessions occurring every 1 to 2 weeks. Sleep medications can be continued during CBT-I, through reducing or eliminating sleep medication use may be a goal of treatment and can be addressed during the course of CBT-I. Similar to other applications of CBT, CBT-I is time-limited, collaborative, present-focused, and includes key elements of education, self-monitoring, symptom tracking, and between-session homework. Typical components of CBT-I sessions include reviewing sleep diaries, reviewing adherence to recommendations, discussing difficulties with adherence and troubleshooting barriers, adjusting recommendations based on progress (*e.g.*, adjusting the sleep schedule, setting a goal for decreasing medication use), assessing current symptoms either through discussion or administering standardized questionnaires, introducing new skills, and providing instructions for new between-session tasks (*e.g.*, daily relaxation practice, completing thought records).

As noted above in the discussion of CBT-I efficacy, the treatment consistently improves sleep continuity but does not necessarily change sleep duration. Reasonable expectations for treatment include improving the consolidation of one's sleep, improving sleep consistency (*i.e.*, reducing night-to-night variability in sleep), improving sleep quality, and reducing sleep-related anxiety. CBT-I achieves these goals by targeting underlying biological and psychological processes, particularly the homeostatic sleep drive, circadian rhythm, physiological arousal, classical conditioning, operant conditioning, and unhelpful thought patterns. It is important to note that CBT-I does not teach patients how to fall asleep (though strategies such as guided relaxation may be perceived as such). Sleep is a natural process that occurs on its own when conditions—external and internal—are conducive. Thus, while some patients may have the expectation that CBT-I will teach them how to sleep, in actuality CBT-I facilitates the natural process of sleep by regulating the aforementioned processes and eliminating factors that interfere with sleep.

TREATMENT COMPONENTS

Sleep Education

Education about sleep and insomnia is a pivotal initial component of CBT-I. Sufficient knowledge about sleep and insomnia processes primes the patient for the cognitive and behavioral changes that are central to CBT-I. Moreover, this education base enables patients to collaborate with the CBT-I provider to tailor their treatment. Typical components of education include theories of why we sleep, the two-process model of sleep, and expectations for sleep across the lifespan. Sleep architecture and sleep stages are reviewed, emphasising the benefits of a consolidated sleep period. Reviewing these topics serves to correct misconceptions about sleep and explain normal phenomena which patients may have perceived as problematic. For example, patients may have an unrealistic goal of sleeping continuously without waking, though brief awakenings are a normal part of healthy sleep.

During this initial education, definitions of acute and chronic insomnia are reviewed. In explaining how chronic insomnia develops, it is helpful to discuss the 3-P model of chronic insomnia both in a general sense and in relation to the individual patient by identifying their personal predisposing, precipitating, and perpetuating factors. An emphasis on the role of perpetuating factors is essential, as CBT-I primarily targets these variables. This discussion facilitates a patient's understanding of how their insomnia developed and why previous attempts to fix insomnia have not worked (or may have even exacerbated the problem). Doing so lays the groundwork for subsequent discussion of necessary cognitive and behavioral changes.

Sleep Hygiene

Sleep hygiene recommendations and the details of implementation vary widely according to different sources [63, 64]. Moreover, items that overlap with other elements of CBT-I are sometimes included. Recommendations for sleep hygiene commonly focus on substances (caffeine, alcohol, nicotine), exercise, diet, bedroom environment, sleep timing regularity, naps, and evening exposure to light/electronics (see Table **1**). Evidence to support the impact of these recommendations on sleep is mixed, and good sleep hygiene is typically insufficient for the treatment of chronic insomnia. For individuals without insomnia, adherence to these recommendations will help to maintain good sleep. For individuals with chronic insomnia, sleep hygiene is considered a good foundation in order for other CBT-I strategies to be effective. However, sleep hygiene alone is insufficient as a treatment for chronic insomnia [2]. It is beneficial to review sleep hygiene with patients early in treatment to ensure these factors do not negatively impact their sleep. By the time they are engaged in CBT-I, most patients have already implemented some if not all sleep hygiene recommendations. It is important to clarify that sleep hygiene is not equivalent to CBT-I and to reassure patients that failure to significantly improve their insomnia is not evidenced that CBT-I will be ineffective for them.

Stimulus Control

Stimulus control therapy addresses an often concealed perpetuating factor of insomnia: the person's conditioned responses to the bed and bedroom. Difficulty falling asleep or resuming sleep leads to a conditioned association between the bed and wakefulness rather than the bed and sleep. Moreover, months or years of insomnia can also condition the person with insomnia to associate the bed with negative emotions such as anxiety, frustration, anger, and even despair. Additionally, the person may introduce other activities into the bed or bedroom that promote wakefulness (*e.g.*, reading, work, exercising, watching television). Over time, the bedroom will become associated with those activities. The goal of stimulus control therapy is to strengthen the relationship between the bed and the experience of successful sleep onset and maintenance. The original stimulus control instructions proposed by Bootzin included four components [65] which have subsequently undergone slight revision and expansion. The guidelines discussed herein are based on those described by Bootzin and Perlis [66].

(1) Do not lie down to sleep until sleepy. Following this instruction will strengthen the association of sleepiness with the bed. Getting into bed and trying to sleep before experiencing the physiological sensation of sleepiness is a key perpetuating factor for chronic insomnia; patients commonly go to bed at a certain time dictated by the sleep duration they hope to achieve (*i.e.*, "I want 8 hours of sleep and I have to wake at 6 AM, so I need to go to bed by 10 PM"). It is important to go to bed only when sleepy, and education on what it means to be sleepy versus tired, fatigued, or exhausted is typically necessary.

(2) Do not use the bed for anything but sleep or intimacy. Activities such as reading, watching television or working in bed weaken the association between bed and sleep.

(3) If you are unable to fall asleep, get out of bed and go to another room. When out of bed, patients may engage in an activity that is pleasant, calming, and mildly engaging but not stimulating or alerting. These will tend to be the same types of activities that help patients wind down prior to initially going to bed. In order to prevent clock-watching, Bootzin's original instruction did not include guidance on the length of time one should wait before getting out of bed. Bootzin and Perlis subsequently [66] advised getting out of bed if not asleep within "about 10 minutes" and CBT-I protocols (for example, the therapist's manual developed by the U.S. Department of Veterans Affairs [67]) often include suggestions within the range of 15-20 minutes, but it is important to emphasize alertness or the subjective sense of being unable to sleep as the primary cue to get out of bed [68]. Patients should also be advised that this instruction will not necessarily put them back to sleep quickly; instead, it helps to achieve the longer-term goal of strengthening the association between bed and sleep. In order to strengthen this association, patients are instructed to return to bed when sleepy rather than trying to sleep in another location.

(4) If still unable to sleep upon returning to bed, repeat step 3. Do this as many times as needed during the night.

(5) Wake at the same time every day regardless of the amount of sleep obtained the prior night. Bootzin and Perlis advise having at most a 1 hour discrepancy in the wake time of work days and days off, noting that "irregular schedules weaken the association between the cues of the bed and bedroom and sleep."

(6) Avoid napping or dozing. Avoiding sleeping during the day increases the likelihood of falling asleep quickly at night, and this experience strengthens the association of bed/bedroom with falling asleep. Moreover, napping/dozing can associate sleep with places other than the bed. This is a particularly important instruction for patients who find themselves dozing while reading or watching television at night. If needed, steps should be taken to prevent dozing, such as engaging in a more stimulating activity, avoiding prolonged sedentary periods, and adjusting body position or posture.

For some patients, strict adherence to stimulus control therapy is not possible or advised. For example, space limitations such as living in a dorm room or studio apartment may make it impossible to leave the bedroom when unable to sleep. Individuals with mobility limitations or at risk of falls will likely need to remain in the bed in order to ensure safety, though some may be able to safely move to a chair adjacent to the bed. CBT-I providers should take into account an individual patient's barriers or limitations and modify instructions accordingly. Counter control is an alternative to stimulus control which recommends sitting up in bed and engaging in a calming activity until feeling sleepy. Like stimulus control, counter control breaks the unhelpful pattern of lying in bed trying to sleep and dissociates the bed from negative emotions which accompany insomnia. Counter control may also be indicated for patients who experience significant anxiety in reaction to getting out of bed or who tend to get out of bed immediately after waking, which eliminates the opportunity to resume sleeping [68].

Sleep Restriction

Sleep restriction is a technique used to quickly increase homeostatic sleep pressure by limiting patients' time in bed to an amount of time closer to their actual total sleep time [69, 70]. It is a data-driven approach guided by the individual patient's sleep diaries. The goal of sleep restriction is to maximize sleep efficiency and have a patient sleep in a more consolidated period by reducing sleep onset latency and wake after sleep onset. This technique also addresses several perpetuating factors of insomnia, including spending excess time in bed, lack of consistent bed/wake times, and anxiety about falling asleep.

After the patient keeps 1-2 weeks of sleep diaries (2 weeks is ideal but not always available), sleep parameters are calculated, including time in bed (TIB), total sleep time (TST), and sleep efficiency (SE). The calculations for the restricted time in bed are derived from the sleep diaries. There are several approaches to calculate the recommended sleep window. The most commonly used calculation is TIB + 30 minutes (with a 5 hour lower limit of TIB) [71]. The addition of 30 minutes normalizes for patients that some time awake at night is expected, while also providing an adequate sleep window given that individuals with insomnia tend to over-estimate wake time during the night. In follow-up sessions, the sleep window is adjusted based on the most recent week of sleep diaries. Formulas for when and how the sleep window is adjusted vary slightly according to different sources. In actuality, the process of adjusting the sleep window is a collaborative decision taking into account the patient's preferences and willingness to make changes. In common practice, if sleep efficiency < 85%, TIB remains the same or is reduced (the latter particularly if sleep efficiency is lower than 80%). When sleep is well consolidated and sleep efficiency ≥ 85%, TIB can be increased in 15-30 minute intervals every 1-2 weeks. The sleep window is increased only if the patient reports a need for more sleep.

Simulated patient graphs of TST, TIB, and SE can be found in Figs. (**1** and **2**). In weeks 1 and 2, there is a clear disparity between TIB and TST. Based on their most recent TST (5.49 hours) and SE (70%) their TIB for the next 2 weeks was restricted from 8 hours to 6 hours (5.5 hours + 30 minutes). After weeks 3 and 4, their SE was 85% and 92%, respectively, and their TIB was increased 30 minutes to 6.5 hours. After weeks 5 and 6, SE was 92% and 96%, respectively, and TIB was increased to 7 hours. The figure demonstrates that after the initial implementation of sleep restriction, the patient made incremental gains in TST while slowly increasing TIB.

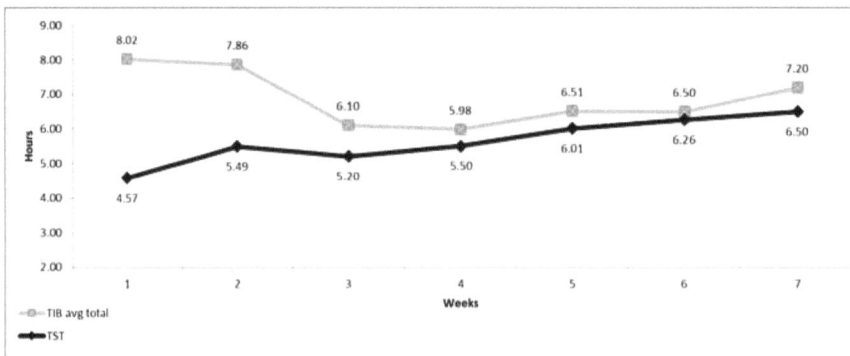

Fig. (1). Simulated sleep diary illustrating changes in time in bed (TIB) and total sleep time (TST) while implementing sleep restriction.

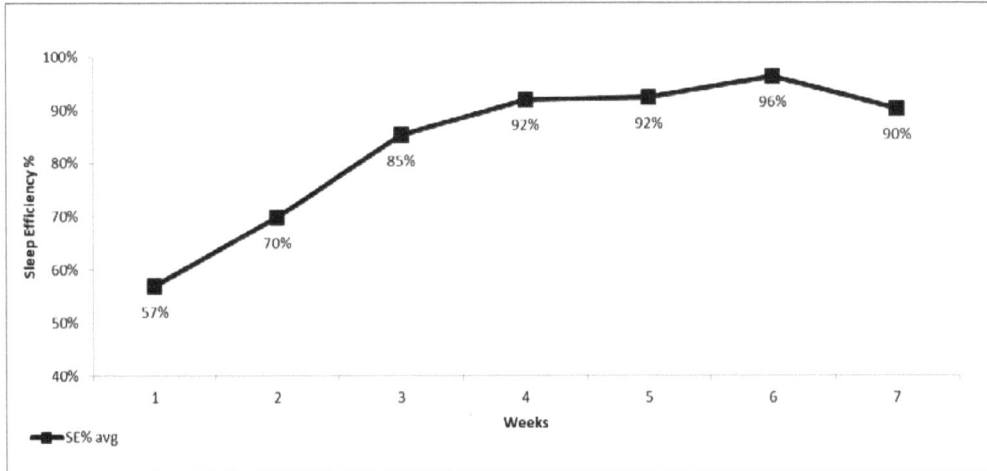

Fig. (2). Simulated sleep diary illustrating changes in sleep efficiency (SE%) while implementing sleep restriction.

It is important to be clear with patients regarding the expectations for future adjustments of sleep and wake times with a thorough explanation of the plan to constrict then expand TIB. The patient should also be made aware of the potential for short-term sleep deprivation at the outset of implementing sleep restriction and to avoid situations where it may be dangerous to be drowsy (*e.g.*, avoid drowsy driving). Short naps should be encouraged if needed for safety, such as before driving or to ensure alertness for caregiving.

Because of the potential for initial sleep deprivation and increased daytime sleepiness, there are several contraindications for sleep restriction. Even temporary sleep deprivation should be avoided in individuals for whom this would likely exacerbate an underlying condition such as epilepsy, bipolar disorder, panic disorder, migraines, or parasomnias. It is also important to avoid exacerbating pre-existing severe daytime sleepiness, for example, with individuals who have comorbid narcolepsy or sleep apnea. Caution in implementing sleep restriction should also be taken when sleep deprivation would be hazardous due to their jobs or daily activities (*e.g.*, truck drivers, machinery workers, ride-share drivers, caregivers). Finally, some patients will report anxiety about the process of sleep restriction or a strong preference to try a more gradual approach. For these and other similarly suited patients, sleep compression is an acceptable alternative to sleep restriction.

In sleep compression [72, 73], the discrepancy between TIB and TST is reduced slowly over the weeks of treatment. Reducing TIB gradually rather than with an initial sharp decrease minimizes the risk of sleep deprivation. The rate at which

TIB is reduced depends on clinical judgment and patient preference. Reducing TIB by 30 minutes per week is a common approach [67]. Lichstein and colleagues [73] proposed reducing the excess TIB in equal increments over a 6-week treatment course, though they note that the length of treatment may be adjusted depending on the magnitude of the TIB-TST discrepancy. If sleep compression was implemented for the patient in the simulated sleep diary in Figs. (1 and 2), TIB could be decreased 30 minutes per week, starting with an initial decrease from 8 hours to 7.5 hours. Fig. (3) shows how TIB and TST would gradually change over time with sleep compression. For both sleep compression and sleep restriction, the end result is the same—highly consolidated sleep as evidenced by sleep efficiency in the goal range of 85-90%.

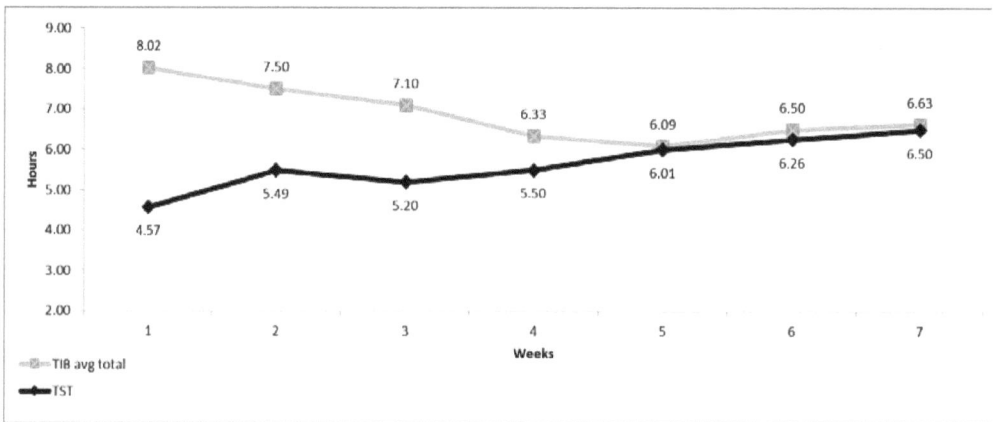

Fig. (3). Simulated sleep diary illustrating changes in time in bed (TIB) and total sleep time (TST) while implementing sleep compression.

Cognitive Therapy

The rationale for the use of cognitive therapy in treating insomnia is that thoughts, beliefs, and attitudes about sleep can be significant perpetuating factors for chronic insomnia. A negative appraisal of the situation (poor sleep, insomnia) leads to emotions that are wake-promoting, which results in a vicious cycle of insomnia and negative thoughts/emotions.

There are often numerous negative or unhelpful thoughts about sleep and insomnia to address during cognitive therapy. Some of the most common are assumptions about the cause of their insomnia ("My insomnia was caused by a chemical imbalance"), unrealistic expectations for sleep ("I keep hearing 8 hours is the magic number for sleep so I need 8 hours"), and worry about sleep's influence on daytime functioning ("I won't be able to go to work if I don't sleep well tonight").

Often dysfunctional cognitions that were present initially during treatment are effectively addressed during education about sleep and insomnia. Unhelpful thoughts may also improve spontaneously while implementing stimulus control and sleep restriction. For example, stimulus control provides a behavioral experiment that challenges the belief "If I get out of bed I'll be awake the rest of the night." Likewise, improvement in sleep quality during sleep restriction provides evidence to counter the belief "I need to be in bed 8 hours in order to get enough sleep." Conversely, there are also patients for whom dysfunctional beliefs and negative emotions are so severe that addressing those thoughts must take precedence over behavioral changes. Sleep diaries may even be counterproductive if these significantly increase sleep-related anxiety. For such patients, cognitive therapy should be prioritized as the initial component of CBT-I.

It is important at the outset of cognitive therapy to introduce a basic framework of the cognitive behavioral model. Situations elicit thoughts or appraisals that lead to an emotional reaction, influencing behavior. Thoughts, emotions, and behaviors are simultaneously interrelated and impact one another. This may lead to an unstructured conversation about unhelpful thoughts the clinician has heard the patient express thus far in treatment.

Often it is valuable for patients to keep a log of thoughts and emotions related to their sleep to discuss in session. For patients with limited awareness of their thoughts, self-monitoring is also a tool to increase awareness. The Dysfunctional Beliefs and Attitudes about Sleep scale [74, 75], which quantifies the extent of these thoughts, can also be useful for identifying specific thoughts which need to be targeted. A typical thought record would have the patients write down thoughts and emotions about sleep throughout the week, including the situations in which they occurred and the behaviors which followed. During sessions, thought records are reviewed and the clinician encourages patients to consider alternative explanations and outcomes using Socratic questioning. Examples include: "What is the evidence for this outcome?", "What is the evidence against this outcome?", "What is the worst possible outcome?", "What is the best possible outcome?", "How would you advise a friend who told you the same thing?", "Can you live through this outcome?", and "Even if this thought is true, is it helpful or unhelpful to focus on it?".

Relaxation

Relaxation techniques are included in CBT-I to reduce somatic and cognitive arousal [76]. Persons with insomnia characteristically experience arousal both at bedtime and during the day. Practice at least twice per day—during the daytime and at bedtime—is typically recommended. Daytime practice should be during a time of low stress in order to facilitate skill development, and it may even be advisable to have patients practice only during the daytime for the first couple of weeks [76]. Explaining the importance of practice and framing relaxation as a skill helps to create an expectation for patients that this technique will help them over time even if it does not appear to have an immediate benefit. Depending on patient preference and clinical judgment, a variety of types of relaxation can be explored, including autogenic relaxation, progressive muscle relaxation, and guided imagery.

CONCLUSION

Multicomponent CBT-I is the first line treatment for chronic insomnia. It produces sustained improvement in insomnia symptoms, including in individuals with psychiatric and medical comorbidities. CBT-I effectively addresses the underlying maladaptive behaviors and thought patterns that perpetuate chronic insomnia. CBT-I typically is delivered over the course of 4-8 sessions and includes the components of sleep education, sleep hygiene instructions, stimulus control, sleep restriction, cognitive therapy, and relaxation training. However, the length of treatment, order of interventions, and emphasis on specific components can be modified to suit the needs of individual patients.

CONSENT FOR PUBLICATION

Not applicable.

CONFLICT OF INTEREST

The authors declare no conflict of interest, financial or otherwise.

ACKNOWLEDGEMENT

Declared none.

REFERENCES

[1]   Schutte-Rodin S, Broch L, Buysse D, Dorsey C, Sateia M. Clinical guideline for the evaluation and management of chronic insomnia in adults. J Clin Sleep Med 2008; 4(5): 487-504.
       [http://dx.doi.org/10.5664/jcsm.27286] [PMID: 18853708]

[2]   Edinger JD, Arnedt JT, Bertisch SM, *et al.* Behavioral and psychological treatments for chronic insomnia disorder in adults: an American Academy of Sleep Medicine clinical practice guideline. J Clin Sleep Med 2021; 17(2): 255-62.
       [http://dx.doi.org/10.5664/jcsm.8986] [PMID: 33164742]

[3]   Riemann D, Baglioni C, Bassetti C, *et al.* European guideline for the diagnosis and treatment of insomnia. J Sleep Res 2017; 26(6): 675-700.
       [http://dx.doi.org/10.1111/jsr.12594] [PMID: 28875581]

[4]   Qaseem A, Kansagara D, Forciea MA, Cooke M, Denberg TD. Management of chronic insomnia

disorder in adults: A clinical practice guideline from the american college of physicians. Ann Intern Med 2016; 165(2): 125-33.
[http://dx.doi.org/10.7326/M15-2175] [PMID: 27136449]

[5]   Himelfarb M, Shatkin JP. Pediatric Insomnia. Child Adolesc Psychiatr Clin N Am 2021; 30(1): 117-29.
[http://dx.doi.org/10.1016/j.chc.2020.08.004] [PMID: 33223056]

[6]   Lunsford-Avery JR, Bidopia T, Jackson L, Sloan JS. Behavioral treatment of insomnia and sleep disturbances in school-aged children and adolescents. Child Adolesc Psychiatr Clin N Am 2021; 30(1): 101-16.
[http://dx.doi.org/10.1016/j.chc.2020.08.006] [PMID: 33223055]

[7]   Morin CM, Jarrin DC. Epidemiology of Insomnia. Sleep Med Clin 2013; 8(3): 281-97.
[http://dx.doi.org/10.1016/j.jsmc.2013.05.002]

[8]   Brown KM, Malow BA. Pediatric Insomnia. Chest 2016; 149(5): 1332-9.
[http://dx.doi.org/10.1378/chest.15-0605] [PMID: 26378738]

[9]   International Classification of Sleep Disorders. 3rd ed., Darien, IL: American Academy of Sleep Medicine 2014.

[10]   World Health Organization (2020) International classification of diseases for mortality and morbidity statistics (11th Revision). https://icd.who.int/browse11/l-m/en

[11]   Patel D, Steinberg J, Patel P. Insomnia in the Elderly: A Review. J Clin Sleep Med 2018; 14(6): 1017-24.
[http://dx.doi.org/10.5664/jcsm.7172] [PMID: 29852897]

[12]   Miner B, Kryger MH. Sleep in the Aging Population. Sleep Med Clin 2017; 12(1): 31-8.
[http://dx.doi.org/10.1016/j.jsmc.2016.10.008] [PMID: 28159095]

[13]   Suh S, Cho N, Zhang J. Sex Differences in Insomnia: from Epidemiology and Etiology to Intervention. Curr Psychiatry Rep 2018; 20(9): 69.
[http://dx.doi.org/10.1007/s11920-018-0940-9] [PMID: 30094679]

[14]   Zhang B, Wing Y-K. Sex differences in insomnia: a meta-analysis. Sleep 2006; 29(1): 85-93.
[http://dx.doi.org/10.1093/sleep/29.1.85] [PMID: 16453985]

[15]   Bethea TN, Zhou ES, Schernhammer ES, Castro-Webb N, Cozier YC, Rosenberg L. Perceived racial discrimination and risk of insomnia among middle-aged and elderly Black women. Sleep 2020; 43(1): zsz208.
[http://dx.doi.org/10.1093/sleep/zsz208] [PMID: 31555803]

[16]   Cheng P, Cuellar R, Johnson DA, *et al.* Racial discrimination as a mediator of racial disparities in insomnia disorder. Sleep Heal 2020.
[http://dx.doi.org/10.1016/j.sleh.2020.07.007]

[17]   Butler ES, McGlinchey E, Juster RP. Sexual and gender minority sleep: A narrative review and suggestions for future research. J Sleep Res 2020; 29(1): e12928.
[http://dx.doi.org/10.1111/jsr.12928] [PMID: 31626363]

[18]   Patterson CJ, Potter EC. Sexual orientation and sleep difficulties: a review of research. Sleep Heal. 2019; 5: pp. (3)227-35.
[http://dx.doi.org/10.1016/j.sleh.2019.02.004]

[19]   Raglan GB, Swanson LM, Arnedt JT. Cognitive Behavioral Therapy for Insomnia in Patients with Medical and Psychiatric Comorbidities. Sleep Med Clin 2019; 14(2): 167-75.
[http://dx.doi.org/10.1016/j.jsmc.2019.01.001] [PMID: 31029184]

[20]   Hoang HTX, Molassiotis A, Chan CW, Nguyen TH, Liep Nguyen V. New-onset insomnia among cancer patients undergoing chemotherapy: prevalence, risk factors, and its correlation with other symptoms. Sleep Breath 2020; 24(1): 241-51.

[http://dx.doi.org/10.1007/s11325-019-01839-x] [PMID: 31016572]

[21]   Finan PH, Goodin BR, Smith MT. The association of sleep and pain: an update and a path forward. J Pain 2013; 14(12): 1539-52.
[http://dx.doi.org/10.1016/j.jpain.2013.08.007] [PMID: 24290442]

[22]   Malhotra RK. Neurodegenerative Disorders and Sleep. Sleep Med Clin 2018; 13(1): 63-70.
[http://dx.doi.org/10.1016/j.jsmc.2017.09.006] [PMID: 29412984]

[23]   Mayer G, Jennum P, Riemann D, Dauvilliers Y. Insomnia in central neurologic diseases--occurrence and management. Sleep Med Rev 2011; 15(6): 369-78.
[http://dx.doi.org/10.1016/j.smrv.2011.01.005] [PMID: 21481621]

[24]   Barshikar S, Bell KR. Sleep Disturbance After TBI. Curr Neurol Neurosci Rep 2017; 17(11): 87.
[http://dx.doi.org/10.1007/s11910-017-0792-4] [PMID: 28933033]

[25]   Javaheri S, Redline S. Insomnia and risk of cardiovascular disease. Chest 2017; 152(2): 435-44.
[http://dx.doi.org/10.1016/j.chest.2017.01.026] [PMID: 28153671]

[26]   Ogilvie RP, Patel SR. The Epidemiology of Sleep and Diabetes. Curr Diab Rep 2018; 18(10): 82.
[http://dx.doi.org/10.1007/s11892-018-1055-8] [PMID: 30120578]

[27]   Mindell JA, Owens JA. A clinical guide to pediatric sleep: diagnosis and management of sleep problems. 3rd ed., Philadelphia, PA: Wolters Kluwer 2015.

[28]   Taylor DJ, Mallory LJ, Lichstein KL, Durrence HH, Riedel BW, Bush AJ. Comorbidity of chronic insomnia with medical problems. Sleep 2007; 30(2): 213-8.
[http://dx.doi.org/10.1093/sleep/30.2.213] [PMID: 17326547]

[29]   Stewart R, Besset A, Bebbington P, *et al.* Insomnia comorbidity and impact and hypnotic use by age group in a national survey population aged 16 to 74 years. Sleep 2006; 29(11): 1391-7.
[http://dx.doi.org/10.1093/sleep/29.11.1391] [PMID: 17162985]

[30]   Khurshid KA. Comorbid Insomnia and Psychiatric Disorders: An Update. Innov Clin Neurosci 2018; 15(3-4): 28-32.
[PMID: 29707424]

[31]   Bishop TM, Walsh PG, Ashrafioun L, Lavigne JE, Pigeon WR. Sleep, suicide behaviors, and the protective role of sleep medicine. Sleep Med 2020; 66: 264-70.
[http://dx.doi.org/10.1016/j.sleep.2019.07.016] [PMID: 31727433]

[32]   Carney CE, Segal ZV, Edinger JD, Krystal AD. A comparison of rates of residual insomnia symptoms following pharmacotherapy or cognitive-behavioral therapy for major depressive disorder. J Clin Psychiatry 2007; 68(2): 254-60.
[http://dx.doi.org/10.4088/JCP.v68n0211] [PMID: 17335324]

[33]   Belleville G, Guay S, Marchand A. Persistence of sleep disturbances following cognitive-behavior therapy for posttraumatic stress disorder. J Psychosom Res 2011; 70(4): 318-27.
[http://dx.doi.org/10.1016/j.jpsychores.2010.09.022] [PMID: 21414451]

[34]   Spielman AJ, Caruso LS, Glovinsky PB. A behavioral perspective on insomnia treatment. Psychiatr Clin North Am 1987; 10(4): 541-53.
[http://dx.doi.org/10.1016/S0193-953X(18)30532-X] [PMID: 3332317]

[35]   Buysse DJ, Germain A, Hall M, Monk TH, Nofzinger EA. A neurobiological model of insomnia. Drug Discov Today Dis Models 2011; 8(4): 129-37.
[http://dx.doi.org/10.1016/j.ddmod.2011.07.002] [PMID: 22081772]

[36]   Harvey C-J, Gehrman P, Espie CA. Who is predisposed to insomnia: a review of familial aggregation, stress-reactivity, personality and coping style. Sleep Med Rev 2014; 18(3): 237-47.
[http://dx.doi.org/10.1016/j.smrv.2013.11.004] [PMID: 24480386]

[37]   Morin CM, Davidson JR, Beaulieu-Bonneau S. Cognitive and behavioral therapies for insomnia I: Approaches and efficacy.Princ Pract Sleep Med. 6th ed. Philadelphia, PA: Elsevier 2017; pp. 804-13.

[http://dx.doi.org/10.1016/B978-0-323-24288-2.00085-4]

[38]   Arnedt JT, Conroy DA, Mooney A, Furgal A, Sen A, Eisenberg D. Telemedicine versus face-to-face delivery of cognitive behavioral therapy for insomnia: a randomized controlled noninferiority trial. Sleep 2021; 44(1): zsaa136.
[http://dx.doi.org/10.1093/sleep/zsaa136] [PMID: 32658298]

[39]   Koffel EA, Koffel JB, Gehrman PR. A meta-analysis of group cognitive behavioral therapy for insomnia. Sleep Med Rev 2015; 19: 6-16.
[http://dx.doi.org/10.1016/j.smrv.2014.05.001] [PMID: 24931811]

[40]   Soh HL, Ho RC, Ho CS, Tam WW. Efficacy of digital cognitive behavioural therapy for insomnia: a meta-analysis of randomised controlled trials. Sleep Med 2020; 75: 315-25.
[http://dx.doi.org/10.1016/j.sleep.2020.08.020] [PMID: 32950013]

[41]   Zachariae R, Lyby MS, Ritterband LM, O'Toole MS. Efficacy of internet-delivered cognitive-behavioral therapy for insomnia - A systematic review and meta-analysis of randomized controlled trials. Sleep Med Rev 2016; 30: 1-10.
[http://dx.doi.org/10.1016/j.smrv.2015.10.004] [PMID: 26615572]

[42]   Taylor DJ, Pruiksma KE. Cognitive and behavioural therapy for insomnia (CBT-I) in psychiatric populations: a systematic review. Int Rev Psychiatry 2014; 26(2): 205-13.
[http://dx.doi.org/10.3109/09540261.2014.902808] [PMID: 24892895]

[43]   Geiger-Brown JM, Rogers VE, Liu W, Ludeman EM, Downton KD, Diaz-Abad M. Cognitive behavioral therapy in persons with comorbid insomnia: A meta-analysis. Sleep Med Rev 2015; 23: 54-67.
[http://dx.doi.org/10.1016/j.smrv.2014.11.007] [PMID: 25645130]

[44]   Wu JQ, Appleman ER, Salazar RD, Ong JC. Cognitive Behavioral Therapy for Insomnia Comorbid With Psychiatric and Medical Conditions: A Meta-analysis. JAMA Intern Med 2015; 175(9): 1461-72.
[http://dx.doi.org/10.1001/jamainternmed.2015.3006] [PMID: 26147487]

[45]   Zhou F-C, Yang Y, Wang Y-Y, *et al.* Cognitive Behavioural Therapy for Insomnia Monotherapy in Patients with Medical or Psychiatric Comorbidities: a Meta-Analysis of Randomized Controlled Trials. Psychiatr Q 2020; 91(4): 1209-24.
[http://dx.doi.org/10.1007/s11126-020-09820-8] [PMID: 32860556]

[46]   Ye Y-Y, Zhang Y-F, Chen J, *et al.* Internet-Based Cognitive Behavioral Therapy for Insomnia (ICBT-i) Improves Comorbid Anxiety and Depression-A Meta-Analysis of Randomized Controlled Trials. PLoS One 2015; 10(11): e0142258.
[http://dx.doi.org/10.1371/journal.pone.0142258] [PMID: 26581107]

[47]   Ho FY-Y, Chan CS, Tang KN-S. Cognitive-behavioral therapy for sleep disturbances in treating posttraumatic stress disorder symptoms: A meta-analysis of randomized controlled trials. Clin Psychol Rev 2016; 43: 90-102.
[http://dx.doi.org/10.1016/j.cpr.2015.09.005] [PMID: 26439674]

[48]   Harvey AG, Soehner AM, Kaplan KA, *et al.* Treating insomnia improves mood state, sleep, and functioning in bipolar disorder: a pilot randomized controlled trial. J Consult Clin Psychol 2015; 83(3): 564-77.
[http://dx.doi.org/10.1037/a0038655] [PMID: 25622197]

[49]   Selvanathan J, Pham C, Nagappa M, *et al.* Cognitive behavioral therapy for insomnia in patients with chronic pain - A systematic review and meta-analysis of randomized controlled trials. Sleep Med Rev 2021; 60: 101460.
[http://dx.doi.org/10.1016/j.smrv.2021.101460] [PMID: 33610967]

[50]   Ho KKN, Ferreira PH, Pinheiro MB, *et al.* Sleep interventions for osteoarthritis and spinal pain: a systematic review and meta-analysis of randomized controlled trials. Osteoarthritis Cartilage 2019; 27(2): 196-218.
[http://dx.doi.org/10.1016/j.joca.2018.09.014] [PMID: 30342087]

[51]   Ballesio A, Aquino MRJV, Feige B, *et al.* The effectiveness of behavioural and cognitive behavioural therapies for insomnia on depressive and fatigue symptoms: A systematic review and network meta-analysis. Sleep Med Rev 2018; 37: 114-29.
[http://dx.doi.org/10.1016/j.smrv.2017.01.006] [PMID: 28619248]

[52]   Mitchell LJ, Bisdounis L, Ballesio A, Omlin X, Kyle SD. The impact of cognitive behavioural therapy for insomnia on objective sleep parameters: A meta-analysis and systematic review. Sleep Med Rev 2019; 47: 90-102.
[http://dx.doi.org/10.1016/j.smrv.2019.06.002] [PMID: 31377503]

[53]   Bastien CH, Vallières A, Morin CM, Vallières A, Morin CM. Validation of the Insomnia Severity Index as an outcome measure for insomnia research. Sleep Med 2001; 2(4): 297-307.
[http://dx.doi.org/10.1016/S1389-9457(00)00065-4] [PMID: 11438246]

[54]   Buysse DJ, Reynolds CF III, Monk TH, Berman SR, Kupfer DJ. The Pittsburgh Sleep Quality Index: a new instrument for psychiatric practice and research. Psychiatry Res 1989; 28(2): 193-213.
[http://dx.doi.org/10.1016/0165-1781(89)90047-4] [PMID: 2748771]

[55]   Trauer JM, Qian MY, Doyle JS, Rajaratnam SMW, Cunnington D. Cognitive Behavioral Therapy for Chronic Insomnia: A Systematic Review and Meta-analysis. Ann Intern Med 2015; 163(3): 191-204.
[http://dx.doi.org/10.7326/M14-2841] [PMID: 26054060]

[56]   van Straten A, van der Zweerde T, Kleiboer A, Cuijpers P, Morin CM, Lancee J. Cognitive and behavioral therapies in the treatment of insomnia: A meta-analysis. Sleep Med Rev 2018; 38: 3-16.
[http://dx.doi.org/10.1016/j.smrv.2017.02.001] [PMID: 28392168]

[57]   van der Zweerde T, Bisdounis L, Kyle SD, Lancee J, van Straten A. Cognitive behavioral therapy for insomnia: A meta-analysis of long-term effects in controlled studies. Sleep Med Rev 2019; 48: 101208.
[http://dx.doi.org/10.1016/j.smrv.2019.08.002] [PMID: 31491656]

[58]   Johns MW. A new method for measuring daytime sleepiness: the Epworth sleepiness scale. Sleep 1991; 14(6): 540-5.
[http://dx.doi.org/10.1093/sleep/14.6.540] [PMID: 1798888]

[59]   Carney CE, Buysse DJ, Ancoli-Israel S, *et al.* The consensus sleep diary: standardizing prospective sleep self-monitoring. Sleep 2012; 35(2): 287-302.
[http://dx.doi.org/10.5665/sleep.1642] [PMID: 22294820]

[60]   American   Academy   of   Sleep   Medicine   Two   week   sleep   diary
http://sleepeducation.org/docs/default-document-library/sleep-diary.pdf

[61]   Roehrs TA, Randall S, Harris E, Maan R, Roth T. MSLT in primary insomnia: stability and relation to nocturnal sleep. Sleep 2011; 34(12): 1647-52.
[http://dx.doi.org/10.5665/sleep.1426] [PMID: 22131601]

[62]   Zhang Y, Ren R, Lei F, *et al.* Worldwide and regional prevalence rates of co-occurrence of insomnia and insomnia symptoms with obstructive sleep apnea: A systematic review and meta-analysis. Sleep Med Rev 2019; 45: 1-17.
[http://dx.doi.org/10.1016/j.smrv.2019.01.004] [PMID: 30844624]

[63]   Stepanski EJ, Wyatt JK. Use of sleep hygiene in the treatment of insomnia. Sleep Med Rev 2003; 7(3): 215-25.
[http://dx.doi.org/10.1053/smrv.2001.0246] [PMID: 12927121]

[64]   Irish LA, Kline CE, Gunn HE, Buysse DJ, Hall MH. The role of sleep hygiene in promoting public health: A review of empirical evidence. Sleep Med Rev 2015; 22: 23-36.
[http://dx.doi.org/10.1016/j.smrv.2014.10.001] [PMID: 25454674]

[65]   Bootzin RR. Effects of self-control procedures for insomnia. Am J Clin Biofeedback 1972; 2: 70-7.

[66]   Bootzin RR, Perlis ML. 2011; pp. Stimulus Control Therapy.In: Perlis ML, Aloia MS, Kuhn B (eds)

Behav Treat Sleep Disord Academic Press. 21-30.
[http://dx.doi.org/10.1016/B978-0-12-381522-4.00002-X]

[67] Manber R, Friedman L, Siebern AT, *et al.* Cognitive Behavioral Therapy for Insomnia in Veterans: Therapist Manual. Washington, D.C.: U.S. Department of Veterans Affairs 2014.

[68] Manber R, Carney C. Treatment plans and interventions for insomnia: A case formulation approach. New York: Guilford Press 2015.

[69] Spielman AJ, Saskin P, Thorpy MJ. Treatment of chronic insomnia by restriction of time in bed. Sleep 1987; 10(1): 45-56.
[PMID: 3563247]

[70] Spielman AJ, Yang CM, Glovinsky PB. 2011; pp. Sleep Restriction Therapy.In: Perlis M, Aloia MS, Kuhn B (eds) Behav Treat Sleep Disord Academic Press. 9-19.
[http://dx.doi.org/10.1016/B978-0-12-381522-4.00001-8]

[71] Edinger JD, Carney CE. Overcoming Insomnia: A Cognitive-Behavioral Therapy Approach, Therapist Guide. 2nd ed., Oxford University Press 2014.

[72] Lichstein KL, Riedel BW, Wilson NM, Lester KW, Aguillard RN. Relaxation and sleep compression for late-life insomnia: a placebo-controlled trial. J Consult Clin Psychol 2001; 69(2): 227-39.
[http://dx.doi.org/10.1037/0022-006X.69.2.227] [PMID: 11393600]

[73] Lichstein KL, Thomas SJ, McCurry SM. 2011; pp. Sleep Compression.In: Perlis M, Aloia MS, Kuhn B (eds) Behav Treat Sleep Disord Academic Press. 55-9.
[http://dx.doi.org/10.1016/B978-0-12-381522-4.00005-5]

[74] Morin CM. Dysfunctional beliefs and attitudes about sleep: Preliminary scale development and description. Behav Ther 1994; 17: 163-4.

[75] Morin CM, Vallières A, Ivers H. Dysfunctional beliefs and attitudes about sleep (DBAS): validation of a brief version (DBAS-16). Sleep 2007; 30(11): 1547-54.
[http://dx.doi.org/10.1093/sleep/30.11.1547] [PMID: 18041487]

[76] Lichstein KL, Taylor DJ, McCrae CS, Thomas SJ. Relaxation for Insomnia. In: Perlis M, Aloia M, Kuhn B. Behavioral Treatments for Sleep Disorders. Practical Resources for the Mental Health Professional. 2011, pp. 45-54.
[http://dx.doi.org/10.1016/B978-0-12-381522-4.00004-3]

CHAPTER 10

Silver Sleepers: Sleep and Ageing

Sonia Ali Malik[1,*]

[1] *University of Utah, Salt Lake City, Utah. USA*

Abstract: Sleep difficulties and disorders are among the most prevalent problems of ageing. In addition to changes in sleep duration and quality, sleep architecture also changes as age progresses. Age by itself does not result in sleep disorders; rather, these changes are associated with psychosocial and health factors in the elderly such as the existence of multiple comorbidities, polypharmacy, and age-related changes in circadian rhythm. Older adults have increased prevalence of various primary sleep disorders, including restless leg syndrome, insomnia, sleep-disordered breathing, circadian rhythm disturbances and periodic limb syndrome. Challenges in identifying, diagnosing, and treating sleep disorders in older adults with dementia also exist, which further complicates the management of sleep disorders in these patients. Poor sleep not only impacts the quality of life and cognitive functioning but is also associated with increased morbidity and mortality and thus requires careful screening and assessment in the elderly population.

Keywords: Ageing, Comorbidities, Dementia, Depression, Geriatric, Insomnia, Restless leg Syndrome, Sleep disorders, Sleep, Sleep Stages, Sleep-disordered breathing.

INTRODUCTION

The population of older adults continues to grow rapidly. In the U.S., there are more than 46 million older adults age 65 and older and the number is expected to grow to almost 90 million by 2050 [1]. Sleep disorders in an ageing society constitutes a significant public health problem. Fifty percent of people aged 55 years and older have trouble sleeping, including initiating and maintaining sleep [2]. Sleep disorders and sleeping difficulty are among the most poorly addressed problems of ageing. In a National Institute on Ageing study of over 9,000 individuals aged 65 years and older, over one-half of the men and women reported at least one chronic sleep complaint [3]. Another cross-sectional study conducted on 360 people aged 60 or older, which utilized a self-made structured

---

* **Corresponding author Sonia Ali Malik:** University of Utah, Salt Lake City, Utah. USA; Tel: 8015872865; Fax: +8015873349; E-mail: u6033036@utah.edu

Imran H. Iftikhar and Ali I. Musani (Eds.)

questionnaire and interview, concluded that 70.3% of subjects suffered from sleep disorders and 81.81% of them had primary insomnia [4]. While increasing age is associated with changes in sleep architecture, age by itself does not result in sleep disorders; rather, these changes are associated with psychosocial and health factors in the elderly [5]. There are several factors that increase sleep disturbance with age, including polypharmacy, the prevalence of various medical and psychiatric conditions, age-related changes in circadian rhythms, and other environmental factors [6]. Although sleep disorders are prevalent in all age groups, older adults are particularly at higher risk with increased prevalence of sleep-disordered breathing, restless legs syndrome, periodic limb movements of sleep, sleep behaviour disorders, insomnia, and circadian rhythm disturbances [6]. Given the impact of sleep on quality of life, cognitive functioning and a growing body of research linking poor sleep with adverse health outcomes in the elderly; identifying sleep disorders in older adults is crucial to their overall wellbeing. Sleep disorders not only affect the overall quality of life, these disorders are also associated with increased mortality in the elderly [7].

AGE-RELATED CHANGES IN SLEEP

Ageing is associated with well-characterized changes in sleep architecture, sleep quality and sleep timing. Ageing is linked to a decreased ability to maintain sleep (increased awakening after sleep onset), advanced sleep timing (early to bed, early to rise), decreased sleep duration, increased sleep latency (increases time to sleep onset), sleep fragmentation, decreased sleep efficiency and decrease in deep sleep (slow-wave sleep).

Sleep Initiation and Maintenance

Various studies suggest a decrease in the ability to initiate and maintain sleep with ageing. Sleep in the older population is believed to be more disrupted [increased wake after sleep onset (WASO)] with an increase in duration to initiate and resume sleep after an awakening (increased sleep latency) (Fig. **1**). A meta-analysis by Floyd *et al.* that pooled 41 published studies indicated that the ability to initiate sleep decreases with age; however, the magnitude of this change is small. Majority of the studies included in Floyd *et al.* meta-analysis utilized polysomnography (PSG) to measure the objective increase in sleep latency (SL) [8]. The meta-analysis also supported a positive correlation between age and increased waking frequency and duration [8]. Another meta-analysis by Ohayon *et al.* demonstrated a modest but significant change in sleep latency with age; however, these changes were subtle when compared over different age groups [9]. A mathematical model that represented 258 subjects aged 17 to 91 years, indicated a non-linear increase in sleep latency with age, suggesting an increase in sleep latency until about age 30, remaining steady from ages 30 until about 50 years, and then increasing progressively after the age of 50 years [10].

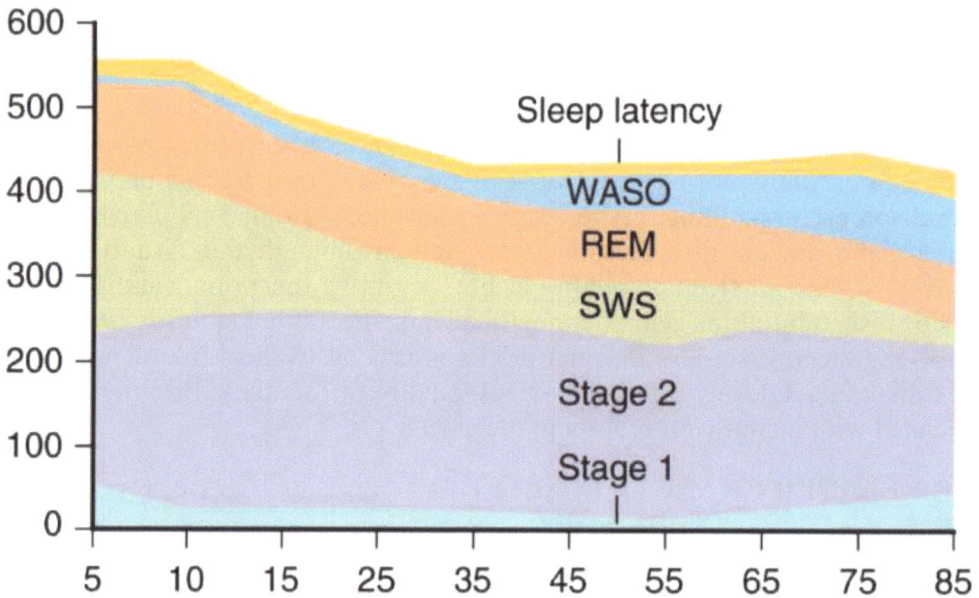

Fig. (1). Age-related trends for stage 1 sleep, stage 2 sleep, slow wave sleep (SWS), rapid eye movement (REM) sleep, wake after sleep onset (WASO) and sleep latency (in minutes).From Ohayon M, Carskadon MA, Guilleminault C, Vitiello MV. Meta-Analysis of Quantitative Sleep Parameters From Childhood to Old Age in Healthy Individuals: Developing Normative Sleep Values Across the Human Lifespan Maurice. Sleep. 2004;27:1255-1273.

Sleep Efficiency

Sleep efficiency declines slowly with age. A meta-analysis by Ohayon and colleagues found a larger effect size of this decline in studies that compared young with elderly adults and young with middle-aged subjects [8].

Total Sleep Time

Compared with younger adults, older adults are known to have a decrease in total sleep time (TST) with age. Campbell and Murphy used the disentrainment protocol to study spontaneous sleep across young, middle-aged, and older adults, with the goal of determining the duration of spontaneous sleep. An effect of age was identified on total sleep time with older subjects obtaining 2.4 hours (hr) less sleep per 24hr compared with young subjects (old: 8.13h/24hr versus young: 10.53h/24 hr *versus* middle-age subjects 9.06 h/24 hr) [11]. Numerous meta-analyses further support the evidence of a substantial decline in TST over the adult lifespan [8, 12]. SIESTA project gathered data from ages 20-90 and found a reduction in total sleep time objectively as measured by polysomnography [13]. Their data showed a strong reduction in total sleep time with an age of about 8 minutes per decade for males and 10 minutes for females [13] (Fig. **2**). The decrease in sleep duration has also been linked with a decline in cognitive function in older adults [14].

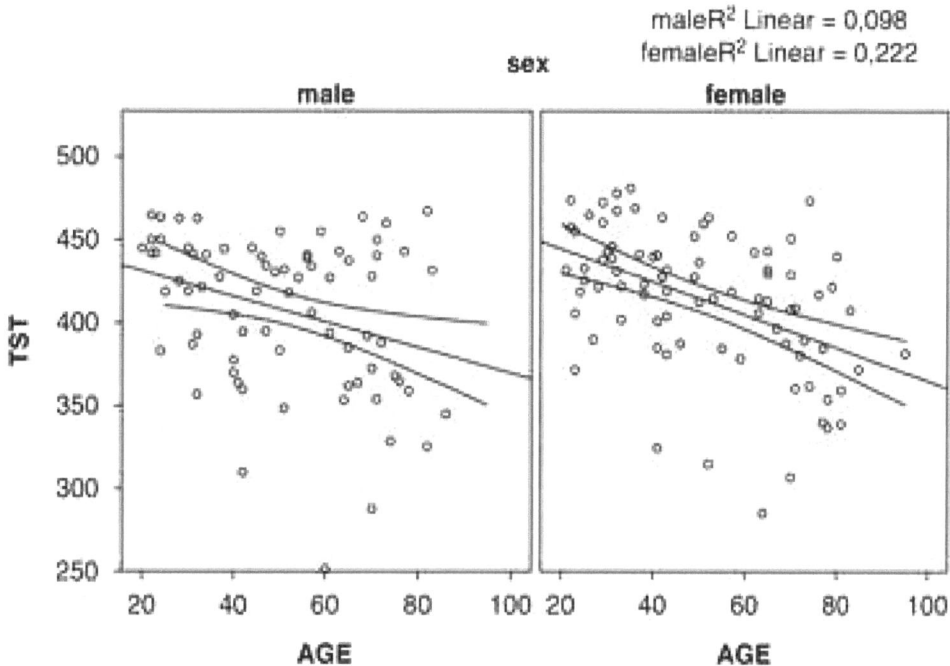

Fig. (2). Age-dependency of total sleep time (TST, in minutes) for male (left) and female (right) subjects. Lines show the estimated regression lines with 95% confidence intervals.From Dorffner G, Vitr M, Anderer P. The effects of aging on sleep architecture in healthy subjects. Adv Exp Med Biol. *2015;821:93-100.*

Sleep Schedule

Older adults tend to have sleepiness earlier in the evening, wake up earlier in the morning and normally encounter a phase advance of sleep schedule [15]. A reduction in responsiveness and exposure to light has been hypothesized as a possible reason for the advanced circadian phase in older adults [16]. Additionally, with age, there is a reduced amplitude of circadian rhythmicity in endogenous core body temperature and melatonin release. Circadian rhythm of plasma melatonin secretion occurs at a significantly earlier clock hour in older subjects than in young adults [17] (Fig. **3**). This phase advance in circadian pacemaker timing may not be the only factor affecting the early bedtimes and wake times. In addition to the usual age-related phase advance in the timing of the circadian plasma melatonin rhythm, older subjects, in comparison to young adults not only wake up earlier relative to clock time but also earlier relative to the phase of the melatonin rhythm [17 - 19].

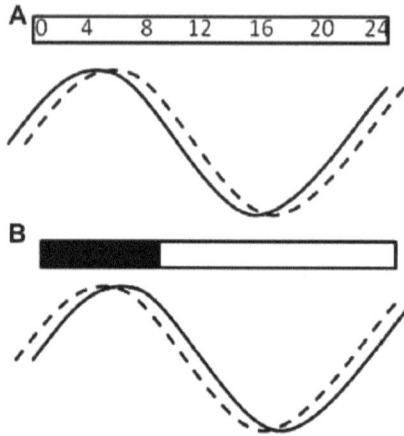

Fig. (3). Schematic illustrating the altered phase in older adults. A. When compared with clock time, the phase of both core body temperature and plasma melatonin is earlier in older adults (solid line) than it is in young adults (dashed line). B. When compared with their usual sleep-wake and dark-light timing, the phase of both core body temperature and plasma melatonin is later with respect to sleep/darkness in older adults (solid line) than it is in young adults (dashed line).From Duffy JF, Zitting K–M, Chinoy ED. Aging and circadian rhythms. Sleep medicine clinics. 2015; 10(4):423–434.

SLEEP STAGES

Sleep architecture evolves with ageing. Based on current literature, the following changes in sleep stages is typically observed with ageing (Table **1**). 1) The proportion of time spent in NREM sleep stage N1 and N2 increases with age [20]. 2) Restorative slow wave sleep (SWS) stage N3 decreases with age [20]. 3) Decrease in REM sleep percentage and REM latency is observed with ageing [20]. The proportion of REM sleep typically declines with ageing; however, this decline is not significant after age 60 [9]. A meta-analysis by Ohayon's *et al.* concluded that the percentage of REM sleep first increases from childhood to adolescence, then decreases between young and middle-aged adults, and remains unchanged in subjects aged 60 years of age or more. Stage N1 sleep increases across all of adulthood. There was a decrement observed by investigators in REM latency with age which was found to be very prone to drug/alcohol use, psychiatric and sleep disorders. The magnitude of this decrement in REM latency was larger in elderly women compared to elderly men which may point towards a gender-related difference in sleep stages. Likewise, the effect size of the decrease in stage N1 sleep was larger in women compared to men. SWS was similar in both genders [9].

Table 1. Age Related Changes in Sleep.

Changes in Sleep Parameters with Age	
Sleep Latency	Increase
Sleep Maintenance	Decrease
Total Sleep Time (TST)	Decrease
Sleep Efficiency	Decrease
Stage N1 sleep %	Increase
Stage N2 sleep %	Increase
Stage N3 sleep %	Decrease
REM sleep % and REM Latency	Decrease
Wake after sleep onset	Increase

COMMON SLEEP DISORDERS IN THE ELDERLY

Insomnia

Introduction

Insomnia is the most prevalent sleep disorder in the older population [3]. More than half of the older adults complain about difficulty initiating or maintaining sleep. Among older individuals with insomnia, difficulty in sleep maintenance is most prevalent (50% to 70%), followed by difficulty in initiating sleep (35% to 60%) and nonrestorative sleep (20% to 25%) [21]. The prevalence of insomnia is difficult to determine despite vast literature as epidemiological studies have used variable criteria to define insomnia [22]. In a review of more than 50 epidemiological studies, the prevalence of insomnia symptoms in the community-dwelling general population was estimated at 10–48% [22 - 24]. In comparison, the prevalence of insomnia in community-dwelling older population was as high as 11.7% to 70%. The prevalence of insomnia in the older population is much higher in institutional settings compared to community-living older adults. The Established Populations for Epidemiologic Studies of the Elderly (EPESE) included 9,282 community-dwelling adults aged 65 and older and found that 43% of participants reported difficulty with sleep onset or maintenance, while 25% reported napping [22]. These findings were confirmed in the National Sleep Foundation's (NSF) 2003 Sleep in America Poll, which reported one or more symptoms of insomnia in 46% of individuals aged 65–74 years and 50% of those aged 75–84 years, with corresponding rates for napping of 39% and 46%.In the elderly wide ranging age-related medical/psychiatric conditions, polypharmacy, as well as age-related changes in sleep structure and sleep disorders, may explain the higher prevalence of insomnia. It is estimated that 93% of the elderly have one or more comorbid conditions contributing to insomnia most commonly depression, chronic pain, cancer, chronic obstructive pulmonary disease, cardiovascular diseases, medication use, and other factors associated with ageing [25, 26] (Table **2**). A 2003 National Sleep Foundation survey of community-dwelling men and women aged 55-84 years found sleep complaints common in older adults resulting from their comorbidities and not ageing per se [27].

Table 2. Causes of Insomnia in the older population.

Causes of Insomnia in Older Population
1) Medical Conditions
o Lung and Heart disorders affecting breathing such as chronic obstructive pulmonary disease, heart failure, coronary artery disease, *etc* o Gastrointestinal conditions like gastroesophageal reflux disease, constipation/diarrhoea o Urinary problems that cause increased urination at night; such as incontinence, enlarged prostate, overactive bladder o Mood problems such as depression and anxiety o Painful conditions, including osteoarthritis o Neurodegenerative disorders such as Cerebrovascular Disease, Alzheimer's and Parkinson's
2) Medications
o Beta-Blockers (nightmares) o Diuretics(nocturia) o Anti-Parkinson's drugs o Anticholinergics o Anti-depressants (may worsen RLS) o Alcohol (may increase arousal frequency) o Stimulants o Corticosteroids.
3) Psychiatric Conditions
o Depression o Anxiety o Psychosis
4) Primary Sleep Disorders
o Sleep Disordered Breathing o Restless Leg Syndrome o Circadian rhythm disorders (commonly advanced sleep wake phase disorder) o REM behavior disorder
5) Psychosocial and Behavioral
o Daytime Naps o Bereavement o Financial stresses o Lack of exercise o Poor sleep hygiene

Spielman *et al.* proposed the 3P model of insomnia, which includes the following components:

i. Predisposing factors: physiological, psychological, or genetic/biological predispositions that increase the risk of insomnia (gender differences, smoking, alcohol use, *etc.*). Women older than 45 years compared to men are 1.7 times more likely to have insomnia [24, 28].
ii. Precipitating factors: environmental, physiological, or psychological stressors that prompt the onset of insomnia (life events *etc.*). Older individuals with depression and anxiety have a higher prevalence of insomnia [25, 28].
iii. Perpetuating factors: environmental, behavioral, psychological, and physiological factors that maintain insomnia (decrease physical activity in elderly, social isolation).

Consequences of Insomnia in Elderly

Insomnia in the older population is associated with not only increased morbidity and mortality but also impaired physical function and increased fall risk [29, 30]. In various studies presence of insomnia has been associated with poor health outcomes, including cognitive decline, depression, poorer quality of life, and risk of institutionalization [31, 32]. Napping as a result of daytime drowsiness has been identified as a risk factor for cardiovascular disease and death in elderly population [32 - 34]. Older adults with a sleep latency of more than 30 minutes, decreased sleep efficiency (<80%) and a high or low percentage of REM was found to have increased mortality risk [30].

Treatment of Insomnia in Elderly

Treatment for insomnia includes both nonpharmacological and pharmacological interventions. The first attempt for treating insomnia in the elderly should be at introducing adaptive behavior and utilizing techniques with a foundation in behavioral and cognitive interventions. Among behavioural interventions, sleep hygiene education should be the first approach. A 16 week randomized control trial of adults aged >55 found sleep hygiene improved sleep quality in the elderly [35]. Sleep hygiene by itself as a single therapy is, however, unlikely to be successful in treating insomnia and should be used in conjunction with other therapies [36]. Accompanied comorbid sleep disorders or mental/physical illnesses should also be identified and addressed alongside treating primary insomnia.

Non-Pharmacological Interventions

Hygiene measures as follows may serve as the first line of treatment approach for insomnia.

- Increasing exposure to bright light during the day, avoiding heavy meals and caffeine near bedtime, performing exercise during the day, maintaining comfortable room temperature, going to bed when sleepy, avoiding large fluid intake near bedtime.

According to the 2008 AASM guideline [36], psychological and behavioral interventions are effective in adults.

- Per AASM practice parameters, initial approaches to treatment should include at least one behavioral intervention such as stimulus control or the combination of cognitive therapy, stimulus control, sleep restriction with or without relaxation therapy—known as cognitive behavioral therapy for insomnia (CBT-I) [36]. Position papers and guidelines from organizations such American Academy of Sleep Medicine (AASM) and the American College of Physicians (ACP) recommend CBT-I as the initial treatment for adults with chronic insomnia [36, 37].
- Other common therapies include sleep restriction, paradoxical intention, and biofeedback therapy.
- Table **3** lists non-pharmacological treatment for insomnia.

Table 3. Non-pharmacological treatment for insomnia.

Cognitive behavioral therapy *Identifying negative thoughts and beliefs about sleep and challenging these emotions and behaviors. This intervention focuses on cognitive beliefs that may interfere with sleep. This is the first line recommended treatment for insomnia [37].*
Sleep Hygiene *Interventions that promote sleep and limit behaviors that disrupt sleep like avoiding caffeine, maintaining comfortable room temperature, going to bed when sleepy, and avoiding large fluid intake near bedtime.*
Stimulus Control *Bed should be used for sleep only. This therapy involves re-associating bed with sleep. If the patient is unable to fall asleep within 20 min, it is suggested they get up and go to another room to do something non-stimulating. Limit time spent awake in bed.*
Sleep Restriction *Time in bed is restricted to the actual time spent sleeping. Time in bed may be adjusted based on sleep efficiency.*
Relaxation technique *These may include guided imagery, muscle relaxation and meditation. The goal is to reduce mental arousal that may interfere with sleep.*

Pharmacological Interventions

Pharmacological interventions have proven to be a challenge in the elderly mainly due to age-related changes in pharmacodynamics and pharmacokinetics, which along with changes in homeostatic mechanisms in the elderly may contribute to an increase in adverse drug side effects [38]. It is well known that with ageing, there is an increased absorption of fat-soluble drugs (benzodiazepines) due to the increase in body fat storage with age resulting in an increased volume of distribution for lipid-soluble drugs [39]. Polypharmacy is a problem amongst elderly people and the degree of polypharmacy has been shown to increase with advancing age. Current literature recommends avoiding the use of sedative-hypnotics to treat insomnia in the elderly. Such prescribing practice elevates the risk of drug interactions and adverse drug reactions.

Adverse Drug Reaction in the Elderly: Hypnotics which are potential treatment options for insomnia may in elderly contribute to higher risk of falls, fractures, sedation, daytime drowsiness, disorientation, amnesia and rebound insomnia. Since elderly also commonly suffer from insomnia due to comorbid medical conditions and other sleep disorders, such treatment may additionally worsen underlying breathing issues and further contribute to hypoxemia.

Compliance: Accidental errors in drug compliance are common in elderly people. Incidence of mistakes increased 15-fold in elderly due to polypharmacy [39, 40]. Compliance may be deliberate or non-deliberate and can take the form of failing to take prescribed medication as directed; taking a larger dose in the mistaken belief that it will be more therapeutic or lead to a faster cure or taking an un-prescribed dose just out of memory trouble.

Drug Interactions are common in the elderly due to polypharmacy. Ageing is also known to be associated with changes in renal function, which can reduce the clearance of drugs. Careful dose adjustments may be required for prescribing such medications.

Medications

Available hypnotic drugs (Z-drugs, benzodiazepines, low-dose doxepin, and suvorexant) all have significant risks in the elderly, and only short-term or intermittent use of such medications should be considered. Benzodiazepines have been associated with an increased risk of falling in the elderly [41]. Falls appear to be related to not just the use of long-acting BZDs but also the short-acting BZDs [42]. Newer nonbenzodiazepine hypnotics like zolpidem, zaleplon, and eszopiclone do not cause rebound insomnia at discontinuation and have fewer ADRs. However, some adverse effects are similar to benzodiazepines (e.g. hip fracture, cognitive impairment) [43]. Dependency also remains an issue. In 2011, approximately 3233 ER visits by the elderly in the United States were associated with zolpidem abuse [44]. Beers criteria strongly advise avoiding short and intermediate acting non-benzodiazepine receptor agonists (*e.g.*, eszopiclone, zaleplon) and BZDs (*e.g.*, temazepam) in the elderly [45].

Various antidepressants, including tricyclic antidepressants (doxepin), phenylpiperazine compounds (trazodone) and serotonergic antidepressants (mirtazapine) are often used for the treatment of insomnia. American Academy of Sleep Medicine clinical guideline suggests against the use of trazodone for sleep onset or maintenance insomnia because it's harms outweigh benefits [46]. Low-dose doxepin (1 mg and 3 mg) improves sleep continuity and sleep duration and appears to be a good substitute for the elderly with sleep maintenance problems [47]. Melatonin receptor agonists like ramelteon are approved at a dose of 8 mg 30 minutes before bed for sleep-onset and sleep maintenance insomnia with no dependency [48]. In a study, ramelteon reduced patient reports of sleep latency over 5 weeks of treatment with no significant rebound insomnia or withdrawal effects [49]. Suvorexant, the first FDA approved dual orexin receptor antagonist at a dose of 5-20 mg, has been studied in the elderly (age 65 years or older) with demonstrated efficacy in decreasing sleep latency and increasing total sleep time; however, long term data is lacking (Table **4**) [50, 51].

Table 4. Pharmacokinetics of medications commonly used in the elderly.

Class	Drug Name	Elderly Dose (mg)	Half Life (hr)
Nonbenzodiazepines	Zolpidem (Short-acting)	5-10	~2.8
	Zaleplon (ultra-short acting)	5-10	1
	Eszopiclone (intermediate)	1-2	5-7
Benzodiazepines	Triazolam (ultra-short acting)	0.125-0.25	2-5
	Temazepam (intermediate acting)	7.5-15	8-20
	Flurazepam (long acting)	7.5-15	47-100
Melatonin Receptor Agonist	Ramelteon (short acing)	8	1-2
Dual Orexin Receptor Antagonist	Suvorexant	10-15	12

Sleep Disorder Breathing in Older Adults

Prevalence and Pathophysiology

Sleep disorder breathing (SDB) is an umbrella term that includes disorders of respiration (obstructive sleep apnea, central sleep apnea, hypoventilation) during sleep. It is estimated that the prevalence of sleep apnea in the elderly may be as high as 30%-80% [52] although estimates vary widely due to population studies. Data from Ancoli-Israël *et al.* study of 427 elderly community-dwelling persons showed the prevalence of an Apnea-Hypopnea Index (AHI) >5 was 24%, and that of an AHI>10 was 62% [53]. Prevalence was also noted to gradually increase with advancing age, with a plateau between age 60 and 65 years [54, 55]. Data showed that the severity of sleep apnea characterized by AHI increased across decades [56]. Current data supports changing anatomy and physiological mechanisms with ageing that may predispose the elderly to sleep disorder breathing. There is a higher susceptibility towards airways collapse in the elderly due to age-related changes in the pharyngeal airway for both men and women [57]. This, along with the decrease in response of the muscles to negative pressure during sleep and crowding of the posterior oropharynx, may explain the higher prevalence of SDB in the elderly [57]. There is also an increase in pharyngeal fat pads with age which is not dependent on the body mass index(BMI) [57]. Known changes in sleep architecture with increased arousal frequency may additionally lead to hyperventilation and subsequently hypocapnia and respiratory instability [58] during sleep. Central sleep apnea (CSA) is seen in the setting of congestive heart failure due to increased sensitivity to carbon dioxide levels.

Associated Comorbidities and Risks

Sleep apnea in the elderly is associated with multiple comorbidities, including metabolic syndrome, diabetes, hypertension, stroke and cardiovascular events [59]. It is also associated with an increased risk of automobile accidents and mortality rates independent of age and BMI, however, this increased mortality has not been consistently proven [60]. An increased risk for all-cause mortality and stroke has also been seen in patients with moderate-to-severe OSA. The use of long-term CPAP therapy improves cardiovascular outcomes [61]. In a study of SDB and nocturnal cardiac arrhythmias in older men, an increase in severity of SDB was associated with an increased risk of complex ventricular ectopy (CVE) and atrial flutter/fibrillation. Different forms of SDB were associated with different types of arrhythmias [62]. Data from another longitudinal cohort demonstrated declining cognitive function associated with increasing severity of SDB and self-reported increasing daytime sleepiness [63]. This has been further supported by anecdotal reports that have linked dementia with SDB [64]. Sleep apnea may accelerate cognitive decrement in patients with dementia [65].

Clinical Manifestation and Diagnosis

While snoring is a common presenting complaint of obstructive sleep apnea in the middle age population, it is less common in the elderly. Elderly commonly present with a multitude of distinctive symptoms like refractory atrial fibrillation, complaints of nocturia, fall, frequent daytime naps and confusion [66]. Older people also commonly experience difficulty maintaining sleep and early morning awakenings. Association between elevated BMI and severity of SDB is less common in the elderly. The elderly with obstructive sleep apnea typically have lower BMI and neck circumference compared with the middle age population [67]. The elderly should be screened for sleep apnea. Screening tools like the Epworth sleepiness scale and Berlin Questionnaire may be utilized to screen patients at risk of sleep apnea, but the validity of these tools in the elderly have not been tested [68]. The gold standard diagnostic tool for sleep apnea remains nocturnal polysomnography (PSG); however, it presents particular challenges in the elderly due to functional limitation(*e.g*, pain, arthritis, mobility issues).

Treatment

Positive airway pressure (PAP) therapy can be effectively utilized for treatment in the elderly. The Centers for Medicare and Medicaid Services currently covers PAP therapy with an AHI >5 and symptoms such as sleepiness or comorbid medical/psychiatric conditions such as hypertension and mood disorders. Regardless of symptoms, individuals with an AHI >15 are covered [68]. The use of long-term CPAP therapy improves cardiovascular outcomes [61]. Data from a retrospective analysis revealed a higher prevalence of overlap syndrome (OSA and COPD) in elderly patients and the use of PAP therapy led to significant improvement of blood gases [69, 70]. Similarly, adherence to PAP therapy in patients with Alzheimer's and Parkinson's disease led to improvement in daytime sleepiness and cognition [71].

Following recommendations for the elderly on expert consensus was made by the International Geriatric Sleep Medicine Task Force.

1. *"PAP should be used routinely for the treatment of SDB in older persons and in the frail elderly, particularly those with stroke but without major heart failure with an ejection fraction ≤45% (GRADE: strong).*
2. *While additional RCTs are needed in patients with Alzheimer's or Parkinson's disease, as well as other frail elderly, these patients do tolerate PAP and treatment should be considered (GRADE: strong).*
3. *PAP leads to a significant improvement of oxygenation in patients with SDB and COPD (overlap syndrome), and should be routinely used in these patients. More studies are needed to assess if additional oxygen further improves results (GRADE: weak).*
4. *Due to the results of the large RCT SERVE-HF, and the recommendations of all major pulmonary and sleep societies to abstain from servo-ventilation*

treatment in patients with heart failure (New York Heart Association functional class 2–4) with an ejection fraction ≤45%, no recommendation can be given regarding PAP treatment for this patient group until further trials have shown that CPAP, in comparison to servo-ventilation, has no negative outcome on mortality".

Restless Leg Syndrome

Prevalence and Pathophysiology

Restless leg syndrome (Ekbom's syndrome) is a common neurological sensorimotor disorder characterized by a creeping sensation in the legs that develop at rest and is relieved by movement [72]. The exact prevalence of the disorder is unknown, but it is suggested that its prevalence increases strongly with age. Though uncertain due to population studies and varied definitions used, current literature estimates the prevalence anywhere between 2.7%-35% [73, 74]. The disease is thought to be more prevalent in the elderly population of western countries compared to the Asian population [75, 76]. An increasing prevalence of comorbid medical conditions with age (such as diabetes, neurodegenerative conditions, stroke, chronic liver and kidney disease, rheumatoid arthritis, sleep disorders and iron deficiency) may predispose the elderly to the higher prevalence of restless leg syndrome (RLS). An earlier study found an increased prevalence of RLS in those with Alzheimer's disease, Parkinson's and mild cognitively impaired [77, 78]. Iron deficiency, the most common anemia in the elderly, is known to be a risk factor for RLS. Factors predisposing to iron deficiency in the elderly may include a poor diet, reduced absorption, occult blood loss, chronic inflammatory conditions, common intakes of medication like aspirin and non-steroidal anti-inflammatory drugs [79].

Diagnosis

Given that the diagnosis of RLS is a clinical diagnosis, appropriate detailed clinical history, especially in the elderly, can be a challenge leading to an underdiagnosis of this condition. The ability to express particularly sensory symptoms may be further diminished due to comorbid conditions in the elderly like dementia and/or cognitive impairment [80]. The syndrome is characterized by four essentials. An urge to move the leg begins that worsens during periods of rest, partially or totally relieved by movement or worsened due to symptoms in the evening or at night [81]. International Restless Legs Syndrome Study Group executive committee in 2003 proposed a revised diagnostic criterion for RLS that also addressed the needs of cognitively impaired elderly. The key difference for cognitively impaired adults is recognizing complaints of rubbing, kneading, pounding and excessive motor activity of the leg (pacing, fidgety) as a substitute for "sensation" and "urge" to move. Additionally, careful family history and exclusion of other conditions that may mimic RLS is encouraged [81]. Other supportive features of RLS in the elderly may include response to dopaminergic agents, iron deficiency, sleep-onset problems, diabetes, improved sleep during daytime compared to the night and higher periodic limb movement of sleep index (PLM recorded by polysomnography) [81]. Differential diagnoses of RLS to be considered carefully in elderly with cognitive impairment include arthritis, anxiety, painful neuropathy, nocturnal leg cramps, drug induced akathisia and radiculopathy. There may also be a possibility that these differentials may coexist in the elderly along with RLS making a diagnosis challenging. Careful history of patient's most updated medications should be obtained as drugs like anti-depressants, anti-psychotics and anti-emetics may worsen RLS.

Treatment

Treatment of RLS can be divided into pharmacological and non-pharmacological interventions (Fig. **4**).

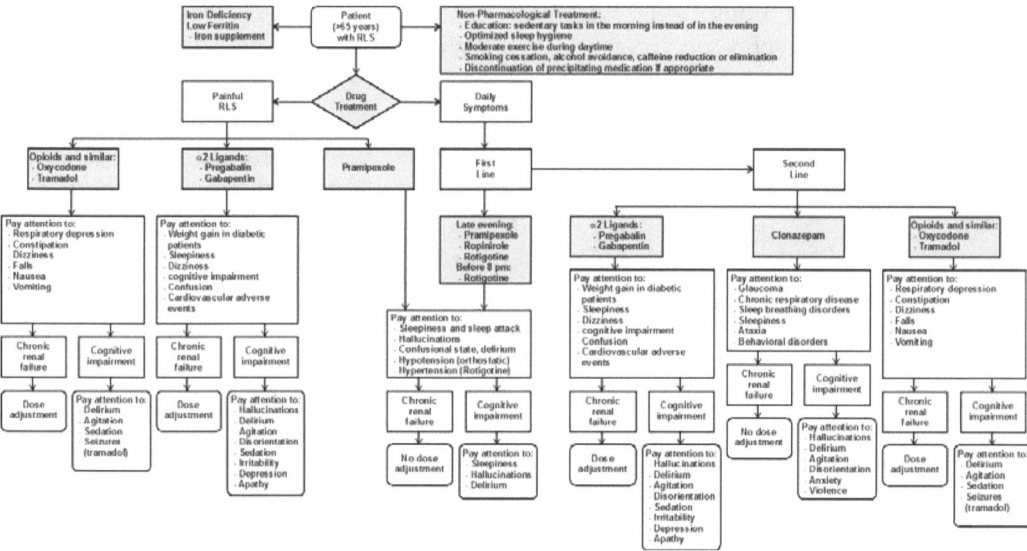

Fig. (4). Treatment algorithm of (restless legs syndrome) RLS, in older patients.From Figorilli M, Puligheddu M, Ferri R. Restless legs syndrome/Willis–Ekbom disease and periodic limb movements in sleep in the elderly with and without dementia. Sleep Med Clin. 2015;10 [3]:331–342.).

Non-Pharmacological Options

Data from a double blinded study revealed pneumatic compression device (PCD) and transcutaneous spinal direct current stimulation as effective treatment options for primary RLS [82]. Exercise training in moderation has also shown benefits. Additionally, acupuncture and other interventions like transcranial magnetic stimulation and mental activity (puzzles) significantly reduced RLS symptoms [82]. Endovenous laser ablation (ELA) may relieve RLS symptoms in patients with RLS and superficial venous insufficiency (SVI) [82]. PCDs and yoga may also be considered options to improve the quality of sleep in primary RLS patients with insomnia [82]. Restiffic, an FDA cleared prescriptional compressive foot wrap, has shown benefits in clinical settings. A good sleep hygiene and avoiding alcohol are equally important. Utilization of non-pharmacological options in the elderly can contribute to fewer side effects given elderly are on multiple medications and are at risk for drug interactions. It can also prevent augmentation, a common side effect of dopaminergic agents.

Iron therapy in treating RLS can be helpful when serum ferritin levels are low. A serum ferritin concentration lower than 45 mcg/L has been associated with increased severity of RLS. Clinical practice guidelines (2018) for the iron treatment of RLS in adults suggest oral iron (65 mg elemental iron) with Vitamin C as possibly effective in those with serum ferritin ≤75 µg/L [83]. IV iron may be considered whenever serum ferritin levels are too high for oral iron absorption, when oral iron is not tolerated or contraindicated, or when there is an unsatisfactory response of serum levels to oral iron [83].

Pharmacological Options

Drug therapy for RLS treatment encompasses alpha-2-delta ligands, dopaminergic drugs, benzodiazepines and opioids (Table **5**). Dopaminergic agonists (pramipexole, ropinirole, transdermal rotigotine) are widely prescribed for the treatment of RLS and are approved by the FDA. Until recently, dopaminergic agents were the gold standard for RLS treatment; however, there are now concerns of augmentation for many patients, potentially causing earlier daily onset or worsening symptoms. Notably, as many as 50% to 70% of patients using dopamine agonists may develop drug-induced augmentation over 10 years [84]. In current literature, the efficacy of pramipexole and ropinirole is well supported by several studies; however, their use in the elderly is not without significant adverse effects [85]. Side effects include orthostatic hypotension, sleepiness, nausea, headaches, augmentation and impulsive behavior (*e.g.,* gambling). Drug inter-actions should be considered carefully [85]. Dose adjustment of dopamine agonists is needed in the elderly. In the elderly, ropinirole has a shorter half-life of

6 hrs, compared to 12 hrs of pramipexole. Additionally, ropinirole is excreted by the liver, while pramipexole is excreted by the kidney, making ropinirole the drug of choice for those with renal disease [86].

Alpha-2-ligands include gabapentin, pregabalin and gabapentin enacarbil. These drugs are excreted by the kidneys and thus should be used carefully in the elderly population with impaired renal function. Side effects of these drugs include sedation, weight gain, sleepiness, confusion, depression, peripheral edema, hypotension and constipation [86, 87]. Starting dose of these medication should be lower in the elderly. In this class gabapentin enacarbil is the only FDA approved drug for RLS treatment. The American Geriatric Society (AGS) recommends cautious use of gabapentinoids and recommends a dose adjustment in those with creatinine clearance < 60 mL/min. AGS also warns against the risk of overdose when combined with opioids.

Benzodiazepine such as clonazepam may be utilized for treatment of RLS; however, clinical trials are lacking. Among the BZDs, clonazepam is best studied for this purpose. In a randomized double blinded trial, clonazepam 1mg was superior to placebo in treating RLS [88]. Caution should be exercised with its use in elderly patients given multiple side effects. It should be avoided in patients with renal failure, chronic respiratory disease, sleep-related breathing disorders, and dysphagia [87]. Use of BZDs is typically limited to an add-on agent for treating refractory RLS rather than sole therapy. Side effects to consider include memory impairment, agitation and confusion.

Current data demonstrate considerable effectiveness of opioids in treating refractory RLS and in instances where augmentation develops in response to dopaminergic agents. A 12-week double-blinded randomized placebo control trial demonstrated prolonged released oxycodone-naloxone was efficacious for short term treatment of severe RLS [89]. Another small, randomized trial showed efficacy in terms of improving sensory and motor symptoms [90]. In addition to oxycodone; methadone and tramadol are also used in clinical practice to treat refractory RLS. Due to risk of prolonged QT, electrocardiogram is suggested before initiating methadone. Before initiating any opioid, careful clinical history including past and current history of drug abuse, addiction, alcohol misuse and current medications should be obtained. Low doses should be given at first with titration to successful doses based on effectiveness and side effects.

Table 5. Suggested dose (after literature review by the author) for treatment of RLS in the elderly.

Drug Dose	Starting Dose in Elderly	Usual Effective Dose
Opioids		
Tramadol	50 mg	50-200 mg
Oxycodone	5-10 mg	10-30 mg
Hydrocodone	10 mg	10-45 mg
Methadone	2.5-5 mg	5-10 mg
Dopaminergic Agents		
Pramipexole	0.125 mg	0.25-0.5 mg
Ropinirole	0.25 mg	0.5-4 mg
Alpha-2-Delta Ligands		
Gabapentin	100 mg	300-2400 mg
Gabapentin Enacarbil	300 mg	600-1200 mg
Pregabalin	75 mg	75-450 mg

PSYCHIATRIC DISODERS AND SLEEP IN OLDER ADULTS

Sleep and Psychiatric Conditions

Different types of psychiatric problems have been associated with sleep disturbances in the elderly. The established viewpoint has been that sleep problems routinely are symptoms of psychiatric disorders. In fact sleep disorders and psychiatric conditions have a bidirectional relationship [91]. Data suggest more than 30% of the older population with insomnia have comorbid psychiatric conditions [92]. Below is a brief review of age-related changes in sleep and psychiatric conditions such as depression, anxiety and psychosis.

Depression

Depression is the most prevalent mental disorder in the elderly. The World Health Organization estimated the prevalence of depression among the elderly to be between 10-20%. Per the Centers of Disease Control and Prevention (CDC), the prevalence of depression among older adults ranges from 15-20% of adults older than 65 years. This percentage is much higher among those adults in nursing homes [93]. One of the diagnostic features of major depression is sleeping disruption, either insomnia or hypersomnia. Epidemiological studies indicate that depression shares a strong relationship with sleep disturbances, and this relationship is likely bi-directional. Depressive symptomatology in the elderly is frequently associated with insomnia, both sleep initiating and maintenance type [94]. Early morning awakenings is a frequent finding with late-life depression

[95]. It has also been observed that patients with major depression who have a poor sleep have slower treatment responses and lower remission rates than those without sleep disturbance [96]. Sleep disturbance is also independently correlated with poorer quality of life in those with major depression [97]. Data suggest that treating insomnia improves not only overall sleep but also non-sleep aspects of depression. As such thorough history and assessment for depression are indicated in the elderly presenting with sleep disruptions.

Anxiety

Anxiety disorders in late-life, especially generalized anxiety disorder, are linked with sleep disturbances even when controlling for co-morbid psychiatric disorders. A study of 1328 subjects aged 55-79 years found that 45.2% of the respondents who had definite anxiety also had sleep difficulties [98]. Another study in the elderly population with the presence of anxiety disorder found nighttime awakenings to be the most common sleep disruption followed closely by increased sleep onset latency [95, 99]. Anxiety was also linked to poor quality of sleep and daytime sleepiness. The degree of sleep disturbance has been correlated with anxiety severity [9]. CBT-I may be utilized to treat co-existing anxiety disorder and sleep disturbances, especially insomnia. The success of this combination therapy is unknown.

Psychosis

Polysomnographic studies confirm that the nighttime sleep of patients with psychosis is highly fragmented [100]. In a study of the elderly population, Martin *et al.* found that schizophrenia is related to increased time in bed, increased daytime sleep, more disrupted nighttime sleep, greater wake after sleep onset, more and longer naps compared to gender and age-matched controls [101]. Similarly, it also found that sleep disruptions are much more frequent and severe with schizophrenia in later life than normal aging [101]. It is suggested that multicomponent interventions focusing on behavioral factors contributing to poor nighttime sleep (*e.g.*, sleep hygiene training), decreased activity during the day (*e.g.*, behavioral therapies), circadian rhythm abnormalities (*e.g.*, light therapy) may help to reduce sleep/wake disturbances [101].

OTHER COMMON CONDITION AND SITUATIONS AFFECTING SLEEP IN THE ELDERLY

Sleep in Dementia

Current literature supports that elderly with dementia are particularly prone to sleep disorders. The relationship between sleep disorders and the cognitive decline appears to be bi-directional. While the underlying degenerative process of dementia contributes to sleep disturbances, patients with dementia may also have primary sleep disorders, such as obstructive sleep apnea, restless leg syndrome and altered circadian rhythm. Furthermore, these sleep disturbances are associated with an increased risk of adverse cognitive outcomes, suggesting a possible causal link [102]. It is also likely that the diffuse brain damage that defines dementia might contribute to changes in cognitive brain areas, which may lead to the involvement of the neural networks that control sleep function (*i.e.,* the anterior hypothalamus, reticular activating system, suprachiasmatic nucleus, and pineal gland) [103]. It is estimated that 60 to 70% of people with cognitive impairment or dementia have sleep disturbances and this is linked to poorer disease prognosis, neuropsychiatric symptoms and overall poorer quality of life [102, 104]. Individuals suffering from Lewy bodies (DLB) and Parkinson's disease (PD) dementia have a prevalence of sleep disturbance as high as 90% of patients affected [105]. Laboratory sleep studies of demented patients have found increased sleep fragmentation and sleep onset latency and decreased sleep efficiency, total sleep time and slow wave sleep. Data from an analysis that studied 235 individuals older than 65 years showed a strong relationship between dementia and sleep apnea when both are severe. The study estimated about 70% of people with dementia might have sleep apnea, and SDB severity increases with dementia severity suggesting a bidirectional relationship [65]. In fact there appears to be a U-shaped curve when it comes to sleep length and cognitive decline. Researchers found a relationship between sleep deprivation (less than 7 hrs) and accelerated development of amyloid plaques which are the protein found to have a role in the pathogenesis of Alzheimer's disease. Longer sleep (>10 hrs) also raises the chances of dementia, though the reason is less known.

Treatment and assessment of individuals with sleep disturbances should first include screening and addressing secondary causes, including underlying medical and psychiatric conditions, medication side-effects, and sleep disorders [106]. Examples of such treatment options include PAP therapy for OSA, light therapy for circadian rhythm disorder, increased physical activity during the day, careful evaluation of medications, improving sleep hygiene, avoiding caffeine and alcohol. Various sleep aids (*e.g.,* BZDs, non-BZDs) have significant side effects and have a negative impact on memory; thus, their use for sleep disturbances should be avoided if possible. Amongst pharmacological agents, low dose trazodone (25-50mg) has commonly been prescribed for insomnia in Alzheimer's disease [107]. However, given the side effects of trazodone (*e.g.,* sedation and orthostatic hypotension) it should be used judiciously with close follow up. Antipsychotic medications have often been used for sleep in dementia patients; however, its use is controversial due to increased mortality risk [108]. A meta-analysis comparing melatonin to placebo has shown melatonin efficacy in improving sleep efficiency in people with dementia with minimal side effects [108]. On the other hand, additional studies have not supported melatonin use and have failed to show any benefits in demented patients [109, 110]. As light is a zeitbeiger, or "cue" for wakefulness, exposure to light may be helpful in decreasing daytime sleepiness and is recommended for patients with dementia. In the elderly with dementia, non-pharmacological interventions are safer with fewer side effects. Pharmacological options should be used after careful consideration of side effects.

SLEEP IN HOSPITALIZED ELDERLY

During hospitalization, older patients face acute sleep deprivation along with the fragmented and poor quality of sleep. The reasons are multifactorial, including medical, patient and environmental factors during the hospital stay. Numerous activities during nighttime revolving around nursing care, medication administration, clinician visits, monitoring of vital signs, leads to frequent awakenings and fragmented sleep. Environmental factors like noise and light exposure also lead to disrupted sleep. A study in the intensive care unit (ICU) setting found that 49% of noise was modifiable (staff conversation and television noise) [111]. Patient factors like pain, chronic conditions (*e.g.*, chronic obstructive pulmonary disease), anxiety and depression also contribute to sleep disturbances in hospitalized patients [112, 113]. As non-pharmacological interventions are preferred for older adults, addressing environmental factors should be the first step. A Cochrane review of 1569 participants showed non-pharmacological interventions like use of earplugs or eye masks or both might have beneficial effects on sleep and the incidence of delirium in ICU settings [114].

CONCLUSION

Sleep disorders are common among elderly persons but are under recognized and under diagnosed even by geriatricians. These disorders can be due to a multitude of factors. Many sleep disorders are attributable to underlying medical conditions and medications and as such, require careful history and assessment. Management of these disorders requires a multifaceted treatment approach and can result in significant improvement in quality of life and daytime functioning in the elderly.

CONSENT FOR PUBLICATION

Not applicable.

CONFLICT OF INTEREST

The author declares no conflict of interest, financial or otherwise.

ACKNOWLEDGEMENTS

Declared none.

REFERENCES

[1]   RHI. Demographic Changes and Aging Population. https://www.ruralhealthinfo.org/toolkits/aging/1/demographics

[2]   Cybulski M, Cybulski L, Krajewska-Kulak E, Orzechowska M, Cwalina U, Kowalczuk K. Sleep disorders among educationally active elderly people in Bialystok. Poland: a cross-sectional study 2019; 19: p. (1)225, 08.
[http://dx.doi.org/10.1186/s12877-019-1248-2]

[3]   Foley DJ, Monjan AA, Brown SL, Simonsick EM, Wallace RB, Blazer DG. Sleep complaints among elderly persons: an epidemiologic study of three communities. Sleep 1995; 18(6): 425-32.
[http://dx.doi.org/10.1093/sleep/18.6.425] [PMID: 7481413]

[4]   Torabi S, Shahriari L, Zahedi R, Rahmanian S, Rahmanian K. "A survey the prevalence of sleep disorders and their management in the elderly in Jahrom City jmj 2012 2008; 10(4): 35-41.

[5]   Roepke S, Ancoli-Israel S. Although changes in sleep architecture are to be expected with increasing age, age itself does not result in disturbed S leep disorders in the elderly. 2010; 131: pp. 302-10.

[6]   Phillips B, Ancoli-Israel S. Sleep disorders in the elderly. Sleep Med 2001; 2(2): 99-114.

[7]   Fu Y, Xia Y, Yi H, Xu H, Guan J, Yin S. Meta-analysis of all-cause and cardiovascular mortality in obstructive sleep apnea with or without continuous positive airway pressure treatment. Sleep Breath 2017; 21(1): 181-9.
[http://dx.doi.org/10.1007/s11325-016-1393-1] [PMID: 27502205]

[8]   Floyd JA, Medler SM, Ager JW, Janisse JJ. Age-related changes in initiation and maintenance of sleep: a meta-analysis. Res Nurs Health 2000; 23(2): 106-17.
[http://dx.doi.org/10.1002/(SICI)1098-240X(200004)23:2<106::AID-NUR3>3.0.CO;2-A] [PMID: 10782869]

[9]   Ohayon MM, Carskadon MA, Guilleminault C, Vitiello MV. Meta-analysis of quantitative sleep parameters from childhood to old age in healthy individuals: developing normative sleep values across the human lifespan. Sleep 2004; 27(7): 1255-73.
[http://dx.doi.org/10.1093/sleep/27.7.1255] [PMID: 15586779]

[10]   Floyd J A, Janisse J J, Marshall Medler S, Ager J W. Nonlinear components of age-related change in sleep initiation. (in eng), Nurs Res 2000; 49(5): 290-4.
[http://dx.doi.org/10.1097/00006199-200009000-00008]

[11]   Campbell SS, Murphy PJ. The nature of spontaneous sleep across adulthood. J Sleep Res 2007; 16(1): 24-32.
[http://dx.doi.org/10.1111/j.1365-2869.2007.00567.x] [PMID: 17309760]

[12]   Floyd JA, Janisse JJ, Jenuwine ES, Ager JW. Changes in REM-sleep percentage over the adult lifespan. Sleep 2007; 30(7): 829-36.
[http://dx.doi.org/10.1093/sleep/30.7.829] [PMID: 17682652]

[13]   Dorffner G, Vitr M, Anderer P. The effects of aging on sleep architecture in healthy subjects. Adv Exp Med Biol 2015; 821: 93-100.
[http://dx.doi.org/10.1007/978-3-319-08939-3_13] [PMID: 25416113]

[14]   Ohayon MM, Vecchierini MF. Normative sleep data, cognitive function and daily living activities in older adults in the community. Sleep 2005; 28(8): 981-9.
[PMID: 16218081]

[15]   Ishihara K, Miyake S, Miyasita A, Miyata Y. Morningness-eveningness preference and sleep habits in

Japanese office workers of different ages. (in eng), Chronobiologia 1992; 19(1-2): 9-16.

[16]   Kim SJ, Benloucif S, Reid KJ, *et al.* Phase-shifting response to light in older adults. J Physiol 2014; 592(1): 189-202.
[http://dx.doi.org/10.1113/jphysiol.2013.262899] [PMID: 24144880]

[17]   Duffy JF, Zeitzer JM, Rimmer DW, Klerman EB, Dijk DJ, Czeisler CA. Peak of circadian melatonin rhythm occurs later within the sleep of older subjects. Am J Physiol Endocrinol Metab 2002; 282(2): E297-303.
[http://dx.doi.org/10.1152/ajpendo.00268.2001] [PMID: 11788360]

[18]   Dijk DJ, Duffy JF. Circadian regulation of human sleep and age-related changes in its timing, consolidation and EEG characteristics. Ann Med 1999; 31(2): 130-40.
[http://dx.doi.org/10.3109/07853899908998789] [PMID: 10344586]

[19]   Monk TH, Thompson WK, Buysse DJ, Hall M, Nofzinger EA, Reynolds CF III. Sleep in healthy seniors: a diary study of the relation between bedtime and the amount of sleep obtained. J Sleep Res 2006; 15(3): 256-60.
[http://dx.doi.org/10.1111/j.1365-2869.2006.00534.x] [PMID: 16911027]

[20]   Pótári A, Ujma PP, Konrad BN, *et al.* Age-related changes in sleep EEG are attenuated in highly intelligent individuals (in eng), Neuroimage 2017; 146: 554-60.
[http://dx.doi.org/10.1016/j.neuroimage.2016.09.039]

[21]   Buysse DJ. Insomnia. JAMA 2013; 309(7): 706-16.
[http://dx.doi.org/10.1001/jama.2013.193] [PMID: 23423416]

[22]   Miner B, Kryger MH. Sleep in the Aging Population. Sleep Med Clin 2017; 12(1): 31-8.
[http://dx.doi.org/10.1016/j.jsmc.2016.10.008] [PMID: 28159095]

[23]   Chung KF, Yeung WF, Ho FY, Yung KP, Yu YM, Kwok CW. Cross-cultural and comparative epidemiology of insomnia: the Diagnostic and statistical manual (DSM), International classification of diseases (ICD) and International classification of sleep disorders (ICSD). Sleep Med 2015; 16(4): 477-82.
[http://dx.doi.org/10.1016/j.sleep.2014.10.018] [PMID: 25761665]

[24]   Ohayon MM. Epidemiology of insomnia: what we know and what we still need to learn. Sleep Med Rev 2002; 6(2): 97-111.
[http://dx.doi.org/10.1053/smrv.2002.0186] [PMID: 12531146]

[25]   Foley DJ, Monjan A, Simonsick EM, Wallace RB, Blazer DG. Incidence and remission of insomnia among elderly adults: an epidemiologic study of 6,800 persons over three years. Sleep 1999; 22 (Suppl. 2): S366-72.
[PMID: 10394609]

[26]   Patel D, Steinberg J, Patel P. Insomnia in the Elderly: A Review (in eng), J Clin Sleep Med 2018; 14(6): 1017-24.
[http://dx.doi.org/10.5664/jcsm.7172]

[27]   Foley D, Ancoli-Israel S, Britz P, Walsh J. Sleep disturbances and chronic disease in older adults: results of the 2003 National Sleep Foundation Sleep in America Survey. J Psychosom Res 2004; 56(5): 497-502.
[http://dx.doi.org/10.1016/j.jpsychores.2004.02.010] [PMID: 15172205]

[28]   Suzuki K, Miyamoto M, Hirata K. Sleep disorders in the elderly: Diagnosis and management (in eng), J Gen Fam Med 2017; 18(2): 61-71.
[http://dx.doi.org/10.1002/jgf2.27]

[29]   Brassington GS, King AC, Bliwise DL. Sleep problems as a risk factor for falls in a sample of community-dwelling adults aged 64-99 years. J Am Geriatr Soc 2000; 48(10): 1234-40.
[http://dx.doi.org/10.1111/j.1532-5415.2000.tb02596.x] [PMID: 11037010]

[30]   Dew MA, Hoch CC, Buysse DJ, *et al.* Healthy older adults' sleep predicts all-cause mortality at 4 to 19

years of follow-up (in eng), Psychosom Med 2003; 65(1): 63-73.
[http://dx.doi.org/10.1097/01.PSY.0000039756.23250.7C]

[31]   Cricco M, Simonsick EM, Foley DJ. The impact of insomnia on cognitive functioning in older adults.
         J Am Geriatr Soc 2001; 49(9): 1185-9.
         [http://dx.doi.org/10.1046/j.1532-5415.2001.49235.x] [PMID: 11559377]

[32]   Newman AB, Spiekerman CF, Enright P, *et al.* Daytime sleepiness predicts mortality and
         cardiovascular disease in older adults. J Am Geriatr Soc 2000; 48(2): 115-23.
         [http://dx.doi.org/10.1111/j.1532-5415.2000.tb03901.x] [PMID: 10682939]

[33]   Bursztyn M, Ginsberg G, Hammerman-Rozenberg R, Stessman J. The siesta in the elderly: risk factor
         for mortality? Arch Intern Med 1999; 159(14): 1582-6.
         [http://dx.doi.org/10.1001/archinte.159.14.1582] [PMID: 10421281]

[34]   Bursztyn M, Ginsberg G, Stessman J. The siesta and mortality in the elderly: effect of rest without
         sleep and daytime sleep duration. Sleep 2002; 25(2): 187-91.
         [http://dx.doi.org/10.1093/sleep/25.2.187] [PMID: 11902427]

[35]   Reid KJ, Baron KG, Lu B, Naylor E, Wolfe L, Zee PC. Aerobic exercise improves self-reported sleep
         and quality of life in older adults with insomnia. Sleep Med 2010; 11(9): 934-40.
         [http://dx.doi.org/10.1016/j.sleep.2010.04.014] [PMID: 20813580]

[36]   Schutte-Rodin S, Broch L, Buysse D, Dorsey C, Sateia M. Clinical guideline for the evaluation and
         management of chronic insomnia in adults. J Clin Sleep Med 2008; 4(5): 487-504.
         [http://dx.doi.org/10.5664/jcsm.27286] [PMID: 18853708]

[37]   Qaseem A, Kansagara D, Forciea MA, Cooke M, Denberg TD, Physicians CGCAC. Management of
         Chronic Insomnia Disorder in Adults: A Clinical Practice Guideline From the American College of
         Physicians. Ann Intern Med 2016; 165(2): 125-33.
         [http://dx.doi.org/10.7326/M15-2175] [PMID: 27136449]

[38]   Hughes SG. Prescribing for the elderly patient: why do we need to exercise caution? Br J Clin
         Pharmacol 1998; 46(6): 531-3.
         [http://dx.doi.org/10.1046/j.1365-2125.1998.00842.x] [PMID: 9862240]

[39]   Greenblatt DJ, Sellers EM, Shader RI. Drug therapy: drug disposition in old age. N Engl J Med 1982;
         306(18): 1081-8.
         [http://dx.doi.org/10.1056/NEJM198205063061804] [PMID: 7040951]

[40]   Parkin DM, Henney CR, Quirk J, Crooks J. Deviation from prescribed drug treatment after discharge
         from hospital. BMJ 1976; 2(6037): 686-8.
         [http://dx.doi.org/10.1136/bmj.2.6037.686] [PMID: 974539]

[41]   Sorock GS, Shimkin EE. Benzodiazepine sedatives and the risk of falling in a community-dwelling
         elderly cohort. Arch Intern Med 1988; 148(11): 2441-4.
         [http://dx.doi.org/10.1001/archinte.1988.00380110083017] [PMID: 2903726]

[42]   Ensrud KE, Blackwell TL, Mangione CM, *et al.* Central nervous system-active medications and risk
         for falls in older women. J Am Geriatr Soc 2002; 50(10): 1629-37.
         [http://dx.doi.org/10.1046/j.1532-5415.2002.50453.x] [PMID: 12366615]

[43]   Berry SD, Lee Y, Cai S, Dore DD. Nonbenzodiazepine sleep medication use and hip fractures in
         nursing home residents. JAMA Intern Med 2013; 173(9): 754-61.
         [http://dx.doi.org/10.1001/jamainternmed.2013.3795] [PMID: 23460413]

[44]   Huang CY, Chou FH, Huang YS, *et al.* The association between zolpidem and infection in patients
         with sleep disturbance. J Psychiatr Res 2014; 54: 116-20.
         [http://dx.doi.org/10.1016/j.jpsychires.2014.03.017] [PMID: 24721551]

[45]   American Geriatrics Society 2015 Updated Beers Criteria for Potentially Inappropriate Medication
         Use in Older Adults. J Am Geriatr Soc 2015; 63(11): 2227-46.
         [http://dx.doi.org/10.1111/jgs.13702] [PMID: 26446832]

[46] Sateia MJ, Buysse DJ, Krystal AD, Neubauer DN, Heald JL. Clinical Practice Guideline for the Pharmacologic Treatment of Chronic Insomnia in Adults: An American Academy of Sleep Medicine Clinical Practice Guideline. J Clin Sleep Med 2017; 13(2): 307-49.
[http://dx.doi.org/10.5664/jcsm.6470] [PMID: 27998379]

[47] Krystal AD, Lankford A, Durrence HH, *et al.* Efficacy and safety of doxepin 3 and 6 mg in a 35-day sleep laboratory trial in adults with chronic primary insomnia. Sleep 2011; 34(10): 1433-42.
[http://dx.doi.org/10.5665/SLEEP.1294] [PMID: 21966075]

[48] Neubauer DN. A review of ramelteon in the treatment of sleep disorders. Neuropsychiatr Dis Treat 2008; 4(1): 69-79.
[http://dx.doi.org/10.2147/NDT.S483] [PMID: 18728808]

[49] Roth T, Seiden D, Sainati S, Wang-Weigand S, Zhang J, Zee P. Effects of ramelteon on patient-reported sleep latency in older adults with chronic insomnia. Sleep Med 2006; 7(4): 312-8.
[http://dx.doi.org/10.1016/j.sleep.2006.01.003] [PMID: 16709464]

[50] Rhyne DN, Anderson SL. Suvorexant in insomnia: efficacy, safety and place in therapy. Ther Adv Drug Saf 2015; 6(5): 189-95.
[http://dx.doi.org/10.1177/2042098615595359] [PMID: 26478806]

[51] Wilt TJ, MacDonald R, Brasure M, *et al.* Pharmacologic Treatment of Insomnia Disorder: An Evidence Report for a Clinical Practice Guideline by the American College of Physicians. Ann Intern Med 2016; 165(2): 103-12.
[http://dx.doi.org/10.7326/M15-1781] [PMID: 27136278]

[52] Young T, Peppard PE, Gottlieb DJ. Epidemiology of obstructive sleep apnea: a population health perspective. Am J Respir Crit Care Med 2002; 165(9): 1217-39.
[http://dx.doi.org/10.1164/rccm.2109080] [PMID: 11991871]

[53] Ancoli-Israel S, Kripke DF, Klauber MR, Mason WJ, Fell R, Kaplan O. Sleep-disordered breathing in community-dwelling elderly. Sleep 1991; 14(6): 486-95.
[http://dx.doi.org/10.1093/sleep/14.6.486] [PMID: 1798880]

[54] Ancoli-Israel S, Gehrman P, Kripke DF, *et al.* Long-term follow-up of sleep disordered breathing in older adults. Sleep Med 2001; 2(6): 511-6.
[http://dx.doi.org/10.1016/S1389-9457(00)00096-4] [PMID: 14592266]

[55] McMillan A, Morrell MJ. Sleep disordered breathing at the extremes of age: the elderly. Breathe (Sheff) 2016; 12(1): 50-60.
[http://dx.doi.org/10.1183/20734735.003216] [PMID: 27064674]

[56] Hoch CC, Reynolds CF III, Monk TH, *et al.* Comparison of sleep-disordered breathing among healthy elderly in the seventh, eighth, and ninth decades of life. Sleep 1990; 13(6): 502-11.
[http://dx.doi.org/10.1093/sleep/13.6.502] [PMID: 2126391]

[57] Malhotra A, Huang Y, Fogel R, *et al.* Aging influences on pharyngeal anatomy and physiology: the predisposition to pharyngeal collapse. Am J Med 2006; 119(1): 72.e9-72.e14.
[http://dx.doi.org/10.1016/j.amjmed.2005.01.077] [PMID: 16431197]

[58] Pack AI, Millman RP. Changes in control of ventilation, awake and asleep, in the elderly. J Am Geriatr Soc 1986; 34(7): 533-44.
[http://dx.doi.org/10.1111/j.1532-5415.1986.tb04247.x] [PMID: 3722671]

[59] Peppard PE, Young T, Palta M, Skatrud J. Prospective study of the association between sleep-disordered breathing and hypertension. N Engl J Med 2000; 342(19): 1378-84.
[http://dx.doi.org/10.1056/NEJM200005113421901] [PMID: 10805822]

[60] Young T, Finn L, Peppard PE, *et al.* Sleep disordered breathing and mortality: eighteen-year follow-up of the Wisconsin sleep cohort. Sleep 2008; 31(8): 1071-8.
[PMID: 18714778]

[61]   Doherty LS, Kiely JL, Swan V, McNicholas WT. Long-term effects of nasal continuous positive airway pressure therapy on cardiovascular outcomes in sleep apnea syndrome. Chest 2005; 127(6): 2076-84.
[http://dx.doi.org/10.1378/chest.127.6.2076] [PMID: 15947323]

[62]   Mehra R, Stone KL, Varosy PD, *et al.* Nocturnal Arrhythmias across a spectrum of obstructive and central sleep-disordered breathing in older men: outcomes of sleep disorders in older men (MrOS sleep) study. Arch Intern Med 2009; 169(12): 1147-55.
[http://dx.doi.org/10.1001/archinternmed.2009.138] [PMID: 19546416]

[63]   Cohen-Zion M, Stepnowsky C, Marler T, Shochat T, Kripke DF, Ancoli-Israel S. Changes in cognitive function associated with sleep disordered breathing in older people. J Am Geriatr Soc 2001; 49(12): 1622-7.
[http://dx.doi.org/10.1111/j.1532-5415.2001.49270.x] [PMID: 11843994]

[64]   Geldmacher DS, Whitehouse PJ. Evaluation of dementia. N Engl J Med 1996; 335(5): 330-6.
[http://dx.doi.org/10.1056/NEJM199608013350507] [PMID: 8663868]

[65]   Ancoli-Israel S, Klauber MR, Butters N, Parker L, Kripke DF. Dementia in institutionalized elderly: relation to sleep apnea. J Am Geriatr Soc 1991; 39(3): 258-63.
[http://dx.doi.org/10.1111/j.1532-5415.1991.tb01647.x] [PMID: 2005339]

[66]   Umlauf MG, Chasens ER, Greevy RA, Arnold J, Burgio KL, Pillion DJ. Obstructive sleep apnea, nocturia and polyuria in older adults. Sleep 2004; 27(1): 139-44.
[http://dx.doi.org/10.1093/sleep/27.1.139] [PMID: 14998251]

[67]   Chung S, Yoon IY, Lee CH, Kim JW. Effects of age on the clinical features of men with obstructive sleep apnea syndrome. Respiration 2009; 78(1): 23-9.
[http://dx.doi.org/10.1159/000218143] [PMID: 19420898]

[68]   Russell T, Duntley S. Sleep disordered breathing in the elderly. Am J Med 2011; 124(12): 1123-6.
[http://dx.doi.org/10.1016/j.amjmed.2011.04.017] [PMID: 21906711]

[69]   Lacedonia D, Carpagnano GE, Aliani M, *et al.* Daytime PaO2 in OSAS, COPD and the combination of the two (overlap syndrome). Respir Med 2013; 107(2): 310-6.
[http://dx.doi.org/10.1016/j.rmed.2012.10.012] [PMID: 23141861]

[70]   Netzer NC, Ancoli-Israel S, Bliwise DL, *et al.* Principles of practice parameters for the treatment of sleep disordered breathing in the elderly and frail elderly: the consensus of the International Geriatric Sleep Medicine Task Force (in eng), Eur Respir J 2016; 48(4): 992-1018.
[http://dx.doi.org/10.1183/13993003.01975-2015]

[71]   Ancoli-Israel S, Palmer BW, Cooke JR, *et al.* Cognitive effects of treating obstructive sleep apnea in Alzheimer's disease: a randomized controlled study. J Am Geriatr Soc 2008; 56(11): 2076-81.
[http://dx.doi.org/10.1111/j.1532-5415.2008.01934.x] [PMID: 18795985]

[72]   Ekbom KA. Restless legs syndrome. Neurology 1960; 10(9): 868-73.
[http://dx.doi.org/10.1212/WNL.10.9.868] [PMID: 13726241]

[73]   O'Keeffe ST, Noel J, Lavan JN. Restless legs syndrome in the elderly. Postgrad Med J 1993; 69(815): 701-3.
[http://dx.doi.org/10.1136/pgmj.69.815.701] [PMID: 8255834]

[74]   Milligan SA, Chesson AL. Restless legs syndrome in the older adult: diagnosis and management. Drugs Aging 2002; 19(10): 741-51.
[http://dx.doi.org/10.2165/00002512-200219100-00003] [PMID: 12390051]

[75]   Allen RP, Walters AS, Montplaisir J, *et al.* Restless legs syndrome prevalence and impact: REST general population study. Arch Intern Med 2005; 165(11): 1286-92.
[http://dx.doi.org/10.1001/archinte.165.11.1286] [PMID: 15956009]

[76]   Tan EK, Seah A, See SJ, Lim E, Wong MC, Koh KK. Restless legs syndrome in an Asian population:

A study in Singapore. Mov Disord 2001; 16(3): 577-9.
[http://dx.doi.org/10.1002/mds.1102] [PMID: 11391765]

[77] Ondo WG, Vuong KD, Jankovic J. Exploring the relationship between Parkinson disease and restless legs syndrome. Arch Neurol 2002; 59(3): 421-4.
[http://dx.doi.org/10.1001/archneur.59.3.421] [PMID: 11890847]

[78] Richards K, Shue VM, Beck CK, Lambert CW, Bliwise DL. Restless legs syndrome risk factors, behaviors, and diagnoses in persons with early to moderate dementia and sleep disturbance. Behav Sleep Med 2010; 8(1): 48-61.
[http://dx.doi.org/10.1080/15402000903425769] [PMID: 20043249]

[79] Lopez-Contreras MJ, Zamora-Portero S, Lopez MA, Marin JF, Zamora S, Perez-Llamas F. Dietary intake and iron status of institutionalized elderly people: relationship with different factors. J Nutr Health Aging 2010; 14(10): 816-21.
[http://dx.doi.org/10.1007/s12603-010-0118-6] [PMID: 21125198]

[80] Spiegelhalder K, Hornyak M. Restless legs syndrome in older adults. (in eng), Clin Geriatr Med 2008; 24(1): 167-80.
[http://dx.doi.org/10.1016/j.cger.2007.08.004]

[81] Allen RP, Picchietti D, Hening WA, Trenkwalder C, Walters AS, Montplaisi J. Restless legs syndrome: diagnostic criteria, special considerations, and epidemiology. A report from the restless legs syndrome diagnosis and epidemiology workshop at the National Institutes of Health. Sleep Med 2003; 4(2): 101-19.
[http://dx.doi.org/10.1016/S1389-9457(03)00010-8] [PMID: 14592341]

[82] Xu X M, Liu Y, Jia S Y, Dong M X, Cao D, Wei Y D. Complementary and alternative therapies for restless legs syndrome: An evidence-based systematic review (in eng), Sleep Med Rev 2018; 38: 158-67.
[http://dx.doi.org/10.1016/j.smrv.2017.06.003]

[83] Allen RP, Picchietti DR, Auerbach M, *et al.* Evidence-based and consensus clinical practice guidelines for the iron treatment of restless legs syndrome/Willis-Ekbom disease in adults and children: an IRLSSG task force report (in eng), Sleep Med 2018; 41: 27-44.
[http://dx.doi.org/10.1016/j.sleep.2017.11.1126]

[84] Lipford MC, Silber MH. Long-term use of pramipexole in the management of restless legs syndrome. Sleep Med 2012; 13(10): 1280-5.
[http://dx.doi.org/10.1016/j.sleep.2012.08.004] [PMID: 23036265]

[85] Bloom HG, Ahmed I, Alessi CA, *et al.* Evidence-based recommendations for the assessment and management of sleep disorders in older persons. J Am Geriatr Soc 2009; 57(5): 761-89.
[http://dx.doi.org/10.1111/j.1532-5415.2009.02220.x] [PMID: 19484833]

[86] During E H, Winkelman J W. Drug Treatment of Restless Legs Syndrome in Older Adults. (in eng), Drugs Aging 2019; 36(10): 939-46.
[http://dx.doi.org/10.1007/s40266-019-00698-1]

[87] Figorilli M, Puligheddu M, Ferri R. Restless legs syndrome/willis-ekbom disease and periodic limb movements in sleep in the elderly with and without dementia (in eng), Sleep Med Clin 10(3): 331-42.2015;
[http://dx.doi.org/10.1016/j.jsmc.2015.05.011]

[88] Montagna P, Sassoli de Bianchi L, Zucconi M, Cirignotta F, Lugaresi E. Clonazepam and vibration in restless legs syndrome. Acta Neurol Scand 1984; 69(6): 428-30.
[http://dx.doi.org/10.1111/j.1600-0404.1984.tb07826.x] [PMID: 6380197]

[89] Trenkwalder C, Beneš H, Grote L, *et al.* Prolonged release oxycodone-naloxone for treatment of severe restless legs syndrome after failure of previous treatment: a double-blind, randomised, placebo-controlled trial with an open-label extension. Lancet Neurol 2013; 12(12): 1141-50.
[http://dx.doi.org/10.1016/S1474-4422(13)70239-4] [PMID: 24140442]

[90]   Walters AS, Wagner ML, Hening WA, *et al.* Successful treatment of the idiopathic restless legs syndrome in a randomized double-blind trial of oxycodone versus placebo. Sleep 1993; 16(4): 327-32.
[http://dx.doi.org/10.1093/sleep/16.4.327] [PMID: 8341893]

[91]   Krystal AD. Psychiatric disorders and sleep. Neurol Clin 2012; 30(4): 1389-413.
[http://dx.doi.org/10.1016/j.ncl.2012.08.018] [PMID: 23099143]

[92]   McCrae CS, Dzierzewski JM, Kay D. Treatment of Late-life Insomnia. Sleep Med Clin 2009; 4(4): 593-604.
[http://dx.doi.org/10.1016/j.jsmc.2009.07.006] [PMID: 23390408]

[93]   CDC Promotes Public Health Approach To Address Depression among Older Adults.

[94]   Maggi S, Langlois JA, Minicuci N, *et al.* Sleep complaints in community-dwelling older persons: prevalence, associated factors, and reported causes. J Am Geriatr Soc 1998; 46(2): 161-8.
[http://dx.doi.org/10.1111/j.1532-5415.1998.tb02533.x] [PMID: 9475443]

[95]   Rodin J, McAvay G, Timko C. A longitudinal study of depressed mood and sleep disturbances in elderly adults. J Gerontol 1988; 43(2): 45-53.
[http://dx.doi.org/10.1093/geronj/43.2.P45] [PMID: 3346525]

[96]   Thase ME, Buysse DJ, Frank E, *et al.* Which depressed patients will respond to interpersonal psychotherapy? The role of abnormal EEG sleep profiles. Am J Psychiatry 1997; 154(4): 502-9.
[http://dx.doi.org/10.1176/ajp.154.4.502] [PMID: 9090337]

[97]   McCall WV, Reboussin BA, Cohen W. Subjective measurement of insomnia and quality of life in depressed inpatients. J Sleep Res 2000; 9(1): 43-8.
[http://dx.doi.org/10.1046/j.1365-2869.2000.00186.x] [PMID: 10733688]

[98]   Mallon L, Broman JE, Hetta J. Sleeping difficulties in relation to depression and anxiety in elderly adults Nordic Journal of Psychiatry 2000; 54(5): 355-60.
[http://dx.doi.org/10.1080/080394800457192]

[99]   Leblanc MF, Desjardins S, Desgagné A. Sleep problems in anxious and depressive older adults. Psychol Res Behav Manag 2015; 8: 161-9.
[http://dx.doi.org/10.2147/PRBM.S80642] [PMID: 26089709]

[100] Tandon R, Shipley JE, Taylor S, *et al.* Electroencephalographic sleep abnormalities in schizophrenia. Relationship to positive/negative symptoms and prior neuroleptic treatment. Arch Gen Psychiatry 1992; 49(3): 185-94.
[http://dx.doi.org/10.1001/archpsyc.1992.01820030017003] [PMID: 1348923]

[101] Martin JL, Jeste DV, Ancoli-Israel S. Older schizophrenia patients have more disrupted sleep and circadian rhythms than age-matched comparison subjects. J Psychiatr Res 2005; 39(3): 251-9.
[http://dx.doi.org/10.1016/j.jpsychires.2004.08.011] [PMID: 15725423]

[102] Wennberg AMV, Wu MN, Rosenberg PB, Spira AP. Sleep disturbance, cognitive decline, and dementia: A review (in eng), Semin Neurol 2017; 37(4): 395-406.
[http://dx.doi.org/10.1055/s-0037-1604351]

[103] Yesavage JA, Friedman L, Ancoli-Israel S, *et al.* Development of diagnostic criteria for defining sleep disturbance in Alzheimer's disease. J Geriatr Psychiatry Neurol 2003; 16(3): 131-9.
[http://dx.doi.org/10.1177/0891988703255684] [PMID: 12967054]

[104] Rongve A, Boeve BF, Aarsland D. Frequency and correlates of caregiver-reported sleep disturbances in a sample of persons with early dementia. J Am Geriatr Soc 2010; 58(3): 480-6.
[http://dx.doi.org/10.1111/j.1532-5415.2010.02733.x] [PMID: 20398116]

[105] Guarnieri B, Adorni F, Musicco M, *et al.* Prevalence of sleep disturbances in mild cognitive impairment and dementing disorders: a multicenter Italian clinical cross-sectional study on 431 patients. Dement Geriatr Cogn Disord 2012; 33(1): 50-8.
[http://dx.doi.org/10.1159/000335363] [PMID: 22415141]

[106]   Cipriani G, Lucetti C, Danti S, Nuti A. Sleep disturbances and dementia. Psychogeriatrics 2015; 15(1): 65-74.
[http://dx.doi.org/10.1111/psyg.12069] [PMID: 25515641]

[107]   Camargos EF, Louzada LL, Quintas JL, Naves JO, Louzada FM, Nóbrega OT. Trazodone improves sleep parameters in Alzheimer disease patients: a randomized, double-blind, and placebo-controlled study. Am J Geriatr Psychiatry 2014; 22(12): 1565-74.
[http://dx.doi.org/10.1016/j.jagp.2013.12.174] [PMID: 24495406]

[108]   Maust DT, Kim HM, Seyfried LS, *et al.* Antipsychotics, other psychotropics, and the risk of death in patients with dementia: number needed to harm. JAMA Psychiatry 2015; 72(5): 438-45.
[http://dx.doi.org/10.1001/jamapsychiatry.2014.3018] [PMID: 25786075]

[109]   Xu J, Wang LL, Dammer EB, *et al.* Melatonin for sleep disorders and cognition in dementia: a meta-analysis of randomized controlled trials. Am J Alzheimers Dis Other Demen 2015; 30(5): 439-47.
[http://dx.doi.org/10.1177/1533317514568005] [PMID: 25614508]

[110]   Gehrman PR, Connor DJ, Martin JL, Shochat T, Corey-Bloom J, Ancoli-Israel S. Melatonin fails to improve sleep or agitation in double-blind randomized placebo-controlled trial of institutionalized patients with Alzheimer disease. Am J Geriatr Psychiatry 2009; 17(2): 166-9.
[http://dx.doi.org/10.1097/JGP.0b013e318187de18] [PMID: 19155748]

[111]   Kahn DM, Cook TE, Carlisle CC, Nelson DL, Kramer NR, Millman RP. Identification and modification of environmental noise in an ICU setting. Chest 1998; 114(2): 535-40.
[http://dx.doi.org/10.1378/chest.114.2.535] [PMID: 9726742]

[112]   Beck-Little R, Weinrich SP. Assessment and management of sleep disorders in the elderly. J Gerontol Nurs 1998; 24(4): 21-9.
[http://dx.doi.org/10.3928/0098-9134-19980401-08] [PMID: 9611561]

[113]   Stewart NH, Arora VM. Sleep in hospitalized older adults. Sleep Med Clin 2018; 13(1): 127-35.
[http://dx.doi.org/10.1016/j.jsmc.2017.09.012] [PMID: 29412979]

[114]   Hu RF, Jiang XY, Chen J, *et al.* Non-pharmacological interventions for sleep promotion in the intensive care unit. Cochrane Database Syst Rev 2015; 2015(10): CD008808.
[http://dx.doi.org/10.1002/14651858.CD008808.pub2] [PMID: 26439374]

SUBJECT INDEX

A

Acid, antiepileptics valproic 12
Acquired long QT-syndrome 81
Activities 7, 80, 111
   abnormal tonic 111
   calcium channel 80
   parasympathetic 7, 80
Adaptive servo ventilation (ASV) 90, 95, 98
Advanced sleep 20, 24, 25, 72
   phase disorder 20, 72
   wake phase disorder (ASWPD) 24, 25
Age 171, 173
   -dependency of total sleep time 171
   -related medical/psychiatric conditions 173
Aging and circadian rhythms 172
AHI and nocturnal oxygen desaturation 84
Airway 95, 136, 141, 142, 179
   collapse 95, 141, 179
   obstruction 136
   pharyngeal 179
Alzheimer's 115, 122, 181, 187
   dementia 115
   disease 115, 122, 181, 187
Apnea-hypopnea index (AHI) 82, 91, 96, 97, 99, 136, 139, 140, 179, 180
Arrhythmias 3, 9, 78, 79, 80, 82, 83, 84, 85, 90, 95, 98, 179
   apnea-induced 79
   cardiac 78, 179
   life-threatening 79
   sinus 83
   susceptibility 80
Arrhythmogenesis 79, 80, 82
Arrhythmogenicity 81
Arthritis 180, 181, 182
   rheumatoid 181

B

Barr virus 12

Benzodiazepine binding site 9
Body mass index (BMI) 82, 135, 179
Bradyarrhythmias 83
Bradycardia 83
Bradykinesia 123
Breathing issues 177
Bright light therapy 28

C

Cardiac 80, 82, 91
   implantable electronic devices (CIED) 82
   surgery 91
   tissues 80
Cardiovascular 78, 90, 94, 135, 174, 175
   diseases 78, 90, 94, 174, 175
   morbidities 135
CDME 70
   certification 70
   guidance 70
Central apnea index (CAI) 96, 99
Cerebrospinal fluid 10
Cerebrovascular disease 174
Cheyne-stokes respiration 91
Chronic 82, 181
   inflammatory conditions 181
   sleep-disordered breathing mechanisms 82
Chronic insomnia 146, 147, 149, 150, 151, 152, 155, 156, 160, 162, 176
   disorder 149
Chronotherapy 23
Circadian 6, 20, 65, 171
   clock genes 20
   dysfunction 6
   influences 65
   rhythmicity 171
Circadian rhythm 20, 21, 22, 27, 29, 30, 32, 64, 72, 73, 153, 154, 168, 169, 171, 172, 174, 187
   age-related changes in 168, 169
   disorders 20, 21, 32, 72, 73, 174, 187
   of plasma melatonin secretion 171

sleep-wake disorders 153
Clarithromycin 3, 4, 9, 10, 12
Cognitive 54, 146, 149, 160, 161, 162, 176
  -behavioral therapy 54
  therapy 146, 149, 160, 161, 162, 176
Collapse, exclusive tongue base 141
Combination 28, 55, 186
  therapy 55, 186
  treatment 28
Commercial driver 64, 70, 72
  license (CDL) 70, 72
  medical examiner (CDME) 64, 70
Comorbid anxiety disorder 48
Comorbidities 40, 43, 54, 84, 94, 146, 150,
  151, 162, 168, 174
  medical 150, 162
  mental 54
  psychiatric 146, 150, 151
Complex ventricular ectopy (CVE) 84, 179
Concentric collapse 140
Constipation 45, 46, 47, 50, 116, 123, 124,
  184
Contraception, hormonal 3
Corticosteroids 174
Cortisol rhythms 6
CPAP 83
  therapy 83
  treatment 83
Craniopharyngioma 12
CRP, plasma 81
Cryptochrome 25

D

Daylight savings time (DST) 72
Daytime 30, 149
  dysfunction 149
  fatigue 30
Default-mode network (DMN) 6
Delayed sleep 20, 21, 22, 23, 26
  phase disorder 20
  -wake phase disorder (DSWPD) 21, 22, 23,
  26

Dementia 106, 107, 114, 115, 116, 168, 179,
  181, 182, 186, 187, 188
Demyelinating diseases 107
Depression 3, 5, 10, 44, 46, 48, 50, 53, 54,
  118, 119, 150, 151, 174, 175, 184, 185,
  186
  comorbid 44
  psychosis 10
  respiratory 3, 10, 50
Depressive symptomatology 185
Device 82, 183
  cardiac implantable electronic 82
  pneumatic compression 183
Disease 3, 53, 115, 116, 123, 124, 174, 181,
  184, 187, 188
  cardiac 3
  chronic obstructive pulmonary 174, 188
  chronic respiratory 184
  coronary artery 174
  gastroesophageal reflux 174
  kidney 181
  limbic-predominant Lewy body 115
  prognosis 187
  progression 53, 116, 123, 124
Disorders 12, 13, 22, 24, 26, 27, 28, 29, 31,
  32, 69, 71, 72, 106, 108, 109, 110, 114,
  118, 119, 124, 150, 153, 159, 168, 169,
  174, 180, 188
  cardiovascular 150
  comorbid 114
  gastrointestinal 150
  mood 13, 180
  neurodegenerative 12, 106, 108, 110, 114,
  124, 174
  neurodevelopmental 27
  neurological 22, 24, 26, 28, 150
  panic 159
  psychotic 118
  trauma-related 119
Distraction osteogenesis maxillary expansion
  (DOME) 138
Dopaminergic 40, 43, 44, 45, 48, 53, 54, 182,
  183, 184, 185
  agents 40, 43, 44, 45, 53, 54, 182, 183, 184,
  185

www.ingramcontent.com/pod-product-compliance
Lightning Source LLC
Chambersburg PA
CBHW050841220326
41598CB00006B/422